STAT DDX

A Systematic Approach to Differential Diagnosis

and Avoiding Diagnostic Error

STAT DDX

A Systematic Approach to Differential Diagnosis and Avoiding Diagnostic Error

LONG H. TU, MD, PHD

*Yale School of Medicine,
New Haven, CT, USA*

STAT DDX

© **Long H. Tu 2025**

All rights reserved. This book is protected by copyright.
No part of this book may be reproduced in any form by any means, including photocopying, or utilized by any information storage and retrieval system without written permission from the copyright owner, except for brief quotations embodied in critical articles and reviews.

First Edition, Salem Publishers, September 2025

ISBN: 979-8-9932318-0-8

Disclaimer

Every effort has been made in preparing this book to provide accurate information in accordance to policies and practice at the time of publication. Nevertheless, the authors, editors, and publishers can make no warranties that the information contained herein is totally free from error, not least because clinical standards are constantly changing through research and regulation.

The authors, editors, and publishers therefore disclaim all liability for direct or consequential damages resulting from the use of material contained in this book.

For my students

Preface

Arriving at the appropriate diagnosis is one of the most important and difficult processes in modern medicine. Once a correct diagnosis is made, patient care may proceed along accepted practice and guidelines. However, without a diagnosis, patient care may be delayed or counterproductive.

Despite the crucial role of diagnosis, errors are common. Large observational studies and systematic reviews have found diagnostic error rates in the range of 5-15% across a variety of care settings. Studies suggest that approximately 5-10% of all outpatient diagnoses and 10-15% of emergency departments diagnoses are incorrect. As many as 10-20% of inpatient diagnoses are incorrect. Similar proportions of error are found in specialty care clinics, long-term care settings, and telemedicine. Error rates of 3-9% are also seen interpretation of diagnostic examinations by radiologists, pathologists, and other specialists. Not all errors impact patient outcomes and not all errors are preventable, yet improving diagnosis remains one of the most powerful ways to ensure the safety and quality of patient care.

Errors or delay in diagnosis are among the leading causes of preventable harm in medicine, resulting in approximately 800,000 cases of serious harm or disability per year in the US. Misdiagnosis is the most common reason for medical malpractice suits, representing a larger proportion of claims than surgical or medication errors. One of the most common reasons for missed diagnosis is cognitive error, e.g., not initially considering the correct entity in a differential diagnosis. Failure or delay in ordering required tests and erroneous interpretation of tests are other common contributors to diagnostic error. There are numerous other context and systems-related factors that influence diagnostic error, such as time pressure, cognitive load, and propagation of mistakes in documentation.

Improving diagnostic accuracy is difficult and is generally most successful via multi-pronged approaches at both the individual and systems levels. This book is primarily focused on what can be done at the individual level – improving the quality and thoroughness of diagnostic reasoning. The early phases of medical education introduce diagnostic reasoning via pattern recognition, typically though "classic" presentations and clinical vignettes. While there is certainly value in teaching typical patient presentations, pattern-matching strategies can fail when patients do not present typically or when clinicians are faced with contradictory or ambiguous information. This sort of approach can lead to "premature closure," a cognitive error where a clinician settles on a single diagnosis too early and fails to consider reasonable alternatives or continue gathering relevant data.

Pattern recognition is useful because it is fast and less mentally taxing. More careful, systematic approaches can help fill in the gaps left by heuristic approaches. In attempts at comprehensiveness, introductory resources on diagnostic reasoning often provide haphazard or uncategorized lists of specific diagnoses, which may be difficult to recall or use in clinical practice. In real-world care, it is more useful to consider checklists of the most serious, most easily missed, and most "likely" explanations for a patient's presentation. When seeking to construct a more comprehensive differential diagnosis, it can be useful to think not just of specific diagnoses, but broader categories of pathologies.

The purpose of this text is to provide tools that can ensure thorough diagnostic reasoning. For common clinical presentations, we provide structured checklists of serious "do-not-miss" etiologies, common, and commonly missed etiologies. We provide further differential possibilities by systems, pathologic process, and/or anatomy – whichever approach is most advantageous for the symptom in question. We also discuss pearls and pitfalls for further evaluation, "red flag" associated symptoms, and considerations for special populations.

This book is meant as an introduction for learners such as medical, physician assistant, and nursing students as well as those in the early stages of post-graduate training. It can also serve as a review for clinicians participating in the diagnostic process in frontline or consultative roles. Improving how healthcare workers and teams approach diagnosis can ensure patient safety, enhance the efficiency of care, and reduce medicolegal risk.

Long H. Tu
9/23/2025

Table of Contents

Introduction 3
    How to Use This Book and Important Caveats 4

The Most Commonly Misdiagnosed Conditions 5
    The Big Three 6
    Commonly Misdiagnosed Serious Conditions Based on Care Setting 7
    Other Commonly Misdiagnosed Conditions 10

Diagnostic Reasoning and Differential Diagnosis 12
    Introduction 13
    Approaches to Generating a Differential Diagnosis 14
    An Update to VINDICATE 19
    A Deeper Dive into Systems-Based Differential Diagnosis 21
    Diagnostic Pauses and Special Scenarios 24
    The Remainder of This Text 28

Constitutional 29
    Fever (including Fever of Unknown Origin) 30
    Chills (without Fever) and Hypothermia 34
    Night Sweats 37
    Weight Loss (Unintentional) 40
    Weight Gain (Increased Adiposity) 43
    Generalized Edema (Pitting Edema) 46

General 49
    Generalized Weakness/Fatigue 50
    Syncope/Loss of Consciousness 53
    Dizziness (Vertigo/Disequilibrium) 56
    Sleep Disturbances 59

Eyes 63
    Red Eye 64
    Eye Pain 67
    Diplopia (Double Vision) 70
    Vision Loss (and Vision Abnormality) 73

Ear, Nose, and Throat 77
    Hearing Loss 78
    Tinnitus 81

Nasal Discharge and Postnasal Drip 84
Mouth Sores 87
Dysphagia 90
Sore Throat (Pharyngitis) 93
Neck Mass 96

Cardiovascular 99
Chest Pain 100
Tachycardia 104
Bradycardia 107
Arrhythmia 110
Murmur 113
Hypotension 117
Cardiac Arrest 120

Pulmonary 123
Shortness of Breath (Dyspnea) 124
Dyspnea on Exertion 129
Wheezing 132
Cough 136
Hemoptysis 140
Snoring 143

Abdominal and Gastrointestinal 146
Abdominal Pain 147
Abdominal Swelling or Distention 155
Nausea/Vomiting 158
Diarrhea 162
Constipation 166
Hematemesis 170
Hematochezia 173
Melena 176

Pelvic and Genitourinary 179
Primary and Secondary Amenorrhea 180
Vaginal Discharge 186
Vaginal Bleeding 189
Testicular Pain 193
Dysuria 196
Hematuria (Blood in Urine) 199
Urinary Incontinence 202
Urethral Discharge 205

Extremities and Musculoskeletal 208
    Joint Pain and Swelling 209
    Muscle Pain 212
    Weakness 215
    Neck Pain 219
    Back Pain (Thoracic, Lumbar, Sacral) 222
    Focal or Uniliteral Extremity Swelling 225
    Non-Pitting Edema 228

Skin and Subcutaneous 230
    Rash (Diffuse, Focal) 231
    Skin Lesion (Focal/Solitary) 237
    Hives 241
    Breast Pain 244
    Breast Lump 248
    Palpable Soft Tissue Abnormality (Other) 252

Neurologic 256
    Headache 257
    Focal Weakness 261
    Focal Paresthesia 265
    Speech Abnormalities 268
    Facial Asymmetry 271
    Ataxia 274
    Delirium 278
    Coma 282

Psychiatric 286
    Depression 287
    Anxiety 291
    Psychosis 294

Endocrine 297
    Heat Intolerance 298
    Cold Intolerance 301
    Excessive Thirst (Polydipsia) 304
    Excessive Hunger (Polyphagia) 308

Hematologic and Lymphatic 312
    Easy Bruising or Bleeding 313
    Pallor 317
    Swollen Glands or Lymph Nodes 321

Allergy 325
    Frequent Sneezing 326
    Seasonal Allergies 329
    Increased/Recurrent Infections 333

Concluding Remarks 337
    Beyond this Text, Contact, and Feedback 338

Acknowledgements

This book has been more than a decade in the making. Its earliest form was a collection of notes and rough outlines I wrote during my intern year at the Kaweah Health Transitional Year program in Visalia, California. I am deeply thankful to the faculty of that program – especially my former program director, Dr. Michael Stanley – for their guidance during my first year as a physician. They introduced me to frameworks for approaching undifferentiated patients across outpatient, urgent, and emergency settings. Experiences during this time stoked my interest in creating a broadly applicable resource for diagnostic reasoning.

This book was made possible through the collaboration of a large team over many years. It represents the work of 25 co-authors, including medical students, research assistants, residents, fellows, and faculty. Among this group, I would like to especially thank Quoc-Huy Ly, who helped get serious writing started with his early, extensive contributions. I would like to also especially thank Dr. Saeed Rahmani, whose efforts were invaluable in filling critical gaps in content that arose in early revisions. I am also indebted to many co-authors from the Yale Department of Emergency Medicine who helped refine this work, particularly at the later stages. All co-authors are acknowledged alphabetically on the following page, as well as at the beginning of relevant chapters.

Aside from these individuals, I am especially appreciative for the help of Dr. Edward (Ted) Melnick, who connected me with many co-authors. I must thank Dr. Jamal Bokhari for his earlier mentorship surrounding educational projects and systematic approaches to diagnostic problem-solving. Finally, I am grateful to Gresi Kello for her early feedback on the scope of this text as well as her aid in copy-editing. To everyone who has contributed along the way – thank you so much!

Contributors

Editor
    Long H. Tu, MD, PhD[1,2]

Co-authors (alphabetical)
    Ahmed Kertam, MD[1,2]
    Ashley A. Jacobson, MD[3]
    Carys Kenny-Howell, BSc[2,4]
    Curtis Xu, MD[3]
    John Sather, MD[3]
    Jonathan Heavey, MD[3]
    Katja Goldflam, MD[3]
    Laura Hanson, DO[3]
    Leah B. Colucci, MD, MS[3]
    Lisa-Qiao MacDonald, MD[3]
    Long H. Tu, MD, PhD[1,2]
    Maad Galal, MD[1,2]
    Nicholas Cochran-Caggiano, MD, MS[5]
    Nickolas Srica, MD[3]
    Nurudeen L. Osumah, MD, MBA[3]
    Omar Zaree, MD[1,2]
    Quoc-Huy Ly, BBA[2,6]
    Ramtin Hajibeygi, MD[1,2,7]
    Richard J. Lozano, BSc[2,4]
    Roshan Singh, MBBS[2,8]
    Saeed Rahmani, MD, MPH, MHPE, HMBA[1,2]
    Samreen Vora, MD[3]
    Suresh K. Pavuluri, MD, MPH[3]
    Susan L. Giampalmo, MD[3]
    Zachary Boivin, MD[3]

[1]Department of Radiology and Biomedical Imaging, Yale School of Medicine
[2]Tu Lab for Diagnostic Research, Yale School of Medicine
[3]Department of Emergency Medicine, Yale School of Medicine
[4]Yale School of Medicine, Yale University
[5]Department of Emergency Medicine, Dartmouth Geisel School of Medicine
[6]College of Medicine, SUNY Downstate Health Sciences University
[7]School of Medicine, Tehran University of Medical Sciences
[8]Department of Surgery, Montefiore Medical Center

Introduction

Long H. Tu

How to Use This Book and Important Caveats

This book is primarily focused on diagnostic thinking and the construction of thorough differential diagnoses. Information about disease epidemiology, underlying pathophysiology, and management are omitted for brevity. This text provides differential considerations for individual symptoms. Symptom clusters and means by which to narrow differential diagnoses based on clinical evaluation and testing are not specifically addressed. Familiarity with these topics (or the ability to look them up) is considered a prerequisite for understanding this text.

The contents of this book are curated to focus on what is most useful to have in working memory. In modern clinical practice, it is always possible to gather further information from internet searches, dedicated medical applications, or artificial intelligence-based systems. Having a core of critical information in memory however can improve the ease and speed of problem solving in practice. We also consider what information would be most critical to have quickly recalled when further resources are less accessible, such as during emergencies or unexpected scenarios occurring outside of professional settings (e.g., in day-to-day life, during flights, in the wilderness, etc.)

The first few chapters, focused on differing approaches to diagnostic reasoning and avoiding diagnostic error are likely to be useful to most or all readers. Each of the following chapters focuses on chief concerns or symptoms that could be revealed by a "review of systems." These chapters can be consulted out of order, or on an as-needed basis.

While we provide differential considerations for many common clinical presentations, it does not encompass every symptom or potential diagnosis. Rare conditions, especially those that are not urgent or immediately actionable, may be mentioned only within broader pathologic categories. Instead of appending "etc." to each line where additional, uncommon etiologies could be considered, we leave to the reader to recognize that the contents of this book are curated, not necessarily exhaustive. ("Etc." is still used in select instances where only a few of very numerous pathologies are listed.) The most important take-aways are the patterns of reasoning and the generalizable lessons.

The Most Commonly Misdiagnosed Conditions

Long H. Tu

Suresh K. Pavuluri

Lisa-Qiao MacDonald

The Big Three

Research literature highlights three major categories of pathology responsible for the majority of serious harm attributable to misdiagnosis. The "big three" are:

1. **Cancers**: malignancies and/or locally aggressive neoplasia (e.g., lung, breast, prostate, colorectal, and skin cancers)
2. **Vascular events**: infarct, ischemia, and other acute vascular pathologies (e.g., strokes, heart attacks/myocardial infarction, aortic aneurysms and dissections, and venous thromboemboli)
3. **Infections**: fulminant/aggressive infectious processes (e.g., sepsis, meningitis, encephalitis, pneumonia, and spinal infections)

These categories are not necessarily those that are most commonly misdiagnosed, but rather those in which misdiagnosis can result in serious disability or death. It is therefore important, in all differential diagnoses, to consider whether vascular, infectious, or neoplastic possibilities have been sufficiently addressed, to avoid committing the most serious diagnostic errors.

We can consider expansive definitions of these categories, to include arterial, venous, as well as central cardiac pathologies within the "vascular" grouping. Similarly, "infection" may be considered together (e.g. "infectious/inflammatory") with less common fulminant non-infectious etiologies, such as autoimmune, allergic, and systemic inflammatory processes. Neoplasia includes both malignancies as well as locally aggressive even if histologically "benign" processes.

Commonly Misdiagnosed Serious Conditions Based on Care Setting

The types of pathology seen in differing care settings may vary, and clinicians may predominately practice in one type of setting. To understand related variation in misdiagnosis, we review the most common serious misdiagnoses in outpatient, emergency, and inpatient care.

Outpatients

The 10 most commonly misdiagnosed conditions leading to serious harm in outpatients are (in order of prevalence):

1. Pneumonia
2. Decompensated congestive heart failure
3. Acute renal failure
4. Cancer (primary: colorectal, lung, breast, prostate)
5. Urinary tract infection or pyelonephritis
6. Myocardial infarction
7. Stroke
8. Sepsis
9. Pulmonary embolism
10. Brain hemorrhage

If we organize these into pathologic groups, the list looks like this:

- **Vascular:** myocardial infarction, stroke, brain hemorrhage, pulmonary embolism
- **Infection/inflammation:** pneumonia, urinary tract infection or pyelonephritis, sepsis
- **Neoplasia:** cancer (primary: colorectal, lung, breast, prostate)
- **Other:** decompensated congestive heart failure, acute renal failure

As expected, most pathologies fit into the "big three." Only heart failure and renal failure fall outside of the big three; both these entities could be considered a form of end-organ dysfunction or failure. Commonly missed vascular conditions mirror the most prevalent causes of death in the general population (i.e., diseases involving the heart, lungs, and brain). The most commonly missed serious infections include common ones (respiratory and urinary tract) as well as sepsis. The most commonly missed serious cancers reflect prevalence, with the caveat that low-morbidity skin cancers are excluded from the list.

Emergency Care

In emergency departments, the 10 most commonly misdiagnosed pathologies producing serious harm are:

1. Stroke
2. Myocardial infarction
3. Aortic aneurysm and dissection
4. Spinal cord compression and injury
5. Venous thromboembolism
6. Meningitis and encephalitis
7. Sepsis
8. Lung cancer
9. Traumatic brain injury and traumatic intracranial hemorrhage
10. Arterial thromboembolism

Other commonly missed serious pathologies in this setting (ranked 11-15 in one study) include spinal and intracranial abscess, cardiac arrhythmia, pneumonia, gastrointestinal perforation and rupture, and intestinal obstruction. If we sort just the top 10 into categories, the list looks like this:

- **Vascular:** stroke, myocardial infarction, aortic aneurysm and dissection, venous thromboembolism, arterial thromboembolism
- **Infection/inflammation:** meningitis and encephalitis, sepsis
- **Neoplasia:** lung cancer
- **Other:** traumatic brain injury and traumatic intracranial hemorrhage (which can also be considered a vascular process).

Trauma is the major category in acute settings outside of the big three. In fact, trauma (e.g., missed fracture) is more common than many of the listed entities, though if missed, is usually quickly diagnosed on follow-up or sufficiently minor that there is low morbidity. It is useful to attempt categorizing not just the top 10, but other commonly misdiagnosed conditions in emergency settings, especially spinal cord pathologies and intestinal obstruction, perforation, or rupture. These can be considered compressive or obstructive pathologies, which form another category of serious, commonly missed diagnoses outside of the big three.

Inpatients

The most commonly misdiagnosed pathologies producing serious harm in the inpatient setting are:

1. Cancer
2. Pulmonary embolism
3. Aortic aneurysm
4. Congestive heart failure
5. Urinary tract infection
6. Gastrointestinal perforation
7. Sepsis
8. Appendicitis
9. Intercranial lesions (subarachnoid hemorrhage, subdural hemorrhage, brain metastasis)
10. Skeletal fractures

If we sort these into categories, the list looks like this:

- **Vascular:** pulmonary embolism, aortic aneurysm, intracranial hemorrhage
- **Infection/inflammation:** urinary tract infection, sepsis, appendicitis
- **Neoplasia:** cancer, intracranial/brain masses
- **Other:** skeletal fractures, gastrointestinal perforation (potentially categorized with infection/inflammation), congestive heart failure

Etiologies outside of the big three include trauma and organ (e.g., cardiac) failure. Other commonly misdiagnosed outside of the top 10 in inpatient care include acute coronary syndrome, alcohol use disorder, and delirium. The first of these is a vascular condition; the remaining two are toxic-metabolic or neurologic.

Other Commonly Misdiagnosed Conditions

Aside from commonly misdiagnosed conditions covered in the big three and mentioned in the preceding lists, there are specific entities which are associated with higher rates of misdiagnosis or delays in diagnosis in general. These may have a more indolent or subacute course than those highlighted in literature focused on serious morbidity and mortality. Selected categories and diagnoses include:

- **Neuropsychiatric diseases:** multiple sclerosis, dementia, depression, functional neurologic disorders (conversion disorder)
- **Gastrointestinal diseases:** inflammatory and functional processes such as irritable bowel syndrome, inflammatory bowel disease, and microscopic colitis (many of these could be also considered under the umbrella of infectious/inflammatory processes or end-organ dysfunction)
- **Rheumatic disorders:** fibromyalgia, rheumatoid arthritis, systemic lupus erythematous
- **Endocrine and metabolic processes**: thyroid conditions, diabetes (especially type 1 in adults), adrenal disorders
- **Genetic conditions:** leukodystrophies, inherited immunodeficiencies, muscular dystrophies, etc.

Many of these conditions have vague, overlapping, or atypical symptoms. There may be variable progression or presentation of symptoms. Many affect multiple organ systems or can be considered systemic processes that can manifest with local symptoms – mimicking a focal process.

The "Little Three" and Everything Else

We have already seen that the "big three" (vascular, infection, and neoplasia) covers the largest share of commonly misdiagnosed serious conditions. For the sake of conceptualizing or easily remembering other conditions that are commonly missed, it can be useful to consider trends in misdiagnosis outside of the big three.

Organ dysfunction, injury, and obstructive/compressive processes represent the next most common categories of life-threatening conditions that are frequently misdiagnosed. These could be considered the "little three" (or "next three") categories to keep in mind in diagnostic dilemmas. Diffuse or non-focal processes affecting multiple organs constitute the last major bucket of differential considerations. This group includes metabolic, endocrinologic, and developmental or genetic conditions, which are often misdiagnosed but may present with lower morbidity or acuity compared to those in the "big three" and "little three" categories.

Further Reading

- Schiff GD, Volodarskaya M, Ruan E, Lim A, Wright A, Singh H, Nieva HR. Characteristics of disease-specific and generic diagnostic pitfalls: a qualitative study. JAMA Network Open. 2022 Jan 4;5(1):e2144531-.
- Singh H, Meyer AN, Thomas EJ. The frequency of diagnostic errors in outpatient care: estimations from three large observational studies involving US adult populations. BMJ quality & safety. 2014 Sep 1;23(9):727-31.
- Newman-Toker DE, Peterson SM, Badihian S, Hassoon A, Nassery N, Parizadeh D, Wilson LM, Jia Y, Omron R, Tharmarajah S, Guerin L. Diagnostic Errors in the Emergency Department: A Systematic Review.
- Gunderson CG, Bilan VP, Holleck JL, Nickerson P, Cherry BM, Chui P, Bastian LA, Grimshaw AA, Rodwin BA. Prevalence of harmful diagnostic errors in hospitalised adults: a systematic review and meta-analysis. BMJ quality & safety. 2020 Dec 1;29(12):1008-18.

Diagnostic Reasoning and Differential Diagnosis

Long H. Tu

Lisa-Qiao MacDonald

Suresh K. Pavuluri

Introduction

Diagnosis is a dynamic process. As a clinician obtains more information about a patient, or the patient's condition evolves, diagnostic hypotheses and differential considerations are further refined. A few nuances are useful to keep in mind as we discuss approaches to diagnostic reasoning and error mitigation.

First, information in medicine can be incomplete or misleading. Patients may be unable or unwilling to share all relevant details, documentation can be imperfect, and diagnostic tests may produce incorrect or inconclusive results. Early in patient evaluation, it is often helpful to use "working diagnoses" or consider a "differential diagnosis" rather than assigning a definitive diagnosis. A formal diagnosis requires meeting diagnostic criteria, confirmatory testing, and possible exclusion of mimicking pathologies. It is important to remember that 5-10% of diagnoses across healthcare settings are incorrect. Throughout care, there are ongoing opportunities to review and revise diagnoses. Recognizing that diagnoses are provisional and evolving encourages continual reassessment and helps prevent diagnostic errors from adversely affecting patients.

Second, constellations of signs and symptoms may arise from one or multiple processes. In many cases, patient presentations occur due to a single disease process. However, patients that meet specific diagnostic criteria may still having overlapping, complicating, or associated pathology. Infection may obscure malignancy; benign diseases can undergo malignant transformation; treatment complications may mimic recurrence. The identification of one explanatory process does not necessarily exclude the presence of others. Keep in mind the pitfall known as "satisfaction of search," in which finding one seemingly satisfactory diagnosis can reduce attention to detecting additional problems.

Third, the consideration of broader differential diagnoses does not necessarily require extensive diagnostic testing or consultation. In many cases, pathology can be excluded based on clinical evaluation or risk-stratification tools. The thoughtful use of diagnostic resources is critical to providing efficient and cost-effective care. Misuse or overuse can inadvertently contribute to misdiagnosis through false reassurance or overextension of specialist input. Keeping this concept in mind can help support diagnostic practices within broader organizations, in addition to serving individual patients.

Finally, diagnostic error is strongly influenced by contextual factors. Distractions during clinical care, greater workload demands, and the complexity and acuity of patients all impact the risk of error. At a broader level, organizational policies, safety culture, and the availability of technological support can influence the diagnostic process. Although systems-level interventions are beyond the scope of this text, it remains crucial to consider what practical steps can be taken to optimize local practice settings, as these factors also play a large role in determining diagnostic accuracy.

Approaches to Generating a Differential Diagnosis

There are a variety of approaches for constructing a differential diagnosis (DDX). Generally, each sign or symptom elicited in a history and physical exam has its own differential diagnosis, as do clusters of such findings. Differential diagnoses also exist for specific lab, imaging, and other testing results (though these are not covered in this text). Approaches to differential diagnosis include pattern recognition and systematic approaches based on checklists, local anatomy, systems, or mechanistic considerations. Each of these has strengths and weaknesses.

Pattern Recognition

Pattern recognition is a diagnostic strategy where clinicians rapidly match a patient's signs and symptoms to familiar disease patterns, often using mental models known as "illness scripts." This strategy is commonly taught early in medical education and is a good introduction to diagnostic reasoning. Pattern matching works particularly well in cases with classic presentations. A few examples of how clusters of symptoms can be used to consider important disease processes:

- Severe left-sided chest pain, exertional, diaphoresis → myocardial infarction
- "Worst headache of my life," sudden onset → subarachnoid hemorrhage
- Shuffling gait, tremor, rigidity in elderly patient → Parkinson's disease

Thinking in terms of patterns or symptom complexes is fast yet may miss atypical presentations and uncommon entities. For example, patients with chest pain and diaphoresis can alternatively have a pulmonary embolism, or in some cases, an aortic dissection. Sudden onset severe headache can also result from cerebral venous sinus thrombosis, cervical arterial dissections, and other etiologies. Shuffling gait and other movement abnormalities can be seen with other neurodegenerative processes such as atypical Parkinsonism or normal pressure hydrocephalus. To avoid errors that may arise from relying on pattern-based approaches, it is advisable to leverage more systematic approaches.

Checklists

One strategy to ensure consideration of the most important potential etiologies for a presentation is the use of checklists. These may include always considering the most serious, most common, and potentially the most commonly misdiagnosed conditions for any given presentation.

For example, for any patient with acute chest pain, there are number of serious diseases which should always be considered or "excluded." These include: acute coronary syndrome/myocardial infarction, aortic dissection, pulmonary embolism, pneumothorax, esophageal rupture (Boerhaave's syndrome), and/or pericardial effusion. A checklist approach can also be used to consider the most common causes: musculoskeletal pain (e.g., costochondritis), gastroesophageal reflux disease (GERD), anxiety/panic disorders, and pleuritis (from infectious/inflammatory processes). Commonly misdiagnosed conditions could also be remembered in a short list, e.g.: pericarditis, pneumonia, pancreatitis, and gallbladder disease. Having such checklists in mind can help a clinician at least consider a broader differential diagnosis than using illness scripts alone.

Checklists are helpful to ensure consideration of the most important or serious pathologies, though can be unwieldy for comprehensive evaluation of the number of included entities is too numerous. Long, uncategorized lists of differential considerations can be difficult to recall. More structured approaches can be helpful in these cases.

Local Anatomic Approach

A local anatomic approach to creating a differential diagnosis involves considering all anatomical structures located in that region and the diseases that can affect them. For example, a differential diagnosis for right upper quadrant pain can be generated by mapping out the organs and tissues present – such as the liver, gallbladder, biliary tree, right kidney, duodenum, colon (hepatic flexure), and right lung base. This list then helps generate potential diagnoses related to each structure. The liver and gallbladder give rise to hepatobiliary conditions like cholecystitis, biliary colic, cholangitis, hepatitis, choledocholithiasis, and liver abscess. Gastrointestinal structures are associated with pathology such as duodenal ulcer or colitis. Pain can from pathology of the right kidney and right lower chest structures can similarly be considered.

When using an anatomic approach, it is important to consider not just viscera and solid organs, but also structures which are present throughout the body: vasculature (arteries, veins, lymphatics), nerves, muscle, joints, bones, other connective tissue, and the skin. The anatomic approach can be useful to consider diseases arising from diverse sites, but has limitations. The anatomic approach can overlook referred pain (e.g., shoulder pain from intra-abdominal pathology). It can also overlook non-local, diffuse, or systemic processes such as metabolic, psychiatric, and central neurological abnormalities.

Mechanistic Approach

The mechanistic approach is useful for specific presentations and involves differential diagnosis guided by the underlying biological or physiological processes that can cause a particular symptom. Potential etiologies are then generated by considering how disruptions in normal physiology can give rise to the patient's presentation. For example, a patient with muscle weakness may have disruptions anywhere along the entire pathway, from the central nervous system, through peripheral nerves, to the neuromuscular junction, and finally the muscle itself. Individual etiologies (e.g., stroke, multiple sclerosis, or spinal cord lesions for central causes) are then generated from points along the mechanistic pathway. Like the anatomic approach, it is important to remember that systemic, metabolic, and other non-local pathologies can also be contributory, and must be included in the differential.

Pathophysiologic Approach

A pathophysiologic approach considers differing processes by which diseases arise, such as infection, inflammation, neoplastic (abnormal cell growth), or developmental anomaly. This approach is very useful, though it can be difficult to recall the many potential pathologic processes that can give rise to disease.

One commonly taught strategy to recall pathophysiologic categories relies on a mnemonic, "VINDICATE," in which each letter stands for a process or collection of processes. The mnemonic prompts consideration of the following major categories:

- V – Vascular
- I – Infectious (or inflammatory)
- N – Neoplastic
- D – Degenerative (or deficiency/drugs)
- I – Idiopathic (or iatrogenic/intoxication)
- C – Congenital
- A – Autoimmune (or allergic)
- T – Traumatic (or toxin)
- E – Endocrine (or metabolic)

There are similar mnemonics such as VITAMIN CDE and VITAMINS ABCDEK, which further expand on these categories (details can found in other resources if interested). One weakness of these mnemonics is that there is little logic to the order of the categories. Some categories are also redundant –

autoimmune and allergic diseases are also technically inflammatory processes. Having multiple unrelated categories correspond to the same letter can also add confusion. Because of these limitations, VINDICATE and related mnemonics are uncommonly used in practice. In real world care, specific categories may be considered based on the patient's presentation, tailored to the degree of clinical suspicion.

Combining Approaches

In some cases, it is useful to combine multiple approaches. For example, a clinician might first consider the most likely causes for a presentation based on pattern recognition. They might then consider a checklist of "do-not-miss" (serious/life-threatening) diagnoses. Beyond the initial diagnostic "hypotheses," the clinician may broaden their differential using a more systematic approach. Each approach therefore helps answer a differing question:

- What is the most *likely* diagnosis?
- What are the "*do not miss*" diagnoses that should be considered?
- What *else* could this be?

In many cases, broadening the differential diagnosis can be done in terms of larger categories, with focus on a few key entities per category. After consideration of the most common and serious differential possibilities for a patient presenting with chest pain (e.g., myocardial infarct, pulmonary embolism, etc.), less emergent possibilities can initially be thought of in broader categories, and then refined to individual diseases as needed (e.g., consideration of gastrointestinal etiologies, then specifically GERD, biliary colic, and pancreatitis.) Combining differing differential approaches with consideration of pathologies at the level of major groups can help ensure greater completeness in diagnostic reasoning.

An Update to VINDICATE

In the prior section, we discussed the use of the VINDICATE mnemonic to provide a systems-based approach to generating a differential diagnosis. Despite its limitations, there are some appealing features to the use of this tool. Chief among these is that the first three letters correspond with the "big three" categories of serious, commonly misdiagnosed conditions: VIN for vascular, infectious, and neoplastic processes. In this section, we suggest a modification to the VINDICATE mnemonic which can improve its utility, capture other commonly misdiagnosed conditions, and improve the ease with which one can commit a systems-based approach to memory.

Many of the most commonly misdiagnosed serious conditions outside of the "big three" can also be grouped into three categories (the "little three"): 1) organ dysfunction, 2) trauma 3) and compressive/obstructive etiologies. If we rename the second portion (DIC) of the mnemonic, we can neatly recall these:

- D – Dysfunction (or failure of organs)
    - Cardiac failure/arrhythmia, renal failure
- I – Injury (e.g., traumatic, post-surgical, etc.)
    - Trauma (e.g., brain, spine, and musculoskeletal)
- C – Compression/obstruction
    - Spinal compression, intestinal obstruction

Similarly, renaming the last three letters (ATE) in the mnemonic allows us to easily recall the remaining non-local and "non-organic" processes that should be included within a differential diagnosis. These include anomalies of development/aging, toxic-metabolic etiologies, as well as "everything else" (exposures, psychiatric conditions, and social factors). Anomalies of aging/development can be thought to include genetic conditions, complications of pregnancy, and degenerative processes. The toxic-metabolic category can be used to capture abnormalities of intrinsic and extrinsic substances that can often be measured by blood tests. "Everything else" can be used to capture other exposures, environmental, psychiatric, and social factors. The last part of the mnemonic would therefore be:

- A – Anomalies (of development/aging),
    - Genetic/congenital, developmental issues, complications of pregnancy, degenerative processes
- T – Toxic-metabolic
    - Metabolic, drugs/toxins, endocrine abnormalities
- E – Everything else
    - Emotional/psychosocial, environmental, etc.

Therefore, a modified VIN-DIC-ATE mnemonic can be used to ensure consideration of all major etiologies, capturing the "big three," (most commonly misdiagnosed serious etiologies) the "little three," (next most common, local pathology) and the "last three" (non-local pathology) categories of disease.

- V – Vascular
- I – Infectious/inflammatory
- N – Neoplastic

- D – Dysfunction
- I – Injury/trauma
- C – Compression/obstruction

- A – Anomalies of development/aging
- T – Toxic-metabolic
- E – Everything else

A Deeper Dive into Systems-Based Differential Diagnosis

It can be useful to recognize that the major categories in a systems-based differential diagnosis can be further broken down into subcategories. Differential diagnoses may use differing degrees of subcategorization to the extent that it aids organization and recollection.

For example, vascular pathologies can be further subdivided by arterial, venous, capillary, and lymphatic abnormalities. These may also be categorized by anatomic size such as large versus small vessels. Pathologies could also be subdivided by pathologic mechanism, such as ischemic/thrombotic/embolic, bleeding, aneurysm/malformation, or inflammatory processes. Vascular pathologies may also be stratified by whether they are acute, chronic, or acute-on-chronic.

Infectious processes can be subdivided by causative organism, such as bacterial, viral, fungal, parasitic, or rare prion pathologies. Other dimensions include site, distribution, and chronicity. Neoplastic processes could be further broken down into benign vs. malignant vs. borderline. Other dimensions that could be considered for subdivision include organ and cell line of origin, as well as stage and distribution of disease.

This approach could be used to provide a more granular categorization of pathology within a differential diagnosis. Having an organizational structure for pathology helps generate differential considerations in challenging cases. What follows is a breakdown of major pathologic categories into example sub-categories. These are provided for illustrative purposes; this list is not intended to be definitive or comprehensive.

- Vascular
    - **Vessel type:** arterial vs. venous vs. capillary vs. lymphatic
    - **Vessel size:** large vs. small vessels (if arterial/venous)
    - **Pathologic process:** ischemia/thrombosis/embolism vs. stenotic/narrowing vs. bleeding vs. aneurysm/malformation vs. inflammation
    - **Chronicity:** acute vs. chronic vs. acute-on-chronic
- Infectious/inflammatory
    - Infectious
        - **Distribution:** superficial vs. deep vs. disseminated
        - **Organism:** bacterial vs. viral vs. fungal vs. parasitic vs. prion
        - **Chronicity:** acute vs. subacute vs. chronic vs. latent vs. subclinical

- o Inflammatory
  - **Mechanism:** autoinflammatory vs. autoimmune vs. allergic vs. mixed; granulomatous vs. non-granulomatous
  - **Chronicity:** acute vs. chronic
  - **Distribution:** organ-specific vs. systemic/multisystem
- Neoplastic
  - o **Histology:** benign vs. borderline/locally aggressive vs. malignant; primary vs. metastatic.
  - o **Origin:** organ and cell line
  - o **Stage:** local vs. regional vs. distant/metastatic
- Dysfunction (or failure of organs)
  - o **Chronicity:** acute vs. chronic
  - o **Distribution/degree:** single vs. multi-organ dysfunction/failure; specific organ involvement, severity
- Injury/trauma
  - o **Mechanism:** blunt vs. penetrating vs. deceleration/acceleration vs. blast; open vs. closed injuries
  - o **Chronicity:** acute vs. chronic
  - o **Intent:** accidental vs. non-accidental
- Compressive/obstructive processes
  - o **By lumen involved:** airway, bowel, CSF flow, blood flow, etc.
  - o **By source:** intrinsic to organ vs. extrinsic vs. functional (neurological, neuromuscular, or metabolic issues)
  - o **Chronicity:** acute vs. chronic
- Anomalies of aging/development
  - o **Timing of onset:** genetic/congenital, prenatal vs. developmental, abnormalities of pregnancy, abnormalities of aging and degenerative processes
  - o **Distribution/degree:** single- vs. multi-system involvement
- Toxic-metabolic (and endocrine)
  - o **Electrolyte abnormalities:** hyper- vs. hypo-
  - o **Nutritional imbalances:** deficiencies vs. excess
  - o **Exposures:** toxic vs. drugs
  - o **Endocrine:** hyposecretion vs. hypersecretion; by hormone/origin
- Everything else
  - o **Psychiatric and related:** psychotic vs. mood vs. trauma-related vs. somatic symptom disorders vs. substance-related vs. behavioral, etc.
  - o **Environmental/social:** socioeconomic factors vs. exposures; lifestyle/cultural factors

In some cases, differential diagnosis may *first* consider chronicity, distribution, morphology or another characteristic, and then sub-divide by the pathologic process. In all cases, it can be useful to consider what approach fits the clinical presentation best, to assist with diagnostic problem solving.

STAT DDX

Diagnostic Pauses and Special Scenarios

Red Flags

In the later chapters of this text, we will highlight associated symptoms for each presentation which should raise suspicion for serious or life-threatening underlying pathology. Some of these "red flags" are specific to differing presentations. Others, which we will highlight here, are common across many scenarios. It can be useful to recognize common signs, which are concerning across diverse patient presentations:

- **Patient and history factors (associated with higher risk pathology)**
    - Age over 50 years with new symptoms
    - History of cancer
    - Immunosuppression
    - Drug or alcohol abuse, especially intravenous drugs
    - Non-adherence to medical therapies
    - Inconsistent/absent primary or preventative care
    - Smoking
    - Recent hospitalization or surgery
    - Pregnancy or postpartum state
    - Family history of hereditary conditions
- **Symptoms which pose an immediate threat to life (the "ABCs")**
    - Airway compromise (e.g., expanding neck hematoma, upper airway edema)
    - Breathing difficulty
    - Circulatory/cardiovascular compromise (chest pain, hypoperfusion, bleeding, etc.)
    - Sudden neurologic deficits (e.g., focal weakness, confusion, altered consciousness, etc.)
- **Systemic symptoms (which can be seen with aggressive infection/inflammation or neoplasia)**
    - Unexplained weight loss
    - Fever
    - Night sweats
    - Unexplained anemia
- **Symptom quality (which may be seen with serious occult pathology)**
    - Signs/symptoms discordant with history
    - Symptoms disproportionate to physical exam
    - Progressive or severe symptoms
    - Persistent or worsening pain (especially at night)

Populations at Higher Risk for Misdiagnosis

Specific demographic groups can be higher risk for misdiagnosis in general. Keeping in mind common pitfalls when caring for specific groups can help minimize the odds of error:

- **Women**
    - More commonly have "atypical" presentations, related to underrepresentation in research or trials and therefore the medical literature
- **Children**
    - May be unable articulate symptoms clearly; many serious conditions are also rare, and therefore potentially unexpected
- **Older adults**
    - Differences in presentation of symptoms related to age; may have multiple conditions, with overlapping presentations
- **Other patients with multiple chronic conditions**
    - Symptom overlap and complex histories increase the risk of diagnostic error
- **Other patients with communication barriers**
    - Language differences, cognitive impairment, or sensory deficits can limit accurate history-taking and assessment; cultural differences can affect articulation of symptoms

Diagnostic Pauses or "Time-Outs"

A number of authors have advocated for the use of diagnostic "time-outs" or deliberate pauses during clinical decision-making, similar to as performed prior to surgery or other invasive procedures. While formal diagnostic time-outs are rarely performed in practice, the concept is a useful one. Even performed as a mental checklist by individual clinicians, such a pause can ensure that appropriately broad differential possibilities have been considered. A framework for such a pause includes the following steps:

- **Stop and reassess the current working diagnosis**
    - Ensure all team members and, if possible, the patient and family, are aware of the presumed diagnosis
- **Systematically review all collected clinical, laboratory, and imaging results**
    - Look for inconsistencies, missing information, or red flag symptoms that may not have been addressed

- **Consider or ask explicitly: what else could this be?**
  - Generate a list of alternative/differential considerations; consider "can't miss" diagnoses, commonly missed diagnoses, and even rare entities
  - Consider whether the working diagnosis and alternatives explain all or most of the findings
  - Consider the possibility of atypical, overlapping, or concurrent disease processes
- **Solicit input from the clinical care team**
  - Consider the contributions of nurses, pharmacists, consultants, and, if appropriate, the patient and family (especially for additional history)
  - Consider whether the input of other specialists or other perspectives would be helpful
- **Plan next diagnostic and management steps**
  - Consider what further testing, repeat assessments, or consultation may be warranted
  - Document reasoning to facilitate communication and care coordination
- **Monitor and reassess**
  - Consider what interval of follow-up or change in clinical status would warrant reassessment

Scenarios involving diagnostic uncertainty or higher stakes for diagnostic error should prompt a clinician to ensure all diagnostic possibilities have been considered, and potentially revise working diagnoses. These include (but are not limited to):

- Situations where the working diagnosis leads to care decisions which are irreversible, e.g., invasive or high-risk procedures
- Patients who are not improving as expected with therapy
- Patients with multiple visits and unexplained or unresolved symptoms
- Testing results which are discordant, non-diagnostic, or technically suboptimal
- Other new or unexpected information, especially when inconsistent with the working diagnosis
- Transitions of care, such as at admission, discharge, or transfer – when information may be lost or miscommunicated
- When any clinical team member, consultant, or other individuals involved in the care of the patient raise concern for potential error

Further Reading

- Cook CE, Décary S. Higher order thinking about differential diagnosis. Brazilian journal of physical therapy. 2020 Jan 1;24(1):1-7.
- Yale S, Cohen S, Bordini BJ. Diagnostic time-outs to improve diagnosis. Critical Care Clinics. 2022 Apr 1;38(2):185-94.
- Trowbridge RL. Twelve tips for teaching avoidance of diagnostic errors. Medical teacher. 2008 Jan 1;30(5):496-500.

The Remainder of This Text

The remainder of this text focuses on the differential diagnosis for specific signs and symptoms, which may represent chief concerns or findings during a review of systems. The structure of each differential is tailored to the symptom in question, highlighting the approach most useful for that presentation. Individual chapters and sections can be reviewed out of order or on an as-needed basis.

Each section concerns a single presenting symptom, rather than a constellation of findings. When patients present with multiple concerns, differentials for the individual symptoms can often be combined, much like overlapping sets in a Venn diagram. Causes that explain more aspects of the presentation are generally more likely than those that account for only a few. Narrowing the differential or arriving at a single diagnosis requires integrating history, exam findings, and test results, guided by an understanding of disease presentations and test characteristics. Complete coverage of these details is beyond the scope of this text, though lies in complementary resources.

We also focus primarily on diagnostic considerations, rather than specifics of work-up or management. The tests and clinical tools used in differing care settings may vary based on resource availability, local expertise, and evolving research. Current guidelines and local policies should be consulted for this information.

In contrast to the specifics of management, the structure of differential diagnosis and diagnostic reasoning is unlikely to change between settings. Differential diagnosis therefore is among the most "universal" aspects of medical care. Readers are encouraged to focus on the recurring patterns and themes that shape diagnostic reasoning across clinical presentations.

Constitutional

Long H. Tu

Ramtin Hajibeygi

John Sather

Fever (including Fever of Unknown Origin)

Introduction

Fever is a nonspecific sign, usually attributable to a specific infection or other pathology based on concurrent signs. Fever is often accompanied by chills or rigors. The differential diagnosis for fever overlaps those of these similar systemic symptoms. When the etiology is unclear ("fever of unknown origin"), occult infection, malignancies, inflammatory conditions, vascular processes, and even medication side effects should be considered. Among the most rapidly fatal conditions are acute vascular processes like pulmonary embolism, fulminant infectious processes such as sepsis or meningitis, and medication side effects like malignant hyperthermia or serotonin syndrome. Concurrent symptoms or context are often more specific than fever for the underlying etiology. Immunocompromised states, prolonged hospitalization, and recent travel are special scenarios with associated specific etiologies for fever.

Checklist DDX

Serious/life-threatening: vascular (pulmonary embolism, deep venous thrombosis, other thromboembolism, bleeding), infectious (sepsis, meningitis, disseminated infections), inflammatory (e.g., giant cell arteritis), neoplastic/oncologic emergencies (e.g., leukemic crisis, tumor lysis syndrome), drug reactions (malignant hyperthermia, serotonin syndrome, neuroleptic malignant syndrome, Stevens-Johnson syndrome/toxic epidermal necrolysis), endocrine (thyrotoxic states, adrenal insufficiency)

Common: upper respiratory tract infections (e.g., common cold, influenza, sinusitis, and pneumonia), urinary tract infections (e.g., cystitis and pyelonephritis), gastroenteritis/gastrointestinal infections

Commonly misdiagnosed: drug-induced fever, occult/intra-abdominal abscesses (cholangitis, hepatic abscess), osteomyelitis, spinal infections (epidural abscess, discitis), endocarditis

Systematic DDX

- **Vascular**
    - Pulmonary embolism, deep venous thrombosis, other thromboembolism, stroke, bleeding

- **Infection**
  - **Sites involved:** upper respiratory, urinary, and gastrointestinal sources, etc.
  - **Infectious agents:**
    - **Bacterial:** occult abscess, endocarditis, bone/joint infection, TB, brucellosis, Q fever, staphylococcal scalded skin syndrome (SSSS)
    - **Viral:** CMV, EBV, HIV, HCV, HBV, HHV, HSV, etc.
    - **Fungal:** cryptococcus, aspergillosis, etc. (especially in the immunocompromised)
    - **Parasitic/other:** malaria, tick borne (Lyme, ehrlichiosis, babesiosis, etc.), worms, arthropods
- **Inflammatory**
  - **Autoimmune and collagen-vascular:** adult Still's disease, juvenile rheumatoid arthritis, systemic lupus erythematosus, rheumatoid arthritis, polymyalgia rheumatica, dermatomyositis/polymyositis, ulcerative colitis/Crohn's disease, Sjögren's syndrome, mixed connective tissue disease, Behcet's disease, etc
  - **Vasculitis:** temporal arteritis, polyarteritis nodosa, Takayasu arteritis, etc.
  - **Auto-inflammatory:** familial periodic fever syndromes
- **Neoplasia and hematologic**
  - **Solid tumors:** malignancy (especially renal cell), brain tumors disrupting thermal homeostasis, atrial myxoma
  - **Lymphoproliferative:** leukemias/lymphomas, malignant histiocytosis, Castleman's disease
  - **Other:** tumor lysis syndrome, cryoglobulinemia, cyclic neutropenia
- **Organ dysfunction**
  - Cirrhosis (from portal endotoxins)
- **Endocrine**
  - Thyrotoxic states, adrenal insufficiency, hypothalamic syndrome/dysfunction
- **Toxic-metabolic**
  - **Medication related:** malignant hyperthermia, serotonin syndrome, neuroleptic malignant syndrome, drug fever, drug induced lupus, Stevens-Johnson syndrome/toxic epidermal necrolysis
  - **Other:** factitious fever

Special scenarios:
- **"Classic" fever of unknown origin (FUO):** most commonly endocarditis, UTI, abscesses (e.g., hepatic), TB, connective tissue diseases.
- **Nosocomial FUO:** drug fever, post-op complications, thromboembolism, transfusion, C. diff
- **Travel associated (overlaps with infection):** malaria, enteric fever, leptospirosis, viral hemorrhagic fevers, typhus, and acute undifferentiated febrile illness of tropical countries
- **Immunocompromised:** opportunistic infections (host-derived, viruses, bacterial, fungal), other transplant related (rejection, graft-versus-host disease, graft intolerance, lymphoma/post-transplant lymphoproliferative disorder (PTLD), hemophagocytic lymphohistiocytosis, ureaplasma-related hyperammonemia syndrome, and immune reconstitution syndrome
- **Idiopathic**

Notes

General considerations: When an infectious source is not readily apparent, evaluation may entail broad testing for occult infections (especially abscesses), malignancies, and rheumatologic conditions. Empiric antibiotics are not always warranted. Approximately half of fevers of unknown origin may ultimately remain undiagnosed or resolve without treatment.

Red flags: (fever is itself often a red flag) hemodynamic compromise, myoclonus/meningismus, muscle rigidity, diffuse skin rash, immunocompromise, vision loss, history of IV drug use

Special populations: In children, fever is often caused by viral and bacterial infections; the most common serious non-infectious diseases include leukemia or autoimmune diseases; infants <3 months of age warrant special consideration. Continuous fever and lethargy usually demand detailed workup to exclude life-threatening diseases. In older patients, fever may be low-grade or even absent even with serious infectious or other systemic illnesses. Fever in pregnant and peripartum patients can be seen as a result of vascular events such as deep venous thrombosis or pulmonary embolism, as well as usual infectious causes.

Further Reading

- Haidar G, Singh N. Fever of unknown origin. New England Journal of Medicine. 2022 Feb 3;386(5):463-77.
- Wright WF, Auwaerter PG. Fever and fever of unknown origin: review, recent advances, and lingering dogma. InOpen Forum Infectious Diseases 2020 May (Vol. 7, No. 5, p. ofaa132). US: Oxford University Press.
- Cunha BA, Lortholary O, Cunha CB. Fever of unknown origin: a clinical approach. The American journal of medicine. 2015 Oct 1;128(10):1138-e1.
- Mourad O, Palda V, Detsky AS. A comprehensive evidence-based approach to fever of unknown origin. Archives of internal medicine. 2003 Mar 10;163(5):545-51.

Chills (without Fever) and Hypothermia

Introduction

The differential for chills (without fever) may differ from that of chills with fever. If fever or rigors are also present, refer to the section regarding fevers. If fevers are absent, the differential diagnosis overlaps that of hypothermia. Most chills/hypothermia results from environmental heat loss (e.g., "primary hypothermia"). Hypothermia resulting from an underlying medical abnormality is termed "secondary hypothermia." Chills and secondary hypothermia may result from a variety process that disrupt heat production or produce greater heat loss via central regulatory or circulatory dysfunction. Sedative-hypnotic drugs, endocrine abnormalities, dermatologic and neuromuscular processes are all potential contributors or etiologies. Like chills with fever, disseminated infection (e.g., sepsis) is a major potential etiology. Neoplastic and inflammatory conditions do not feature highly for isolated chills, however. Immediately life-threatening etiologies include severe primary hypothermia, circulatory collapse/sepsis, drug exposures, and endocrine emergencies (like myxedema coma). Please note that patients may have concurrent primary and secondary etiologies of hypothermia.

Checklist DDX

Serious/life-threatening: severe primary hypothermia, drug toxicity (especially carbon monoxide), sepsis, myxedema coma, acute adrenal crisis, ketoacidosis, hypoglycemia, stroke (rarely)

Common: primary hypothermia, drug intoxication, sepsis, hemodynamic compromise, iatrogenic

Commonly misdiagnosed: drug intoxication (e.g., opioids, alcohol), sepsis, and hypoglycemia

Systematic DDX

- **Vascular**
    - Stroke and intracranial hemorrhage (CNS failure), shock, hemodynamic compromise
- **Infectious/inflammatory**
    - Sepsis
- **Neoplastic**
    - Brain neoplasm, carcinomatosis

- **Neurologic**
    - **Central failure of thermoregulation:** Parkinson's disease, hypothalamic dysfunction, metabolic failure, toxin and pharmacologic effects,
    - **Peripheral failure:** acute spinal cord transection, neuropathy
    - **Other:** anorexia
- **Dermatologic**
    - Erythrodermas, burns
- **Endocrine**
    - Hypopituitarism, hypoadrenalism (including acute adrenal crisis), hypothyroidism (including myxedema coma), hypoglycemia
- **Injury/trauma:**
    - Multisystem trauma (via shock and cerebrospinal injury, destabilizing thermoregulation), burn injuries
- **Toxic-metabolic**
    - **Toxins:** carbon monoxide
    - **Drugs:** opioids, alcohol, barbiturates, benzodiazepines and other sedative-hypnotic medications
    - **Metabolic disorders:** alcoholic or diabetic ketoacidosis, lactic acidosis
    - **Deficiencies:** hypoglycemia, malnutrition (especial of thiamine in alcohol abuse), anemia
- **Environmental and other**
    - **Primary hypothermia:** elderly, homeless, avalanche victims, submersion injuries, etc.
    - **Iatrogenic causes:** emergency childbirth, cold infusion, heat-stroke treatment

Notes

General considerations: Management generally entails rewarming, and as needed: gentle handling, airway control, fluid resuscitate, treatment of dysrhythmias/complications, as well as any superimposed secondary etiologies. Some medications and usual therapies may not function normally if a patient is extremely hypothermic. Isolated chills or hypothermia is usually not a diagnostic dilemma, though it is crucial to recognize the possibility of multiple contributing etiologies, including drug effects or the superimposed effect of dysregulation from trauma to environmental heat loss. Remember that hypothermia is protective against ischemia in cardiac arrest, and that "no one is dead until they are warm and dead."

Red flags: older age (>65), temperature <32°C, hemodynamic instability, shock, cardiac arrest

Special populations: Children are particularly vulnerable to hypothermia from cold exposure. Prevalence of viral infections is high in this population. Hypothermia can be more common in elderly patients as a result of many systemic illnesses which may impair temperature regulation.

Further Reading

- Brown DJ, Brugger H, Boyd J, Paal P. Accidental hypothermia. New England Journal of Medicine. 2012 Nov 15;367(20):1930-8.
- McDaniel L. Hypothermia and Cold Injury in Children. Pediatr Rev. 2022 Jan 1;43(1):58-60. doi: 10.1542/pir.2021-004975. PMID: 35229129.
- Wang X, Zhang Y, Li Z, Wang X, Qiu H. Risk factors for perioperative hypothermia in pregnant women undergoing cesarean section: a systematic review and meta-analysis. Annali Italiani di Chirurgia. 2024 Aug 20;95(4):448-60.

Night Sweats

Introduction

Night sweats is a nonspecific symptom which may portend any number of life-threatening pathologies including malignancies and underlying infection. However, many common, and less serious conditions can cause night sweats. Menopause, mood disorders, reflux disease, and sleep apnea are among the most common causes. Evaluation is generally structured around the consideration/exclusion of serious infectious and neoplastic etiologies, and correlation with clues which may suggest common benign etiologies. Empiric management of alcohol use, smoking cessation, treatment for GERD or OSA, and potential dietary contributors play a role alongside diagnostic testing.

Checklist DDX

Serious/life-threatening: occult infection including HIV/AIDS and TB, malignancy, lymphoma/leukemias

Common: infection (viral, bacterial), menopause, medication side effects (methadone, antidepressants), alcohol use disorder, obesity, reflux disease, hyperthyroidism

Commonly misdiagnosed: medication side effects (e.g., antidepressants, methadone), obesity, and reflux disease

Systematic DDX

- **Vascular**
    - Coronary vasospasm (Prinzmetal angina), chronic arterial dissections (rarely)
- **Infections**
    - **Viral:** HIV, EBV (mono), etc.
    - **Bacterial:** abscess, endocarditis, etc. TB, MAI, Lyme, etc.
    - **Fungal infections:** histoplasmosis, blastomycosis, cryptococcosis, etc. (especially in immunocompromised)
    - **Parasitic:** malaria, tick born (Lyme, ehrlichiosis, babesiosis, etc.)
- **Inflammatory**
    - **Vasculitis:** Takayasu's arteritis, temporal arteritis
    - **Other:** chronic eosinophilic pneumonia, granulomatous diseases (e.g., sarcoid), other autoimmune conditions

- **Neoplastic/hematologic**
    - Malignancy (any, including brain tumors), lymphoma/leukemia, lymphoproliferative processes, large hemangioma (from inflammatory response or necrotic changes)
- **Neurologic/psychiatric**
    - **Autonomic dysregulation:** anxiety, autonomic dysregulation (primary or secondary such as from diabetes)
    - **Neurological conditions:** sympathetic tract lesions, syringomyelia
    - **Psychiatric:** panic disorder, PTSD
- **Endocrine**
    - Menopause/perimenopause, other ovarian failure, pregnancy, peripartum states, hyperthyroidism/thyrotoxicosis, diabetes mellitus or insipidus, endocrine tumors (pheochromocytoma, carcinoid tumor), hypogonadism (e.g., orchiectomy)
- **Drugs**
    - **Psychiatric medications:** SSRIs/serotonin syndrome, clozapine, TCAs
    - **Analgesics/antipyretics:** NSAIDS, acetaminophen
    - **Endocrine:** antiandrogens, corticosteroids, insulin/hypoglycemic agents, SRMs, thyroid medications
    - Antihypertensives, anticholinergics, antihistamines, antitussives
    - **Substances of abuse:** alcohol, heroin, and withdrawal syndromes
- **Other**
    - Obstructive sleep apnea, obesity, gastroesophageal reflux disease, dietary factors (e.g., high-sugar diets), chronic fatigue syndrome

Notes

General considerations: In outpatient settings, if a specific diagnosis is apparent based on initial history and physical examination, specific initial treatment may be offered. Otherwise, further diagnostic evaluation can be pursued. The presence of night sweats in isolation has not clearly been associated with an increased risk of death.

Red flags: easy bruising/bleeding, other constitutional symptoms, unintentional weight loss, travel history, drug abuse, other HIV/TB risk factors, adenopathy

Special populations: Older patients may be particularly at risk of night sweats related to medications/polypharmacy (in addition to infection and malignancy). Hormone fluctuations in pregnancy can contribute to night sweats.

Further Reading

- Bryce C. Persistent night sweats: diagnostic evaluation. American Family Physician. 2020 Oct 1;102(7):427-33.
- Mold JW, Holtzclaw BJ, McCarthy L. Night sweats: a systematic review of the literature. The Journal of the American Board of Family Medicine. 2012 Nov 1;25(6):878-93.
- Viera AJ, Bond MM, Yates SW. Diagnosing night sweats. American family physician. 2003 Mar 1;67(5):1019-24.

Weight Loss (Unintentional)

Introduction

Unintentional weight loss can arise from a variety of factors. Benign gastrointestinal (GI) disorders, psychiatric disorders, and underlying malignancy are the three most common categories of etiology. Medication side effects and neurologic disorders are also common. Cachexia syndromes related to organ failure (e.g., heart failure, chronic obstructive pulmonary disease, renal failure), endocrinopathies, serious infections, drugs of abuse, and social factors may produce unintended weight loss. Serious infection, organ failure cachexia, and endocrine emergencies are among those etiologies with the highest acuity. As usual, underlying cancer and serious etiologies should be excluded alongside consideration of other etiologies.

Checklist DDX

Serious/life-threatening: malignancy, HIV, TB, other serious infections, DKA, adrenal insufficiency, thyrotoxic states, abuse/neglect, serious depression

Common: swallowing disorders, other gastrointestinal issues (e.g., reflux, ulcers, biliary colic/cholecystitis), dental issues, dementia, aging related anorexia, socioeconomic and functional issues (especially in older patients), endocrine abnormalities, medication side effects (including polypharmacy and masking of underlying psychiatric/functional issues), anorexia nervosa, alcoholism

Commonly misdiagnosed: functional gastrointestinal disorders, depression, medication side effects, and social factors such as neglect or poor nutrition

Systematic DDX

- **Vascular**
    - Prior stroke (dysphagia), chronic mesenteric ischemia, other vascular intestinal disorders
- **Infection**
    - **Viral:** HIV, HCV, chronic infectious diarrhea, etc.
    - **Bacterial:** dental disease, chronic infectious diarrhea, small bowel overgrowth
    - **Fungal:** candida, other/disseminated in the immunocompromised
    - **Parasitic:** especially enteric (e.g., Giardia) and worm diseases

- **Inflammatory**
    - Systemic sclerosis, chronic inflammation from lupus, rheumatoid arthritis, vasculitis, Behcet's, etc.
- **Neoplasia and hematologic disorders**
    - **Cancers**: GI tumors, hematologic, sarcomas; other common cancers (breast, prostate, lung)
    - **Paraneoplastic syndromes**: carcinoid, VIPoma, Zollinger-Ellison syndrome, etc.
    - Lymphoproliferative processes
- **Gastrointestinal and malabsorptive conditions**
    - **Functional/painful**: dental problems, chewing/swallowing disfunction, GERD/reflex, ulcer disease, biliary disease
    - **Obstructive**: gastrointestinal strictures, webs, and diverticula; intraluminal masses (benign and malignant); extrinsic compression
    - **Dysmotility**: achalasia, esophageal spasm, eosinophilic esophagitis, Chaga's disease, scleroderma, gastroparesis
    - **Malabsorption**: post-surgical (e.g., gastric bypass or GI resections), ulcerative colitis, Crohn's, celiac, Whipple's disease, cystic fibrosis, functional GI disorders, pancreatic (exocrine) insufficiency
    - **Other**: metabolite intolerance (gluten intolerance, lactose, etc.), inherited metabolic issues
- **Organ dysfunction (other than gastrointestinal)**
    - Cardiac, renal, hepatic, pulmonary, neurologic cachexia states (usually late-stage disease)
- **Drugs**
    - **Medication-related nausea**: chemotherapy, HIV medications, antibiotics
    - **Substance use/abuse**: drugs of abuse: methamphetamines, cocaine, laxative, sorbitol, excessive caffeine use/abuse
    - **Other**: NSAID and other medication related ulcer disease
- **Endocrine disorders**
    - Diabetes, hyperthyroidism, hyperparathyroidism, adrenal insufficiency
- **Neurologic**
    - Dementia, Parkinson's disease, anosmia/gustatory dysfunction (dysgeusia), autonomic dysfunction
- **Psychiatric/psychosocial**
    - **Psychiatric disorders**: anorexia, bulimia, depression, bipolar, etc.

- o **Psychosocial factors**: abuse, neglect, isolation, poverty and other social factors

Notes

General considerations: A specific cause of unintentional weight loss is not identified in approximately one quarter of elderly patients with unintentional weight loss. Treatment is directed at underlying causes, though supportive measures to improve dietary intake can be helpful. Multidisciplinary involvement can be helpful in cases of nutritional or functional decline.

Red flags: (unintentional weight loss is often a red flag itself in combination with other presentations, raising concern for malignancy or other underlying infectious/inflammatory process); smoking, other malignancy risk factors, immunocompromise

Special populations: Unintentional weight loss in children may indicate malignancies, malabsorption syndromes, or chronic illnesses such gastrointestinal ailments. Unintentional weight loss in older patients is most commonly associated with depression, other psychiatric conditions, chronic systemic illness, social factors, and poor nutrition. Pregnant patients can develop weight loss due to hyperemesis gravidarum or underlying metabolic abnormalities.

Further Reading

- Bosch X, Monclús E, Escoda O, Guerra-García M, Moreno P, Guasch N, López-Soto A. Unintentional weight loss: Clinical characteristics and outcomes in a prospective cohort of 2677 patients. PloS one. 2017 Apr 7;12(4):e0175125.
- Huffman GB. Evaluating and treating unintentional weight loss in the elderly. American family physician. 2002 Feb 15;65(4):640-51.
- Gaddey HL, Holder K. Unintentional weight loss in older adults. American family physician. 2014 May 1;89(9):718-22.

Weight Gain (Increased Adiposity)

Introduction

Unintentional weight gain, particularly related to increases in adipose tissue, is most often related to environmental, lifestyle, and social factors, which interact with underlying genetic predisposition. There are a variety of medical conditions, however, that will predispose to unintentional increases in adipose tissue. Endocrine diseases and medication side effects are the major contributory categories. Specific genetic syndromes are a rare cause of obesity. Secondary causes of weight gain may coexist with environmental, social, and lifestyle related factors. Many etiologies for weight gain have a bidirectional effect, wherein obesity further perpetuates the underlying cause, which may lead to further weight gain or adiposity.

Weight gain as a result of increase adiposity must be distinguished from weight gain as a result of edema, which has a differing differential, including more concerning etiologies. Refer also to the separate section on generalized edema for weight gain that is not clearly differentiable between these processes.

Checklist DDX

Serious/life-threatening: hormone secreting tumors, Cushing's disease, co-morbid serious psychiatric illness or abuse

Common: lifestyle, social, and environmental factors; physical deconditioning, psychiatric contributors, medication side effects, pregnancy, menopause, age-related changes

Commonly misdiagnosed: medication side effects (e.g., antidepressants, corticosteroids), hypothyroidism, psychiatric conditions like depression or binge eating disorders

Systematic DDX

- **Neoplastic**
    - Adrenal tumors, insulinoma, growth hormone (GH) secreting tumors
- **Endocrine**
    - **Reproductive and age-related changes:** pregnancy, polycystic ovary syndrome (PCOS), menopause, age-related changes
    - **Hormonal imbalances and disorders:** Cushing's disease, hypothyroidism, growth hormone deficiency,

hypothalamic/pituitary dysfunction, hypogonadism (bidirectional effect in males)
    - **Endocrine tumors and syndromes**: insulinoma, pseudohypoparathyroidism
- **Neurologic**
    - **Hypothalamic disorders**: post-surgical, inflammatory processes (sarcoid, TB), vascular damage, trauma, radiotherapy
- **Psychiatric**
    - **Psychiatric disorders**: anxiety, depression, binge eating disorders
    - **Behavioral health and coping**: smoking-cessation, maladaptive coping, prior trauma, including sexual abuse
- **Medications**
    - **Endocrine**: oral contraceptive pills (possible), progesterone injections, growth hormone, corticosteroids (both systemic and local)
    - **Psychiatric**: SSRIs, TCAs, MOAs, atypical anti-psychotics
    - **Diabetic**: insulin, insulin-secretagogues, sulphonyl urea derivates
    - **Anti-epileptics**: carbamazepine, gabapentin, valproic acid
    - **Antihypertensives**: alpha blockers, beta blockers
    - **Other**: PPIs, protease inhibitors, anti-histamines
- **Genetic**
    - **Monogenetic**: leptin and leptin receptor deficiency, POMC deficiency, melanocortin receptor 4 deficiency, prohormone convertase deficiency, BDNF and TrkB insufficiency, SIM 1 insufficiency, etc.
    - **Syndromic**: Prader-Willi, Bardet–Biedl, 16p11.2 deletion syndrome, Albright hereditary osteodystrophy, other rare named and un-named conditions
    - **Other**: polygenic contributions
- **Environmental, social, and other**
    - **Lifestyle factors**: dietary patterns, physical activity, sleep patterns/quality.
    - **Environmental factors**: poor access to healthy food options, access to spaces/venues for physical activity, peer and social support, health promotion initiatives, work related sleep disruptions, chronic stress
    - **Social factors**: social group norms, cultural expectations, health literacy, weight stigma (bidirectional)
    - **Other**: physical deconditioning, early life adverse events, history of prenatal/perinatal insults, exposure to endocrine disrupting chemicals, microbiome factors

Notes

General considerations: Unintentional weight gain and obesity are complex problems, with numerous contributory factors. A comprehensive diagnostic approach is warranted where a secondary cause is suspected. Lifestyle, environmental, and social factors may also be amenable to modification, and may require counseling or referrals for optimal management.

Red flags: other constitutional symptoms which may correlate with rare underlying neoplasia (night sweats, malaise, unexplained anemia), depressive symptom (depressed mood, anhedonia, hypersomnia, etc.), risk factors for ongoing abuse (social isolation, history of abuse or neglect)

Special populations: Weight gain in children may be due to endocrine-related diseases, excessive food and calorie intake, or genetic disorders such as Prader-Willi syndrome. In elderly patients, weight gain may be linked to a sedentary lifestyle and certain medications. Weight gain in pregnancy is expected; patients with greater than expected weight gain may have gestational diabetes, fluid retention, and excessively high-calorie diets.

Further Reading

- van der Valk ES, van den Akker EL, Savas M, Kleinendorst L, Visser JA, Van Haelst MM, Sharma AM, van Rossum EF. A comprehensive diagnostic approach to detect underlying causes of obesity in adults. Obesity reviews. 2019 Jun;20(6):795-804.
- Panuganti KK, Nguyen M, Kshirsagar RK, Doerr C. Obesity (Nursing). InStatPearls [Internet] 2021 Aug 11. StatPearls Publishing.
- Karam JG. Secondary causes of obesity. Clinical Practice. 2007 Sep 1;4(5):641.

Generalized Edema (Pitting Edema)

Introduction

Generalized edema (anasarca) can be considered a more serious form of pitting edema and often first manifests in the lower extremities. Pitting edema is characterized by swelling that, when pressed, leaves an indentation ("pit") in the skin that persists for a few seconds after the pressure is released. Pitting edema results from an accumulation of fluid in the interstitial space, must be differentiated from *nonpitting* edema, which results from increased interstitial proteins and connective tissue changes. With increasing severity, edema first seen at the lower extremities, can affect the upper extremities, abdomen, and ultimately internal organs. Periorbital edema, in particular, is more commonly seen with systemic conditions. This section covers pitting/anasarca related to fluid accumulation; separate sections discuss non-pitting edema and focal extremity edema.

Three major mechanisms contribute to generalized edema: volume overload (heart failure, iatrogenic), decreased oncotic pressure (hepatic or renal dysfunction, malnutrition), and increased vascular permeability (allergic/infectious/toxin). Etiologies may overlap, especially with regard to multi-organ dysfunction. Many causes are serious, including acute infectious etiologies, cardiovascular events, organ failure, and malignant processes. Infectious etiology and trauma are often apparent from other signs. Neurologic and other miscellaneous etiologies are uncommon contributors to generalized or pitting edema. When edema is an isolated finding, systemic (organ dysfunction related), medication-related, and other chronic issues may be considered.

Checklist DDX

Serious/life-threatening: sepsis, anaphylaxis, acute heart failure, acute renal failure, acute hepatic failure, early malignant nodal/lymphatic obstruction, acute leukemic states

Common: iatrogenic/extrinsic fluid overload, chronic cardiac, renal, or hepatic dysfunction, drugs, pregnancy

Commonly misdiagnosed: iatrogenic fluid overload, chronic organ dysfunction (e.g., heart, kidney, liver), medication side effects (e.g., calcium channel blockers [CCBs], thiazolidinediones [TZDs])

Systematic DDX

- **Fluid overload**
    - **Cardiovascular**: acute coronary syndrome (ACS), congestive heart failure, pericardial effusion, pericarditis/myocarditis, valvular diseases, congenital/structural heart diseases, cardiomyopathies (alcoholic, infectious, medication, thiamine deficiency ["wet beriberi"])
    - **Renal**: acute kidney injury, nephrotic syndromes, nephritic syndromes, intrinsic nephropathies, chronic renal failure, dialysis non-compliance
    - **Hepatic**: cirrhosis (non-alcoholic steatohepatitis, alcoholic, chronic hepatitis)
    - **Endocrine**: pregnancy, pre-menstrual state, Cushing's
    - **Drugs**: side effects, including from calcium channel blockers (CCBs), thiazolidinediones (TZDs), androgenic steroids, growth hormone, etc.
- **Decreased oncotic pressure**
    - Renal and liver disease, protein malnutrition, excessive salt intake
- **Increased vascular permeability**
    - **Infectious**: sepsis, diffuse parasitic diseases
    - **Allergic reactions**: anaphylaxis, angioedema, urticaria, allergic reactions
    - **Burns/trauma**: from fluid shifts or resuscitation
    - **Malignant**: leukemic crises, malignant ascites, malignant lymphatic and venous obstructions (early stages of lymphedema can be pitting)
- **Abnormal vascular tone and stasis**
    - **Autonomic dysfunction**: neuropathies (e.g., diabetic neuropathy, peripheral neuropathies) producing abnormal vascular tone and venous stasis
    - **Spinal cord injury and paralysis**: related immobility and venous stasis
    - Immobility from a variety of etiologies
- **Idiopathic**

Notes

General considerations: In some circumstances, pitting and non-pitting edema can overlap; generalized as well as focal edema and related etiologies may also overlap. Review of context, symptoms, and signs is critical part of patient evaluation. Monitoring fluid balance can help assess volume status and guide management.

Red flags: vascular risk factors for acute/underlying cardiac events, fever, immunocompromise, oncologic history

Special populations: In pediatric patients, consider nephrotic syndromes, congenital heart disease, and protein-losing enteropathies. Elderly patients may be at high risk for venous insufficiency, in addition to edema from organ dysfunction. Generalized edema is often physiologic in pregnant patients; consider hemolysis, elevated liver enzymes, and low platelets (HELLP) and preeclampsia if there are other correlate features.

Further Reading

- Trayes KP, Studdiford J, Pickle S, Tully AS. Edema: diagnosis and management. American family physician. 2013 Jul 15;88(2):102-10.
- Kattula SR, Avula A, Baradhi KM. Anasarca.[Updated 2021 Feb 16]. StatPearls [Internet]. Treasure Island (FL): StatPearls Publishing. 2021.
- Smith CC, Emmett M, Kunins L. Clinical manifestations and evaluation of edema in adults. United States: UptoDate. 2019.

General

Ramtin Hajibeygi

Long H. Tu

Katja Goldflam

Generalized Weakness/Fatigue

Introduction

Fatigue is one of the most common patient concerns, usually attributable to lifestyle and environmental factors like sleep deprivation, extreme stress, or effort. Generalized weakness or fatigue, however, can also be a symptom of underlying illness. The differential is broad and includes neurologic conditions, diseases impacting oxygen delivery or metabolism, sleep disorders, infections, rheumatologic conditions, and medication side effects.

Checklist DDX

Serious/life-threatening: sepsis, heart failure, hypoglycemia, hypothyroidism, myasthenia gravis

Common: dehydration, anemia, hypothyroidism, chronic fatigue syndrome, obesity, sleep apnea, medication side effects (e.g., statins)

Commonly misdiagnosed: chronic fatigue syndrome, depression, hypothyroidism, anemia, occult malignancy

Systematic DDX

- **Neoplastic and hematologic**
    - Anemia, occult malignancy
- **Infection**
    - **Post-viral syndromes:** chronic COVID-19, Epstein Barr virus (EBV), cardiomyopathy
        - **Viral infections:** mononucleosis syndrome, viral hepatitis, HIV
        - **Bacterial infections:** tuberculosis (TB), subacute bacterial endocarditis, pneumonia, staphylococcus aureus infection, meningococcal infection
        - **Fungal infections:** candidiasis, aspergillosis, histoplasmosis
        - **Parasitic infections:** malaria, toxoplasmosis, leishmaniasis, schistosomiasis
        - Sepsis (from a variety of etiologies)
- **Rheumatologic/inflammatory**
    - Fibromyalgia, polymyalgia rheumatica, systemic lupus erythematosus, rheumatoid arthritis, Sjogren's syndrome

- **Organ systemic dysfunction**
    - **Cardiopulmonary conditions:** congestive heart failure, chronic obstructive pulmonary disease, sleep apnea
    - Chronic renal disease, chronic hepatic disease
- **Psychiatric**
    - Depression, anxiety disorder, somatization disorder, stress or grief reaction
- **Neurologic**
    - Multiple sclerosis (MS), Guillain-Barré Syndrome (GBS), critical illness polyneuropathy and myopathy (CIP/CIM), stroke (rate subtypes like bilateral medial medullary infarction), amyotrophic lateral sclerosis (ALS)
- **Toxic-metabolic and nutritional**
    - **Medication toxicities:** benzodiazepines, antidepressants, muscle relaxants, first-generation antihistamines, beta-blockers, opioids, selective serotonin reuptake inhibitors (SSRIs), antipsychotics, caffeine (chronic use/withdrawal), sedative-hypnotics (e.g., Z-drugs), barbiturates
    - **Substance use:** alcohol, marijuana, opioids, benzodiazepines, antihistamines (first-generation), nicotine (chronic use/withdrawal), barbiturates, withdrawal from sympathomimetics (e.g., cocaine and methamphetamine)
    - **Nutritional deficiencies:** B-vitamins (B1, B6, B12), vitamin D, iron
    - **Electrolyte imbalance:** (high/hyper- and low/hypo-) sodium, potassium, calcium, magnesium, phosphate, chloride
    - Acidosis and alkalosis
    - Hyperglycemia and hypoglycemia
- **Endocrinologic**
    - Hypothyroidism, hyperthyroidism, adrenal insufficiency, type 1 diabetes mellitus (T1DM), type 2 diabetes mellitus (T2DM)
- **Lifestyle factors**
    - Sleep deprivation, general frailty/deconditioning, stress

Notes

General considerations: Specific evaluation may not be necessary for patients who have fatigue related to a known stressor, benign medical condition, or psychological disorders. Sudden onset, unexplained, persistent, or progressive weakness does warrant further investigation.

Red flags: unintentional weight loss, easy bruising or bleeding, history of travel to endemic regions (e.g., malaria), substance use history, lymphadenopathy, trauma or falls, fever, abnormal vital signs, new onset of confusion or cognitive impairment

Special populations: In children, other differential considerations include chronic diseases such as malignancies, cystic fibrosis, and juvenile idiopathic arthritis; neuromuscular diseases like cerebral palsy and muscular dystrophies; and post-viral syndromes. Pediatric patients are especially vulnerable to malnutrition and psychosocial stress, which are factors that increase fatigue. Differential considerations in older adults include: frailty syndrome, sarcopenia, and chronic inflammatory conditions (e.g. rheumatoid arthritis, cardiovascular disease). This demographic is vulnerable to nutritional deficiencies and physical deconditioning due to loss of functional reserves and multimorbidity. Considerations in pregnancy and the postpartum period should include anemia, hypothyroidism, postpartum cardiomyopathy, pulmonary embolism, and postpartum depression or anxiety. This group is specifically at heightened risk because of changes in hormonal conditions, increased metabolic demands, and sleep disturbances which accentuate both physical and mental fatigue.

Further Reading

- Perrin, J.M., S.R. Bloom, and S.L. Gortmaker, The increase of childhood chronic conditions in the United States. Jama, 2007. 297(24): p. 2755-2759.
- Varni JW, Limbers CA, Bryant WP, Wilson DP. The PedsQL™ Multidimensional Fatigue Scale in pediatric obesity: Feasibility, reliability and validity. International Journal of Pediatric Obesity. 2010 Jan 1;5(1):34-42.
- Levine, J. and B.D. Greenwald, Fatigue in Parkinson disease, stroke, and traumatic brain injury. Physical Medicine and Rehabilitation Clinics, 2009. 20(2): p. 347-361.
- Ream, E. and A. Richardson, Fatigue: a concept analysis. International journal of nursing studies, 1996. 33(5): p. 519-529.

Syncope/Loss of Consciousness

Introduction

Syncope is a sudden temporary loss of consciousness associated with a loss of postural tone and spontaneous recovery to preexisting neurologic function. Syncope must be distinguished from seizures, which are associated with aura, rhythmic movements, tongue biting, incontinence and a post-ictal state. Syncope should also be differentiated from dizziness/vertigo, presyncope, and drop attacks, which do not involve loss of consciousness. Patients with pre-syncope however, may be evaluated similarly to those with full syncope. Etiologies generally fall into three categories: cardiac, neurally mediated, and orthostatic hypotension.

Checklist DDX

Serious/life-threatening: acute cardiac events, dysrhythmias, pulmonary embolism, acute aortic etiologies (rarely, and generally present with other symptoms), acute neurovascular events (rarely; generally present with other symptoms)

Common: vasovagal/situational, orthostatic hypotension, cardiac arrhythmia

Commonly misdiagnosed: epilepsy, psychogenic episodes (e.g., panic attacks, conversion disorder, psychogenic syncope)

Systematic DDX

- **Cardiovascular**
    - **Arrythmias:** tachyarrhythmias, bradyarrhythmia, heart block, long/short QT syndrome, channelopathies and other inherited etiologies (WPW, Brugada), pacemaker dysfunction
    - **Structural:** valvular diseases (e.g., aortic, mitral, or pulmonary stenosis/regurgitation), hypertrophic obstructive cardiomyopathy (HOCM), arrhythmogenic right ventricular cardiomyopathy, infiltrative diseases (e.g., amyloid, hemochromatosis, sarcoidosis)
    - **Ischemia:** acute coronary syndrome, acute myocardial infarction
    - **Other vascular/obstructive processes:** large pulmonary embolism, pericardial tamponade, gastrointestinal hemorrhage, vascular steal syndromes, pulmonary hypertension, cardiac masses (myxoma, cardiac tumors, other metastatic or tumor-embolic disease); less likely to present as pure syncope but

should be considered: aortic dissection, tension pneumothorax, acute blood loss from ruptured aneurysm, subarachnoid hemorrhage
- **Neurally-mediated (reflex)**
    - **Vasovagal:** stress, fear, noxious stimuli, heat exposure
    - **Situational:** micturition, post-exercise, postprandial, gastrointestinal stimulation, cough
    - **Other:** carotid sinus syndrome/hypersensitivity (extrinsic such as from a tight collar)
- **Orthostatic**
    - **Drug induced:** alcohol, antianginal, antidepressants, antidiabetic, anti-hypertensives, antiparkinsonian, diuretics, insulin, flibanserin
    - **Primary autonomic failure:** multiple sclerosis, multisystem atrophy, Parkinson disease/parkinsonism, Wernicke encephalopathy
    - **Secondary autonomic failure:** amyloidosis, connective tissue diseases, chronic inflammatory demyelinating polyneuropathy, diabetes, Lewy body dementia, spinal cord injury, uremia
    - **Volume depletion:** blood loss, vomiting, diarrhea, inadequate fluid intake, environmental causes
    - **Other:** postural orthostatic tachycardiac syndrome (POTS; associated with chronic fatigue syndrome and mitral valve prolapse)

- **Non-syncopal mimics**
    - Hypoxia, hypocapnia, epilepsy, stroke/TIA, vertebrobasilar insufficiency, cataplexy, drop attacks, psychogenic (panic attacks), metabolic syndromes (e.g., hypoglycemia, anemia), toxic syndromes (drug overdoses), delirium

Notes

General consideration: After differentiation of syncope from seizure, and exclusion of life-threatening etiologies, work-up often depends on other findings in the history and physical examination. An underlying etiology is not found in as many as 39% of cases. Consider the possibility of concurrent trauma, especially if unwitnessed or in older patients. Non-syncopal mimics, if suspected, have their own differential diagnosis.

Red flags: underlying heart disease, associated chest pain or dyspnea, pre-existing systemic diseases, family history of sudden death, recurrent syncope, exertional syncope, neurologic compromise, hemodynamic compromise/hypotension, abnormal ECG findings, older age, anemia, serious electrolyte abnormalities, concern for gastrointestinal bleeding

Special populations: Syncope is most often neurally mediated, while cardiac causes (e.g., aortic stenosis) and orthostatic hypotension are also common, especially in elderly patients. Falls, as precursors to or resulting from syncope, are also more common in the elderly. In children, syncope is mostly benign, though potentially life-threatening cardiovascular conditions should always be considered. In pregnancy, syncope is prevalent due to hemodynamic changes in the body, though causes related to hypercoagulability should be considered. Syncope in the first-trimester is associated with adverse outcomes (e.g., preterm birth, congenital abnormalities).

Further Reading

- Runser LA, Gauer R, Houser A. Syncope: evaluation and differential diagnosis. American family physician. 2017 Mar 1;95(5):303-12.
- Reed MJ. Approach to syncope in the emergency department. Emergency Medicine Journal. 2019 Feb 1;36(2):108-16.
- Grossman SA, Badireddy M. Syncope. 2022 Jun 21. In: StatPearls [Internet]. Treasure Island (FL): StatPearls Publishing; 2022 Jan–. PMID: 28723035.
- Kapoor WN. Current evaluation and management of syncope. Circulation. 2002 Sep 24;106(13):1606-9.

Dizziness (Vertigo/Disequilibrium)

Introduction

"Dizziness" is a nonspecific term may refer to vertigo (a sensation of spinning), disequilibrium, presyncope, or lightheadedness. The evaluation of presyncope or lightheadedness is similar to that of syncope, as discussed in a preceding section. Evaluation of the vertiginous patient largely depends on the timing and triggers of the symptoms. Both "central" (central nervous system [CNS]) and "peripheral" (peripheral nervous system, systemic, non-neurologic) etiologies may produce vertigo. Generally, central etiologies are more serious and may require emergent treatment. Stroke/TIA (transient ischemic attack) is the most acute central etiology and commonly misdiagnosed. Common peripheral etiologies often relate to dysfunction of the vestibular system. Disequilibrium may be caused by the same etiologies that produce vertigo, though can also result from variety of peripheral nervous system, musculoskeletal disorders, and sensory deficits which impair proprioception, posture, or spatial orientation.

Checklist DDX

Serious/life-threatening: stroke/cerebrovascular events, brain tumor, acute intoxication or withdrawal, hypoglycemia, arrythmias, critical valvular disease, adrenal (Addisonian) crisis

Common: benign paroxysmal positional vertigo (BPPV), vestibular neuritis, medication effects, persistent postural-perceptual dizziness (PPPD)

Commonly misdiagnosed: posterior circulation stroke, vestibular neuritis, vestibular migraine

Systematic DDX

- **Central (i.e., central nervous system)**
    - **Cerebrovascular disease:** stroke, transient ischemic attack (TIA), vertebrobasilar insufficiency
    - **Mass lesions:** tumor (e.g., vestibular schwannoma, ependymoma, glioma, medulloblastoma), rarely collection/abscess
    - **Demyelination:** multiple sclerosis, osmotic demyelination, etc.
    - **Other:** vestibular migraine, PPPD
- **Peripheral (i.e., peripheral nervous system/otologic)**
    - BPPV, vestibular neuritis (labyrinthitis), Meniere's disease, otosclerosis, barotrauma, traumatic vestibular dysfunction,

cholesteatoma, medication ototoxicity (e.g., aminoglycosides, antirheumatics)
- **Other (overlapping with syncope DDX)**
    - **Cardiovascular:** cerebral hypoperfusion (see section on syncope for additional details)
    - **Toxic:** carbon monoxide poisoning, acute alcohol intoxication, withdrawal
    - **Metabolic:** hypoglycemia, hyperglycemia, uremia/azotemia
    - **Endocrine:** hypothyroidism, hyperthyroidism
    - **Medication:** cardiovascular side effects and cardiac medications (anti-arrhythmic, anti-hypertensives, etc.), antiepileptics, skeletal muscle relaxants, antidiabetics (hypoglycemia), marrow suppression effects, bleeding from anti-coagulants, anti-cholinergic effects, cerebellar toxicity
    - **Psychiatric:** panic attacks
    - **Other:** orthostatic hypotension

- **Additional DDX for disequilibrium**
    - **Cerebellar and subcortical white matter disease:** cerebellar degeneration, leukoencephalopathy, subcortical ischemic changes
    - **Other CNS degenerative disorders:** progressive supranuclear palsy, multiple system atrophy with predominant imbalance
    - **Peripheral neuropathy:** diabetic neuropathy, alcohol-related neuropathy, vitamin B12 deficiency
    - **Musculoskeletal disorders:** osteoarthritis, cervical spondylosis, joint deformities
    - **Visual impairment:** macular degeneration, cataracts, optic neuropathy
    - **Psychiatric:** anxiety, fear of falling, psychogenic imbalance

Notes

General considerations: In addition to eliciting timing and triggers, evaluation of BPPV via the Dix-Hallpike maneuver, and bedside examinations such as the HINTS exam (Head Impulse, Nystagmus, Test of Skew), HINTS+ (bedside hearing test added to HINTS), or similar strategies may be useful. Medications have been implicated in as many as 23% of cases in older adults. Strokes presenting as dizziness are amongst the most commonly misdiagnosed serious conditions in acute care, often due to overreliance on reported quality of dizziness (patients may have difficulty describing their symptoms with specificity) and CT/CTA (which cannot identify posterior circulation strokes as reliably as MRI).

Red flags: gait disturbance, focal neurologic deficits, especially those suggesting brainstem dysfunction (diplopia, dysarthria, dysphagia, ataxia), altered level of consciousness

Special populations: In children, dizziness is often caused by dehydration, inner ear infections, or orthostatic hypotension. Elderly patients are also susceptible to orthostatic hypotension, vestibular dysfunction, and polypharmacy. In pregnancy, dizziness may be associated with hormonal changes, low blood pressure, or postural changes. Severe or persistent dizziness should raise suspicion for anemia, dehydration, or cardiovascular problems.

Further Reading

- Muncie Jr HL, Sirmans SM, James E. Dizziness: approach to evaluation and management. American family physician. 2017 Feb 1;95(3):154-62.
- Balatsouras DG, Kaberos A, Assimakopoulos D, Katotomichelakis M, Economou NC, Korres SG. Etiology of vertigo in children. International journal of pediatric otorhinolaryngology. 2007 Mar 1;71(3):487-94.
- Casani AP, Gufoni M, Capobianco S. Current insights into treating vertigo in older adults. Drugs & aging. 2021 Aug;38(8):655-70.
- Serna-Hoyos LC, Arango AF, Ortiz-Mesa S, Vieira-Rios SM, Arbelaez-Lelion D, Vanegas-Munera JM, Castillo-Bustamante M. Vertigo in pregnancy: a narrative review. Cureus. 2022 May;14(5).

Sleep Disturbances

Introduction

Sleep disturbances encompass a broad range of conditions which produce difficulty falling or staying asleep, excessive daytime sleepiness, abnormal behaviors during sleep, or altered sleep-wake rhythms. The differential diagnosis for sleep disturbances is broad, encompassing primary sleep disorders as well as secondary causes from psychiatric conditions (depression, anxiety), medical illnesses (pain, thyroid disorders), medications/substances, and situational factors like stress or environmental disruptions. Sleep disorders can be classified broadly into categories such as insomnia disorders (difficulty initiating or maintaining sleep), sleep-related breathing disorders (such as obstructive sleep apnea), central disorders of hypersomnolence (e.g., narcolepsy, idiopathic hypersomnia), circadian rhythm sleep-wake disorders (misalignment between the sleep-wake pattern and the environment), parasomnias (abnormal behaviors or experiences during sleep like sleepwalking or nightmares), sleep-related movement disorders (such as restless legs syndrome). For the purposes of this section, we will provide differing approaches to differential diagnosis, based on the disorder classification as well as pathophysiologic mechanisms with selected etiologies provided for both.

Checklist DDX

Serious/life-threatening: severe obstructive sleep apnea, narcolepsy (Type 1 and 2), REM sleep behavior disorder (potential for injury to self/others), congestive heart failure (CHF), central sleep apnea

Common: chronic insomnia, obstructive sleep apnea (OSA), restless legs syndrome (RLS), circadian rhythm sleep-wake disorders (e.g., delayed sleep phase syndrome, advanced sleep phase syndrome), primary (psychophysiologic) insomnia, poor sleep hygiene (irregular bedtimes, napping, screen exposure, caffeine/alcohol), anxiety, stress

Commonly misdiagnosed: paradoxical insomnia, nocturnal frontal lobe epilepsy, sleep-related eating disorder, nightmare disorder, non-24-hour sleep-wake disorder.

Systematic DDX

Sleep disorder classification
- **Insomnia disorders**
    - Chronic insomnia disorder, short-term insomnia disorder, psychophysiological insomnia, insufficient sleep syndrome
- **Sleep-related breathing disorders**
    - Obstructive sleep apnea, central sleep apnea (idiopathic, Cheyne-Stokes breathing in heart failure or stroke, opioid-induced), sleep-related hypoventilation (obesity hypoventilation syndrome, neuromuscular disease), upper airway resistance syndrome
- **Central disorders of hypersomnolence**
    - Narcolepsy type 1 (with cataplexy and low hypocretin), narcolepsy type 2 (without cataplexy), idiopathic hypersomnia, Kleine-Levin syndrome
- **Circadian rhythm sleep-wake disorders (CRSWD)**
    - Delayed sleep-wake phase disorder, advanced sleep-wake phase disorder, irregular sleep-wake rhythm, non-24-hour sleep-wake rhythm (common in blind individuals), shift work disorder
- **Parasomnias**
    - Non-REM parasomnias (confusional arousals, sleepwalking, sleep terrors), REM parasomnias (REM sleep behavior disorder, nightmare disorder), other parasomnias (sleep enuresis, sleep-related eating disorder, exploding head syndrome)
- **Sleep-related movement disorders**
    - Restless legs syndrome (primary or secondary), periodic limb movement disorder, sleep bruxism, sleep myoclonus, benign sleep myoclonus of infancy
- **Other sleep disorders**
    - Isolated symptoms such as snoring without apnea, normal variants, unresolved sleep problems not meeting criteria for other categories.
- **Sleep disturbances secondary to medical and neurologic conditions**
    - **Neurological:** stroke, Parkinson's disease, multiple sclerosis, epilepsy, dementia, traumatic brain injury
    - **Cardiovascular:** congestive heart failure, myocardial ischemia, arrhythmias
    - **Pulmonary:** COPD, asthma, obesity hypoventilation syndrome
    - **Gastrointestinal:** GERD
    - **Endocrine/metabolic:** diabetes mellitus, hyperthyroidism, chronic renal failure

- o **Rheumatologic/other:** rheumatoid arthritis, fibromyalgia, chronic pain syndromes, migraine
- **Sleep disturbances secondary to substances**
  - o **Stimulants** amphetamines, methylphenidate, cocaine
  - o **Antidepressants:** SSRIs, TCAs
  - o **Other:** corticosteroids, beta-agonists/beta-blockers, benzodiazepines and sedative-hypnotics (rebound insomnia), antipsychotics
  - o **Drugs of abuse:** opioids (central sleep apnea), alcohol (initial sedation then rebound insomnia), nicotine, caffeine, illicit drug
  - o **Withdrawal states:** alcohol, benzodiazepine, caffeine

Pathophysiologic approach
- **Neurological**
  - o Narcolepsy (Type 1 and 2, characterized by excessive daytime sleepiness, sleep attacks, and cataplexy in Type 1), REM sleep behavior disorder, nocturnal frontal lobe epilepsy, restless legs syndrome, periodic limb movement disorder (PLMD)
- **Respiratory**
  - o Obstructive sleep apnea, central sleep apnea, sleep-related hypoventilation.
- **Psychiatric/psychological**
  - o Primary (psychophysiologic) insomnia, chronic insomnia, paradoxical insomnia, nightmare disorder, sleep-related eating disorder.
- **Circadian rhythm disorders**
  - o Delayed sleep phase syndrome, advanced sleep phase syndrome, non-24-hour sleep-wake disorder, shift work disorder: jet lag, social jet lag
- **Medical/organ dysfunction:**
  - o Chronic pain, thyroid dysfunction, heart failure, chronic kidney disease.
- **Toxic-metabolic/medication-related**
  - o **Medication-induced insomnia:** SSRIs, beta-blockers, corticosteroids
  - o **Substance-related sleep disturbances:** caffeine, alcohol, or withdrawal from sedatives
  - o **Drug-induced hypersomnia:** antihistamines, benzodiazepines
  - o **Stimulant-induced sleep fragmentation:** amphetamines
- **Lifestyle and behavioral factors**
  - o **Poor sleep hygiene:** irregular bedtimes, napping, screen exposure, caffeine/alcohol
  - o **Other:** anxiety and stress

Notes

General considerations: Sleep disturbances manifest as a variety of symptoms beyond the sleep phase and can affect waking hours. Excessive sleepiness, impaired concentration, mood changes, or functional impairment can be manifestations of sleep disturbance. Routine polysomnography (overnight sleep study) or multiple sleep latency testing are not needed for many patients with insomnia; indications include suspected sleep apnea, periodic limb movement disorder, REM sleep behavior disorder, treatment resistance, or when there are unusual nocturnal behaviors. Consider the contribution of behavior and lifestyle factors caffeine, alcohol, work habits, exercise habits, diet, and sleep hygiene.

Red flags: excessive daytime sleepiness with sudden sleep episodes (e.g., narcolepsy, severe obstructive sleep apnea), loud snoring with observed apneas or gasping, and complex nighttime behaviors with possible injuries (e.g., REM sleep behavior disorder [RBD], nocturnal frontal lobe epilepsy)

Special populations: In children, insomnia disorders, sleepwalking, night terrors, and sleep-disordered breathing are more common. In older patients, problems with sleep arise mainly due to comorbidities or circadian shifting and these are managed by addressing the underlying problems. In pregnant pate, barriers to sleep can arise from hormonal changes, life stressors, and restless legs syndrome.

Further Reading

- Deshpande P, Salcedo B, Haq C. Common Sleep Disorders in Children. Am Fam Physician. 2022 Feb 1;105(2):168-176. PMID: 35166510.
- Silvestri R, Aricò I. Sleep disorders in pregnancy. Sleep Sci. 2019 Jul-Sep;12(3):232-239. doi: 10.5935/1984-0063.20190098. PMID: 31890101; PMCID: PMC6932848.
- Holder S, Narula NS. Common sleep disorders in adults: diagnosis and management. American family physician. 2022 Apr;105(4):397-405.

Eyes

Quoc-Huy Ly

Long H. Tu

Laura Hanson

Red Eye

Introduction

One of the most common ocular complaints, red or pink eye, occurs when blood vessels on the surface of the eye become enlarged or inflamed. Inflammation commonly involves the conjunctiva, though the eyelids, iris, cornea, sclera, and uvea can also be affected. Red eye may be produced by infectious causes (viral, bacterial, fungal, or parasitic), inflammatory conditions (including allergic reactions and autoimmune-related inflammation), trauma or mechanical irritation, vascular issues (such as subconjunctival hemorrhage), neoplastic causes, and other miscellaneous factors like medication side effects. While many cases are mild and manageable within primary care, certain red flags such as associated vision loss, significant eye pain, or recurrent infections suggest more serious underlying pathology that warrants urgent referral to an ophthalmologist.

Checklist DDX

Serious/life-threatening: acute angle-closure glaucoma, orbital cellulitis, bacterial/fungal endophthalmitis, anterior uveitis, scleritis, corneal ulcers, ocular neoplasms, ocular hemorrhage, cavernous sinus thrombosis, chemical burns, Stevens-Johnson syndrome

Common: conjunctivitis (most common), blepharitis, corneal abrasion, dry eye syndrome, chalazion/stye (hordeolum), episcleritis, scleritis, keratitis, iritis, uveitis, subconjunctival hemorrhage, glaucoma, allergies, foreign body irritation

Commonly misdiagnosed: acute angle-closure glaucoma, uveitis, scleritis, corneal ulcers, subconjunctival hemorrhage, dry eye, blepharitis, iritis

Systematic DDX

- **Vascular**
    - **Bleeding:** subconjunctival hemorrhage, ocular hemorrhage, hyphema
    - **Venous congestion:** carotid-cavernous fistula, cavernous sinus thrombosis, elevated episcleral venous pressure syndromes (e.g., Radius-Maumenee syndrome)
- **Infectious/inflammatory**
    - **Sites of involvement:** conjunctivitis (bacterial, viral, allergic/giant papillary), iritis, uveitis (anterior/posterior), episcleritis/scleritis, keratitis (including neurotrophic, viral,

fungal, acanthamoeba), retinitis, vitritis, choroiditis, endophthalmitis (bacterial/fungal, especially post-op or trauma), orbital cellulitis
- o **Etiologies:**
  - **Viral infection:** Adenovirus (most common), coxsackievirus, VZV, EBV, HSV (dendritic/marginal ulcer), influenza
  - **Bacterial infection:** S. pneumococcus & H. influenzae (children), Staph aureus (adults), N. gonorrhoeae, Pseudomonas, Chlamydia trachomatis serotypes D-K
  - **Other infectious:** fungal keratitis, parasitic infections (Acanthamoeba keratitis)
  - **Allergic:** allergic conjunctivitis (seasonal/perennial), atopic/vernal conjunctivitis, giant papillary conjunctivitis
  - **Inflammatory:** Stevens-Johnson syndrome, rheumatoid arthritis, reactive arthritis, granulomatosis with polyangiitis, sarcoidosis, inflammatory bowel diseases, dry eye syndrome, Behçet syndrome, ocular rosacea

- **Neoplastic**
  - o Ocular surface squamous neoplasia, conjunctival squamous cell carcinoma, conjunctival and uveal melanoma, ocular lymphoma, metastatic disease
- **Dysfunction**
  - o **Adnexal/eyelid disorders:** hordeolum (stye), chalazion, entropion, ectropion, trichiasis, floppy eyelid syndrome, dacryocystitis, canaliculitis, Meibomian gland dysfunction
- **Compressive/obstructive**
  - o Acute angle-closure glaucoma, orbital tumors causing venous congestion
- **Injury/trauma**
  - o **Postoperative:** post-surgical endophthalmitis, LASIK complications
  - o **Other:** foreign body, ruptured globe, corneal abrasion, corneal ulcer, chemical burns (acid/alkali), thermal burns, radiation injury, dry eye, contact lens overwear complications
- **Toxic-metabolic**
  - o **Drugs:** bisphosphonates, topiramate, isotretinoin, chlorpromazine
  - o **Endocrine:** Graves ophthalmopathy

- **Everything else**
    - Cluster headaches

> **Notes**

General considerations. The assessment of a patient presenting with red eye begins with a detailed history that is critical to differentiating benign conditions from those that may threaten vision or require urgent intervention. It is important to discern whether one or both eyes are affected, as bilateral involvement is common in viral conjunctivitis and allergic conditions but less so in serious infections like orbital cellulitis. Pain severity, the presence of photophobia, as well as the presence and type of discharge can also be helpful in distinguishing etiologies. Benign conditions like simple conjunctivitis may be managed conservatively, whereas sight-threatening issues such as acute angle-closure glaucoma, keratitis, or orbital cellulitis require prompt specialist evaluation.

Red flags: severe eye pain, sudden vision changes, unilateral redness with proptosis, sudden onset of flashes or floaters, eye trauma or foreign body sensation, unequal or unresponsive pupils, decreased vision, bleeding or discharge around the eye, corneal opacity or ulceration

Special populations: Infectious conjunctivitis is especially common in pediatric populations, due to exposures from daycare, school, etc.; children however, can still have red eye from systemic diseases like juvenile idiopathic arthritis or leukemia. In older adults, it is especially important to consider sight-threatening causes like acute angle-closure glaucoma, anterior uveitis, or scleritis, and to be alert for complications related to comorbidities and use of systemic medications. In immunocompromised populations (such as those with HIV/AIDS or on immunosuppressants), clinicians must be alert to severe infections and unusual pathogens, as these patients are at higher risk for aggressive ocular disease.

> **Further Reading**

- Narayana S, McGee S. Bedside Diagnosis of the 'Red Eye': A Systematic Review. The American Journal of Medicine. 2015;128(11):1220-1224.e1. doi:10.1016/j.amjmed.2015.06.026
- Leibowitz HM. The Red Eye. New England Journal of Medicine. 2000;343(5):345-351. doi:10.1056/NEJM200008033430507
- Cronau H, Kankanala RR, Mauger T. Diagnosis and Management of Red Eye in Primary Care. afp. 2010;81(2):137-144.

Eye Pain

Introduction

Eye pain is a common and often distressing emergency department symptom that frequently co-presents with red eye, sharing many etiologies. Although it is frequently caused by manageable conditions such as conjunctivitis or hordeolum (stye), eye pain can be the first sign of a serious ophthalmologic condition and should thus be quickly evaluated to rule out vision-threatening causes. Workup should include a detailed vision history, with emphasis on the patient's contact lens use, specifically the wear schedule, duration of use, cleaning practices, and exposure to water such as swimming or hot tub use.

Checklist DDX

Serious/vision-threatening: acute angle-closure glaucoma, orbital cellulitis, orbital compartment syndrome, keratitis (bacterial, viral, fungal, *Acanthamoeba*), endophthalmitis, anterior uveitis, optic neuritis, traumatic injury (globe injury, blunt trauma, corneal foreign body)

Common: conjunctivitis (viral, bacterial, allergic), corneal abrasion, hordeolum, blepharitis, dry eye

Commonly misdiagnosed: migraine, scleritis, keratitis, corneal ulcer

Systematic DDX

- **Vascular**
    - Ocular ischemic syndrome, carotid-cavernous fistula, giant cell arteritis
- **Infectious/inflammatory**
    - **Eyelid/superficial inflammation:** blepharitis, hordeolum, chalazion, preseptal cellulitis, conjunctivitis (viral, bacterial, allergic)
    - **Keratitis:** bacterial, viral (VZV, HSV), fungal, Acanthamoeba, neurotrophic keratopathy
    - **Ocular coating inflammation:** scleritis (anterior/posterior), episcleritis, uveitis (anterior, intermediate, posterior)
    - **Deep infection:** orbital cellulitis, endophthalmitis

- - o **Neurologic inflammation:** optic neuritis, idiopathic intracranial hypertension, multiple cranial nerve palsies (trochleitis, Tolosa-Hunt syndrome)
    - o **Systemic autoimmune disease:** Behçet disease, granulomatosis with polyangiitis, sarcoidosis, rheumatoid arthritis, lupus
- **Neoplastic**
  - o Orbital/ocular tumors, optic nerve glioma, meningioma, metastatic disease
- **Dysfunction**
  - o Dry eye syndrome, meibomian gland dysfunction, temporomandibular joint dysfunction,
- **Injury/trauma**
  - o Foreign body (debris, contact lenses), corneal abrasion, chemical exposure, blunt or penetrating trauma
- **Compression/obstruction**
  - o Acute angle-closure glaucoma, ocular hypertension, neovascular glaucoma, orbital compartment syndrome, sinus-related compression
- **Toxic-metabolic**
  - o **Drugs:** antihistamines, anticholinergics, bisphosphonates, topiramate, isotretinoin
  - o Vitamin A deficiency
- **Everything else**
  - o Functional/idiopathic eye pain
  - o **Referred pain:** sinusitis, trigeminal neuralgia, psychogenic

Notes

General considerations: Eye pain accompanied by a headache or facial pain may be due to primary headache disorders such as migraines, tension headaches, and cluster headaches (often presenting with ptosis and lacrimation), alongside referred pain from temporomandibular joint syndrome and otitis media. It is also essential to evaluate for signs of systemic disease: scleritis and uveitis are frequently associated with autoimmune conditions such as rheumatoid arthritis or lupus, while optic neuritis may be an early indicator of multiple sclerosis. Imaging is not frequently required with eye complaints unless red flags are present (e.g., CT orbits/sinuses for possible abscess in orbital cellulitis, or contrast MRI for suspected optic neuritis). Conjunctivitis, a common and typically non-threatening cause of eye pain, can often be managed with any broad-spectrum topical antibiotics.

Red flags: sudden vision changes or loss, photophobia without a foreign body sensation, severe pain, pain on eye movement, distorted or mid-dilated pupil with impaired reflex, hyphema/hypopyon

Special populations: Younger children can have functional eye pain without pathology, but evaluation should be done to exclude foreign bodies or corneal injury. In older patients, eye pain can be associated with more serious conditions such as giant cell arteritis, glaucoma, or ocular ischemic syndrome.

Further Reading

- Belmonte, C., Acosta, M. C., Merayo-Lloves, J., & Gallar, J. (2015). What Causes Eye Pain? Current Ophthalmology Reports, 3(2), 111–121. https://doi.org/10.1007/s40135-015-0073-9
- Cutarelli, P. E., & Aronsky, M. A. (1999). The painful eye: external and anterior segment causes. Clinics in Geriatric Medicine, 15(1), 103–112, vii. https://pubmed.ncbi.nlm.nih.gov/9855661/
- Dargin, J. M., & Lowenstein, R. A. (2008). The Painful Eye. Emergency Medicine Clinics of North America, 26(1), 199–216. https://doi.org/10.1016/j.emc.2007.10.001
- Jabs, D. A., Mudun, A., Dunn, J. P., & Marsh, M. J. (2000). Episcleritis and scleritis: clinical features and treatment results. American Journal of Ophthalmology, 130(4), 469–476. https://doi.org/10.1016/s0002-9394(00)00710-8
- McGinley TC. (2022). Adult Eye Conditions: Common Eye Conditions. FP Essentials, 519. https://pubmed.ncbi.nlm.nih.gov/35947131/
- Pfilipsen, M., Massaquoi, M., & Wolf, S. (2016). Evaluation of the Painful Eye. American Family Physician, 93(12), 991–998. https://www.aafp.org/pubs/afp/issues/2016/0615/p991.html#afp20160615p991-b20
- Richards, A.-L., Patel, V. S., Simon, J. W., & Zobal-Ratner, J. (2010). Eye pain in preschool children: diagnostic and prognostic significance. Journal of AAPOS : The Official Publication of the American Association for Pediatric Ophthalmology and Strabismus, 14(5), 383–385. https://doi.org/10.1016/j.jaapos.2010.06.014
- Robblee, J., & Patel, J. N. (2025). Approach to Eye Pain: Differential Diagnosis and Work Up for the Neurologist. Current Neurology and Neuroscience Reports, 25(1), 48. https://doi.org/10.1007/s11910-025-01436-4

Diplopia (Double Vision)

Introduction

A common presenting complaint in the emergency room, diplopia (double vision, though patients can sometimes describe it as blurry vision) can have benign etiologies but could be a warning sign for a more serious ocular or neurologic pathology, requiring a thorough evaluation. Double vision can be classified as binocular diplopia, due to eye misalignment which is no longer seen if one eye is obscured, or monocular diplopia, which persists even if one eye is obscured. Normal eye positioning and alignment are dependent on the bilateral function of the extraocular muscles, which in turn are innervated by cranial nerves III, IV, and VI; thus, many cases of diplopia are related to lesions of the anatomic pathways of these structures throughout the subarachnoid space and cavernous sinus, including pathologies of the CSF, sphenoid sinus, nasopharynx, and internal carotid arteries, among others.

Checklist DDX

Serious/life-threatening: ischemic stroke, brainstem/cerebellar lesions, intracrancial aneurysm, orbital cellulitis, traumatic brain injury, vascular malformation

Common: for monocular diplopia: astigmatism, cataracts, uncorrected myopia or hyperopia, and corneal or retinal pathologies are common causes; for binocular diplopia: pathologies related to the extraocular muscles (strabismus), cranial nerve palsies (potentially related to microvascular disease), myasthenia gravis, multiple sclerosis

Commonly misdiagnosed: cranial nerve palsies, giant cell arteritis, brainstem stroke

Systematic DDX

- **Neurologic**
    - **Brainstem/cerebellar lesions:** multiple sclerosis, central vertigo (from lesions affecting vestibular nuclei, demyelination)
    - **Other:** osmotic demyelination syndrome, cranial nerve III, IV, or VI palsies, internuclear ophthalmoplegia (INO), idiopathic intracranial hypertension (IIH), neuromuscular junction disorders (e.g., myasthenia gravis)

- **Ophthalmologic**
  - Astigmatism, cataracts, uncorrected myopia or hyperopia, corneal pathology (keratoconus, scars), lens subluxation, retinal pathology (macular edema, scars)
- **Vascular**
  - Ischemic stroke, idiopathic intracranial hypertension, intracranial aneurysm (cranial nerve compression), vascular malformation, microvascular disease (e.g., diabetes, hypertension) contributing to cranial nerve palsies
- **Infectious**
  - Orbital cellulitis, meningitis/encephalitis
- **Inflammatory**
  - Giant cell arteritis, granulomatosis with polyangiitis, Guillain-Barré syndrome (Fisher-Miller variant), Graves' disease, myopathies (e.g., myasthenia gravis), sarcoid, rheumatoid arthritis, lupus
- **Neoplastic**
  - Intracranial neoplasia (compressing ocular nerves/brainstem), or intraorbital tumors (lymphoma, meningioma, optic nerve glioma), head and neck cancers with cranial nerve involvement or orbital involvement
- **Injury/trauma**
  - Traumatic brain injury, trauma to the orbital region (e.g., orbital fracture, potentially with muscle entrapment)
- **Anomalies of development/aging**
  - Strabismus, mitochondrial disorders, decompensated phorias/tropias
- **Toxic-metabolic**
  - **Drugs:** topiramate, carbamazepine, phenytoin, fosphenytoin
  - Thiamine deficiency (Wernicke encephalopathy), diabetic microangiopathy

Notes

General considerations: Diplopia is often acute in onset and its effects on patients' quality of life prompt a visit to the emergency department, but only uncommonly is linked to a life-threatening pathology. Workup should include a thorough eye exam, including evaluation of visual acuity, visual fields, extraocular movements, pupillary testing, and fundoscopy. Emergent imaging and referral should be considered when diplopia is accompanied by other neurological deficits, pain, or other red flag symptoms.

Red flags: sudden onset, headache, neurological symptoms (particularly those related to the brainstem, such as vertigo, dizziness, and ataxia), head trauma

Special populations: In children, early diagnosis and management of strabismus, is important in preventing vision loss. Pediatric patients may not articulate their symptoms, but instead squint, cover their eye, or tilt their heads to compensate for affected vision. In pregnant patients, idiopathic intracranial hypertension is a key consideration. In older patients, consider microvascular disease contributing to cranial nerve palsies, especially in those with vascular risk factors.

Further Reading

- Najem K, Margolin E. Diplopia. In: StatPearls. StatPearls Publishing; 2023. http://www.ncbi.nlm.nih.gov/books/NBK441905/
- Glisson CC. Approach to Diplopia. CONTINUUM: Lifelong Learning in Neurology. 2019;25(5):1362. doi:10.1212/CON.0000000000000786
- Dinkin M. Diagnostic Approach to Diplopia. CONTINUUM: Lifelong Learning in Neurology. 2014;20(4):942. doi:10.1212/01.CON.0000453310.52390.58

Vision Loss (and Vision Abnormality)

Introduction

Many processes and structures are required to form an image in the brain; therefore, there are many possible causes for vision loss. Whether routine or emergent, the causes of vision loss can often be divided into either ocular or optic nerve categories. When evaluating vision loss, a careful history and description of the visual field defects by the patient is crucial. Eliciting whether the vision loss is partial or total, monocular or binocular, central or peripheral, gradual or sudden, transient or permanent, and painful or painless can help to focus a list of differential diagnoses.

Checklist DDX

Serious/life-threatening: amaurosis fugax, stroke, acute angle-closure glaucoma, giant cell arteritis, retinal detachment

Common: uncorrected refractive error, cataract, macular degeneration, diabetic retinopathy

Commonly misdiagnosed: cognitive decline in older adults, learning or behavioral difficulties in children

Systematic DDX

- **Ophthalmologic**
    - **Refractive/lens:** uncorrected refractive error (myopia, hyperopia, astigmatism, presbyopia), cataract
    - **Cornea/anterior chamber:** corneal ulcer, hyphema, hypopyon
    - **Posterior chamber:** acute angle-closure glaucoma
    - **Vitreous chamber:** vitreous hemorrhage
    - **Retinal:** macular degeneration, retinal detachment, retinitis pigmentosa
    - **Optic nerve:** Papilledema, open-angle glaucoma, non-arterial anterior ischemic optic neuropathy
- **Neurologic/psychiatric**
    - **Demyelinating disease:** multiple sclerosis, neuromyelitis optica
    - **Increased intracranial pressures:** idiopathic intracranial hypertension, central venous sinus thrombosis, intracranial lesion, hemorrhage, hydrocephalus

- **Vascular**
    - **Occlusive/ischemic:** stroke, amaurosis fugax, retinal vascular occlusion (branch/central retinal artery/vein)
    - **Retinopathy:** diabetic, hypertensive, sickle cell, central serous chorioretinopathy
    - **Vasculitis:** Behcet's disease, sarcoidosis, temporal arteritis, giant cell arteritis
    - Choroidal neovascularization
- **Infectious/inflammatory**
    - **Eye infection/inflammation:** keratitis (bacterial, viral, fungal), trachoma (*Chlamydia trachomatis*), uveitis (*Toxoplasma gondii*, tuberculosis, syphilis), retinitis/choroiditis (herpes simplex virus, varicella-zoster virus, cytomegalovirus)
    - **Autoimmune:** sarcoidosis, HLA-B27-associated uveitis (ankylosing spondylitis), giant cell arteritis
    - **HIV-associated:** herpes zoster ophthalmicus, varicella-zoster retinitis, toxoplasmosis retinochoroiditis, cytomegalovirus retinitis
- **Neoplastic**
    - Pituitary tumor, optic pathway glioma (neurofibromatosis type I), vascular tumors (retinal hemangioblastoma, von Hippel-Lindau Syndrome), craniopharyngioma, endocrine tumors, other malignancies/compressive lesions
- **Dysfunction**
    - Functional visual disturbance
- **Injury/trauma**
    - Orbital surgery, non-ocular surgery (highest risk cardiac and spine), cosmetic filler injections
- **Compression/obstruction**
    - Foreign body
- **Toxic-metabolic**
    - **Medication:** antiepileptics, antimalarials, psychiatric medications (antipsychotics, TCAs, SSRIs), corticosteroids, antibiotics (ethambutol, linezolid), cardiovascular medications (amiodarone, hydrochlorothiazide), PDE-5 inhibitors, antineoplastics (VEGF inhibitors, platinum-based agents), selective estrogen receptor modulators (Tamoxifen)
    - **Nutritional:** Vitamin A, B12, or folate deficiency
    - **Other:** diabetic retinopathy, diabetic macular edema, pregnancy/postpartum states (eclampsia)
- **Everything else**
    - Cognitive decline, learning difficulties in children

Notes

General considerations: Evaluation of a patient with vision loss should include a detailed history, visual function assessment, and eye examination. Some pathologies may be readily noticeable upon examination, and most initial evaluation can be performed with basic ophthalmologic equipment. Assessment of vision can be difficult in pediatric patients; special exam methods are used in this patient population. Vision loss often warrants a referral to ophthalmology, especially in patients with serious suspected pathologies or recent eye surgery.

Red flags: red and painful eye, headache with vision loss in one eye, flashes and floaters; jaw pain, temple pain, neck pain, stiff joints

Special populations: In children, consider congenital abnormalities as well as optic nerve disorders, trauma, infections, and nonorganic causes. In pregnant patients, vision loss can result from optic neuritis, pituitary adenomas, preeclampsia-related retinal changes, and cortical blindness from hypertensive complications. In older adults, common causes include age-related macular degeneration, glaucoma, cataracts, diabetic retinopathy, and vascular occlusions. In immunocompromised patients, vision loss frequently stems from opportunistic infections such as cytomegalovirus retinitis, herpesvirus, or toxoplasmosis as well as inflammatory optic neuritis.

Further Reading

- Bourne RR, Stevens GA, White RA, Smith JL, Flaxman SR, Price H, Jonas JB, Keeffe J, Leasher J, Naidoo K, Pesudovs K. Causes of vision loss worldwide, 1990–2010: a systematic analysis. The lancet global health. 2013 Dec 1;1(6):e339-49.
- Raharja A, Whitefield L. Clinical approach to vision loss: a review for general physicians. Clin Med (Lond). 2022;22(2):95-99. https://doi.org/10.7861/clinmed.2022-0057
- Pokhrel PK, Loftus SA. Ocular emergencies. Am Fam Physician. 2007;76(6):829-836.
- Zeeman GG, Twickler DM, Cunningham FG. Postpartum blindness. Lancet. 2002;359(9305):890-891. https://doi.org/10.1016/S0140-6736(02)07931-X
- Mendel E, Stoicea N, Rao R, et al. Revisiting postoperative vision loss following non-ocular surgery: a short review of etiology and legal considerations. Front Surg. 2017;4:34. https://doi.org/10.3389/fsurg.2017.00034

- Baig MN, Lubow M, Immesoete P, Bergese SD, Hamdy EA, Mendel E. Vision loss after spine surgery: review of the literature and recommendations. Neurosurg Focus. 2007;23(5):E15. https://doi.org/10.3171/FOC-07/11/15

- Kapoor KM, Kapoor P, Heydenrych I, Bertossi D. Vision loss associated with hyaluronic acid fillers: a systematic review of literature. Aesthetic Plast Surg. 2020;44(3):929-944. https://doi.org/10.1007/s00266-019-01562-8
- Kansakar P, Sundar G. Vision loss associated with orbital surgery – a major review. Orbit. 2020;39(3):197-208. https://doi.org/10.1080/01676830.2019.1658790
- Miller DG, Singerman LJ. Vision loss in younger patients: a review of choroidal neovascularization. Optom Vis Sci. 2006;83(5):316-325. https://doi.org/10.1097/01.opx.0000216019.88256.eb

Ear, Nose, and Throat

Quoc-Huy Ly

Long H. Tu

Samreen Vora

Hearing Loss

Introduction

Hearing loss is a common condition that increases in prevalence with age but also has clinical relevance in neonates due to several congenital etiologies. It can be classified as sensorineural (related to dysfunction of the inner ear or neurological pathway of sound transmission to the brain), conductive (problems with the outer or middle ear in preventing sound from reaching the inner ear), or mixed. Differentiation is necessary in guiding further evaluation and management, as some causes are readily treatable while others require urgent intervention or specialist referral.

Checklist DDX

Serious/life-threatening: anterior inferior cerebellar artery infarct, bacterial meningitis, vestibular schwannoma or meningioma causing brainstem compression, temporal bone fracture, severe head trauma, platinum compounds (irreversible deafness), heavy metal toxicity

Common: presbycusis, noise-induced hearing loss, ototoxic drug use, otitis media, cerumen impaction, otosclerosis, Ménière disease

Commonly misdiagnosed: Ménière disease, vestibular schwannoma, autoimmune inner ear disease, Lyme disease, otosclerosis, psychogenic/functional hearing loss

Systematic DDX

- **By type of hearing loss**
  - **Sensorineural hearing loss**
    - **Vascular**
      - Cerebrovascular accident/stroke (anterior inferior cerebellar artery infarct), cerebrovascular disease, vasospasm/ischemia from migraine-associated hearing loss
    - **Infectious/inflammatory**
      - **Sites of infection:** labyrinthitis, cochleitis, meningitis
      - **Etiologies:**
        - **Bacterial:** congenital syphilis
        - **Viral:** Rubella, CMV, EBV, HSV, VZV
        - **Fungal:** Aspergillus, Candida

- **Vasculitides:** granulomatosis with polyangiitis
- **Autoimmune disease:** rheumatoid arthritis, lupus
- Neoplastic
  - Vestibular schwannoma, meningioma at cerebellopontine angle
- Dysfunction
  - Ménière disease, presbycusis, multiple sclerosis affecting the cerebellum/brainstem
- Injury/trauma
  - Noise-induced hearing loss, head trauma, temporal bone fracture (e.g., involving the otic capsule), perilymphatic fistula
- Anomalies of development/aging
  - Alport syndrome, osteogenesis imperfecta, Waardenburg syndrome
- Toxic-metabolic
  - **Drug-induced ototoxicity:**
    - **Antineoplastics:** bleomycin, platinum compounds, methotrexate, taxanes, etc.
    - **Antimicrobials:** aminoglycosides, tetracyclines, macrolides
    - Salicylates and NSAIDs (high doses), diuretics (loop)
  - **Heavy metal toxicity:** lead, mercury
- Everything else
  - Psychogenic/non-organic hearing loss, idiopathic/functional hearing loss

- **Conductive hearing loss**
  - **Infectious/inflammatory:**
    - Otitis media (Haemophilus influenzae, Streptococcus pneumoniae, Moraxella catarrhalis), otitis externa (Pseudomonas aeruginosa), lyme disease (Borrelia burgdorferi), cholesteatoma
  - **Dysfunction:**
    - Otosclerosis, benign paroxysmal positional vertigo (vestibular symptoms may indirectly affect hearing)
  - **Injury/trauma:**
    - Ear barotrauma, fractures/dislocation of the ossicular chain
  - **Compression/obstruction:**
    - Cerumen impaction, foreign body impaction

- **Mixed hearing loss**
    - Dysfunction
        - Otosclerosis (can involve conductive and sensorineural components)
    - Injury/trauma
        - Temporal bone fracture (can cause both conductive and sensorineural damage)

Notes

General considerations: Initial diagnostic tests include the whispered voice and finger rub tests, as well as the Rinne and Weber tests, which use a tuning fork to distinguish between conductive and sensorineural hearing loss; some cases may be mixed type. Hearing loss during early childhood can lead to delays in speech, language, and social development, and in the elderly can further a sense of isolation.

Red flags: vertigo, unilateral or asymmetric hearing loss, tinnitus, history of recurrent ear infection, pain, drainage or bleeding from the ear

Special populations: Hearing assessments are important in neonates and infants to detect congenital infections (CMV, rubella, syphilis) and genetic syndromes, as well as young children (where otitis media and foreign bodies are common) to treat reversible hearing loss and prevent delays in speech and learning. Older adults are at greater risk of presbycusis, cerumen impaction, or ototoxicity secondary to polypharmacy, with implications for cognition and quality of life. Occupational exposure groups (military, construction, music) are also at greater risk of preventable noise-related dysfunction and proper ear protection should be used when applicable.

Further Reading

- Anastasiadou S, Al Khalili Y. Hearing loss. In: StatPearls. StatPearls Publishing; 2023. Available from: http://www.ncbi.nlm.nih.gov/books/NBK542323/
- Cunningham LL, Tucci DL. Hearing loss in adults. N Engl J Med. 2017;377(25):2465-73. https://doi.org/10.1056/nejmra1616601
- Lieu JEC, Kenna M, Anne S, Davidson L. Hearing loss in children. JAMA. 2020;324(21):2195. https://doi.org/10.1001/jama.2020.17647
- Michels TC, Duffy MT, Rogers DJ. Hearing loss in adults: differential diagnosis and treatment. Am Fam Physician. 2019;100(2):98-108.

Tinnitus

Introduction

Tinnitus describes perception of noise or ringing in the ears or head when there is no external sound source, which is often linked to conditions related to hearing loss. Most people will experience acute or chronic tinnitus at some point during their lifetime, though it is more prevalent with increasing age, especially in cases of presbycusis. It can be classified as objective (sounds that are coming from within the body, which may be heard by an examiner, such as an aneurysm) or subjective (a more common finding which refers to sounds heard only by the patient). Most cases are benign and acute episodes of tinnitus are common with good prognosis, but some rare causes can be life-threatening. Pulsatile tinnitus in particular can suggest underlying vascular abnormalities.

Checklist DDX

Serious/life-threatening: internal carotid artery or vertebral artery aneurysm, arteriovenous malformations, venous sinus thrombosis/stenosis, vasculitides, (large/locally aggressive) vestibular schwannoma or meningioma

Common: presbycusis, noise-related hearing loss, cerumen impaction, idiopathic, ototoxic medication, Ménière disease, Eustachian tube dysfunction, temporomandibular joint disease, head and neck trauma

Commonly misdiagnosed: temporomandibular joint disease, superior semicircular canal dehiscence, palatal or middle-ear myoclonus, giant cell arteritis, perilymphatic fistula, cholesteatoma, venous sinus thrombosis/stenosis

Systematic DDX

- **Vascular**
    - Internal carotid artery or vertebral artery aneurysm, carotid artery stenosis, arteriovenous malformations, intracranial idiopathic hypertension, venous sinus thrombosis/stenosis
- **Infectious/inflammatory**
    - **Bacterial:** Lyme disease, syphilis (Treponema pallidum), otitis media (Streptococcus pneumoniae, Haemophilus influenzae, Moraxella catarrhalis)
    - **Viral:** CMV, measles, rubella, RSV
    - **Fungal:** otomycosis (Aspergillus, Candida)

- - o **Inflammatory/autoimmune:** rheumatoid arthritis, systemic lupus erythematosus, scleroderma
    - o **Vasculitides:** giant cell arteritis, Takayasu arteritis
- **Neoplastic**
  - o Vestibular schwannoma, endolymphatic sac tumor, meningioma, paraganglioma of the middle ear (glomus jugulare)
- **Dysfunction**
  - o **Inner ear/vestibulocochlear dysfunction:** Ménière disease, superior semicircular canal dehiscence, migraine-associated
  - o **Middle ear dysfunction:** Eustachian tube dysfunction, patulous Eustachian tube
  - o **Musculoskeletal and myogenic:** temporomandibular joint disease, tensor tympani muscle spasm, palatal or middle-ear myoclonus
- **Injury/trauma**
  - o Environmental noise trauma (military, construction, music), head/neck trauma, temporal bone fracture, perilymphatic fistula
- **Compression/obstruction**
  - o Cerumen impaction, otosclerosis, cholesteatoma, vascular compression of cranial nerve VIII
- **Anomalies of development/aging**
  - o Presbycusis, Chiari malformation
- **Toxic-metabolic**
  - o **Drug-induced ototoxicity:**
    - **Antineoplastics:** bleomycin, platinum compounds, methotrexate, taxanes, etc.
    - **Antimicrobials:** aminoglycosides, tetracyclines, macrolides
    - Salicylates and NSAIDs (high doses), diuretics (loop)
  - o **Endocrine:** diabetes mellitus, hypo-/hyper-thyroidism, hypo-/hyper-parathyroidism
  - o **Metabolic:** hyperlipidemia, hypervitaminosis B6, vitamin B12 deficiency, iron deficiency
- **Everything else**
  - o **Neurologic:** increased intracranial pressure (e.g. idiopathic intracranial hypertension), cranial nerve VIII lesions, multiple sclerosis, epilepsy
  - o **Psychiatric:** anxiety, depression, stress
  - o Idiopathic tinnitus

Notes

General considerations: Further evaluation is guided by characteristics of the tinnitus (such as chronicity, location, and associated symptoms) to identify any treatable causes or conditions that warrant urgent evaluation. Audiometry with tympanometry is recommended for almost all patients to assess hearing status. Imaging studies such as MRI of the head and auditory canal with and without contrast can be helpful for patients with unilateral, asymmetric, pulsatile tinnitus, or associated neurological symptoms to exclude structural or vascular lesions. Pulsatile tinnitus often necessitates temporal bone CT or CT angiography to evaluate for vascular abnormalities. Laboratory testing is generally directed by clinical suspicion and is not routinely required. Treatment is focused on addressing underlying medical conditions, devices such as hearing aids, and supportive therapy such as counseling or cognitive behavioral therapy. Tinnitus may be exacerbated by psychiatric conditions such as depression, anxiety, or somatization, so early identification and management of comorbidities is effective in preventing symptom severity and progression.

Red flags: asymmetric or pulsatile tinnitus, history of head or neck trauma, associated hearing loss, vertigo, neurologic deficits

Special populations: In children, evaluation should prioritize hearing assessment and exclude treatable causes such as otitis media, cholesteatoma, or vascular issues, to prevent developmental or educational development. While presbycusis and cumulative noise exposure are frequently associated with older populations, ototoxicity from polypharmacy should also be considered.

Further Reading

- Baguley D, McFerran D, Hall D. Tinnitus. The Lancet. 2013;382(9904):1600-1607. doi:10.1016/S0140-6736(13)60142-7
- Bauer, C. A. (2018). Tinnitus. New England Journal of Medicine, 378(13), 1224–1231. https://doi.org/10.1056/nejmcp1506631
- Dalrymple SN, Lewis SH, Philman S. Tinnitus: Diagnosis and Management. afp. 2021;103(11):663-671.
- Grossan M, Peterson DC. Tinnitus. In: StatPearls. StatPearls Publishing; 2023. http://www.ncbi.nlm.nih.gov/books/NBK430809/
- Tunkel DE, Bauer CA, Sun GH, Rosenfeld RM, Chandrasekhar SS, Cunningham Jr ER, Archer SM, Blakley BW, Carter JM, Granieri EC, Henry JA. Clinical practice guideline: tinnitus. Otolaryngology–Head and Neck Surgery. 2014 Oct;151:S1-40.

Nasal Discharge and Postnasal Drip

Introduction

Nasal discharge and postnasal drip are common clinical symptoms observed across all age ranges and populations. Both are related to the continuity of the nasal cavity and oropharynx, in which mucociliary clearance is maintained by the nasal cavity's production of mucus to trap foreign particles and pathogens, and the transport of that matter towards the nasopharynx and oropharynx for swallowing or expulsion. Disruption of this process, where either excess mucus is produced or ciliary action is impaired, can manifest as nasal discharge or post-nasal drip. The possible etiologies behind either symptom are broad, and encompass infectious, allergic, inflammatory, structural, and neoplastic causes, some of the most common of which are related to rhinitis and sinusitis.

Checklist DDX

Serious/life-threatening: cerebrospinal fluid leak, nasopharyngeal neoplasm/carcinoma, severe bacterial sinusitis infection, HIV/AIDS, Rhizopus/Aspergillus infection, granulomatosis with polyangiitis, eosinophilic granulomatosis with polyangiitis

Common: common cold (viral upper respiratory infections), allergic rhinitis, bacterial sinusitis, vasomotor rhinitis, nasal polyps, chronic rhinosinusitis, chemical or airborne irritants, deviated nasal septum

Commonly misdiagnosed: granulomatosis with polyangiitis, nasopharyngeal carcinoma, cerebrospinal fluid leak, medication-induced rhinitis, GERD-related postnasal drip

Systematic DDX

- Infectious/inflammatory
    - **Viral:** common cold (rhinovirus, influenza, adenovirus, RSV, coronavirus, parainfluenza); viral rhinosinusitis
    - **Bacterial:** Streptococcus pneumoniae, Haemophilus influenzae, Moraxella catarrhalis, Staphylococcus aureus, Escherichia coli, and Pseudomonas aeruginosa
    - **Fungal:** Rhizopus, Aspergillus, Candida
    - **Autoimmune/granulomatous disorders:** granulomatosis with polyangiitis, eosinophilic granulomatosis with polyangiitis, sarcoidosis, systemic lupus erythomatosus

- o **Other:** allergic rhinitis, HIV/AIDS
- Neoplastic
  - o Nasal polyps, nasopharyngeal neoplasm (including carcinoma), juvenile nasopharyngeal angiofibroma
- Dysfunction
  - o Vasomotor rhinitis, gustatory rhinitis
- Injury/trauma
  - o Cerebrospinal fluid leak, sinus barotrauma, postsurgical changes
- Compression/obstruction
  - o Foreign body impaction, deviated nasal septum
- Anomalies of development/aging
  - o Primary ciliary dyskinesia, cystic fibrosis, congenital syphilis, choanal atresia, immotile cilia syndromes (Kartagener syndrome)
- Toxic-metabolic
  - o **Drug-related:** aspirin-exacerbated respiratory disease, rebound nasal decongestant use, cocaine use
  - o **Endocrine/metabolic:** rhinitis of pregnancy
  - o **Environmental:** dust, smoke, industrial chemical irritants (cement, wood, formaldehyde)
- Everything else
  - o Atrophic rhinitis, referred nasal discharge from gastroesophageal or laryngopharyngeal reflux

Notes

General considerations: Evaluation involves a detailed history and physical examination focusing on associated symptoms such as nasal congestion, throat clearing, cough, and the character of the mucus. Imaging studies such as sinus CT may be helpful if anatomical abnormalities or other underlying lesions are suspected. Allergy testing can be helpful if allergic causes are suspected. In some cases, nasal endoscopy can help visualize the nasal cavity and identify the source and nature of discharge; the location and consistency of mucus can suggest specific diagnoses. For example, thin mucus suggests allergic rhinitis, while thick mucus is more typical for sinusitis or reflux-related inflammation.

Red flags: unilateral nasal discharge (particularly if clear and watery or following trauma), recurrent or significant nosebleeds in combination with nasal discharge, persistent headache or facial pain, high fever, other systemic signs

Special populations: In children, viral and allergic rhinitis are common, but foreign body impaction should also be considered especially in the case of unilateral, foul-smelling discharge. Nasal discharge in older populations is more often due to age-related mucosal atrophy or medication-induced rhinitis, but chronic rhinosinusitis and nonallergic rhinitis are also common; sinonasal malignancy should be ruled out. In immunocompromised patients, the risk of life-threatening invasive fungal sinusitis from mucormycosis and aspergillosis is high; patients with poorly managed diabetes are also at a greater risk of mucormycosis from Rhizopus species, which can rapidly progress to orbital or intracranial compartments.

Further Reading

- Akhouri S, House SA. Allergic rhinitis. StatPearls [Internet]. 2023 Jul 16. Available from: https://www.ncbi.nlm.nih.gov/books/NBK538186/
- Bhattacharyya N. Nasal obstruction: diagnosis and management. UpToDate [Internet]. 2024 Jun 6. Available from: https://www.uptodate.com/contents/nasal-obstruction-diagnosis-and-management?search=rhinorrhea&topicRef=7533&source=see_link
- Osguthorpe JD. Adult rhinosinusitis: diagnosis and management. Am Fam Physician [Internet]. 2001 Jan 1. Available from: https://www.aafp.org/pubs/afp/issues/2001/0101/p69.html
- Patel ZM, Hwang PH. Acute sinusitis and rhinosinusitis in adults: clinical manifestations and diagnosis. UpToDate [Internet]. 2023 Feb 23. Available from: https://www.uptodate.com/contents/acute-sinusitis-and-rhinosinusitis-in-adults-clinical-manifestations-and-diagnosis?search=rhinorrhea&topicRef=7533&source=see_link
- Sexton DJ, McClain MT. The common cold in adults: diagnosis and clinical features. UpToDate [Internet]. 2023 Oct 31. Available from: https://www.uptodate.com/contents/the-common-cold-in-adults-diagnosis-and-clinical-features?search=rhinorrhea&topicRef=6871&source=see_link#H11414528
- Smallwood D, Ledford D, Kennedy D, Lockey R. Postnasal drip. J Allergy Clin Immunol Pract. 2024;12(6):1472-8. doi: 10.1016/j.jaip.2024.04.030. Available from: https://doi.org/10.1016/j.jaip.2024.04.030
- Weinberger SE, Saukkonen K. Evaluation and treatment of subacute and chronic cough in adults. UpToDate [Internet]. 2023 Dec 1. Available from: https://www.uptodate.com/contents/evaluation-and-treatment-of-subacute-and-chronic-cough-in-adults?search=post+nasal+drip&source=search_result&selectedTitle=2~58&usage_type=default&display_rank=2

Mouth Sores

Introduction

A common finding both in and outside of the clinical setting, mouth sores (and general oral lesions) can have benign etiologies such as trauma or aphthous stomatitis but may also indicate more serious conditions such as concerning infections and malignancy. Diagnostic considerations include characterizing the duration and recurrence of such lesions as well as associated symptoms such as bleeding/discharge or dysphagia. Based on history taking, workup may involve cultures or biopsy. In cases where severe mouth sores limits intake, patients may suffer from weight loss and nutritional deficiencies requiring supplementation.

Checklist DDX

Serious/life-threatening: Stevens-Johnson syndrome/toxic epidermal necrolysis (SJS/TEN), severe bacterial infections/abscess, pemphigus vulgaris, oral SLE, leukemia/lymphoma, oral cavity squamous cell carcinoma, Kaposi sarcoma, metastatic tumors to oral mucosa

Common: aphthous stomatitis, herpes simplex virus (HSV-1), morsicatio buccarum, trauma from dental procedures, nutritional deficiencies, oral lichen planus, oral candidiasis

Commonly misdiagnosed: oral cavity squamous cell carcinoma, pemphigus vulgaris, granulomatosis with polyangiitis, Crohn disease oral involvement, leukemia/lymphoma

Systematic DDX

- **Vascular**
    - **Malformations:** hemangiomas, vascular malformations
    - **Hemorrhagic:** petechiae, coagulopathy-/vasculitis-related ecchymoses, hereditary hemorrhagic telangiectasia (Osler-Weber-Rendu)
    - **Vasculitis:** granulomatosis with polyangiitis, Behçet disease
- **Infectious/inflammatory**
    - **Viral infection:** Herpes simplex virus, herpes zoster, coxsackie A, mumps, EBV, cytomegalovirus, HIV
    - **Bacterial infection:** secondary syphilis, gingivitis, mastoiditis, parotitis, sinusitis, actinomycosis, dental abscess

- - ○ **Fungal infection:** oral candidiasis, hair leukoplakia, histoplasmosis, blastomycosis, leishmaniasis
    - ○ **Autoimmune:** oral lupus erythematosus, oral lichen planus, pemphigus vulgaris, bullous pemphigoid (rare/less severe), ulcerative stomatitis, Sjögren syndrome, Crohn disease oral involvement, graft-versus-host disease
    - ○ **Drug reaction:** SJS/TEN, immunosuppressant reaction (methotrexate, azathioprine)
- **Neoplastic**
  - ○ **Benign:** salivary gland tumors, gingival overgrowth
  - ○ **Malignant:** oral cavity squamous cell carcinoma, Kaposi sarcoma, leukemia/lymphoma, metastatic spread to oral mucosa
- **Dysfunction**
  - ○ Temporomandibular joint dysfunction, salivary gland hyposecretion
- **Injury/trauma**
  - ○ Traumatic fibroma, morsicatio buccarum (cheek biting), thermal/chemical burns, iatrogenic (dental procedures, intubation)
- **Compression/obstruction**
  - ○ Sialolithiasis, oral changes from obstructive sleep apnea
- **Anomalies of development/aging**
  - ○ Fordyce granules, atrophic mucosa, lingual thyroid
- **Toxic-metabolic**
  - ○ **Drug-related:** chemotherapy, immunosuppressive medications, radiation therapy
  - ○ **Metabolic/nutritional:** vitamin deficiencies (B12, folate, C, iron, zinc), heavy metal toxicity (arsenic, lead)
  - ○ Alcohol- and tobacco-related lesions
- **Everything else**
  - ○ Aphthous stomatitis, stress-related ulcers

Notes

General considerations: Assessment of mouth sores should begin with identifying the onset, duration, number, and distribution of lesion(s) alongside associated symptoms of pain, fever, or dysphagia. History should also address any recent illnesses, medication use, trauma, nutritional status, and risk factors for malnutrition or infection. Biopsy is indicated for sores or ulcers that persist for longer than 2-4 weeks or have signs concerning for malignancy. Oral lesions may be more frequently encountered and identified by dental providers, making them a potentially viable point of screening in addition to primary care settings.

Red flags: dysphagia or odynophagia, spontaneous bleeding from lesions, frequent recurrence, induration or fixation without healing

Special populations: Children are more likely to present with viral stomatitis from herpes simplex and hand-foot-and-mouth disease from coxsackie A virus, while older adults are at a greater risk for denture/dental-related traumatic ulcers. Immunocompromised patients (HIV, post-transplant, chemotherapy) are more likely to develop opportunistic infections such as thrush, herpes simplex virus, and CMV. Patients with autoimmune disorders (Behçet disease, pemphigus vulgaris) also frequently present with recurrent or severe oral mucosal lesions.

Further Reading

- Bilodeau EA, Lalla RV. Recurrent oral ulceration: etiology, classification, management, and diagnostic algorithm. Periodontol 2000. 2019;80(1):49-60. doi: 10.1111/prd.12262. Available from: https://doi.org/10.1111/prd.12262
- Lodi G. Oral lesions. UpToDate. 2024 Apr 1. Available from: https://www.uptodate.com/contents/oral-lesions?search=mouth%2Bsores&source=search_result&selectedTitle=1~150&usage_type=default&display_rank=1
- Randall DA, Westmark NLW, Neville BW. Common oral lesions. Am Fam Physician. 2022 Apr 15;104(7):369-76. Available from: https://www.aafp.org/pubs/afp/issues/2022/0400/p369.html
- Stoopler ET, Villa A, Bindakhil M, Díaz DLO, Sollecito TP. Common oral conditions: a review. JAMA. 2024;331(12):1045-54. doi: 10.1001/jama.2024.0953. Available from: https://doi.org/10.1001/jama.2024.0953
- Watters C. Cancer of the oral mucosa. StatPearls [Internet]. 2024 Mar 15. Available from: https://www.ncbi.nlm.nih.gov/books/NBK565867/

Dysphagia

Introduction

Dysphagia may arise from a wide range of anatomic, muscular, or neurological conditions, reflecting the complex coordination required between the mouth, throat, and esophagus during swallowing. While many causes are benign and respond well to supportive measures such as diet modification to facilitate swallowing and reduce aspiration risk, others may be acutely life-threatening (e.g., epiglottitis, food bolus impaction) or signal a serious underlying illness such as malignancy. In cases where swallowing difficulty limits intake, patients may suffer from weight loss and nutritional deficiencies requiring supplementation.

Checklist DDX

Serious/life-threatening: esophageal and head/neck malignancy, stroke, dysphagia aortica, infectious esophagitis (often in immunosuppressed patients), epiglottitis, esophageal perforation (Boerhaave syndrome), caustic ingestion, reflux esophagitis, amyotrophic lateral sclerosis (ALS)

Common: food bolus impaction, reflux/infectious/pill/eosinophilic esophagitis, mechanical obstructions, peptic strictures, hiatal hernia, Zenker diverticulum, neurodegenerative disorders

Commonly misdiagnosed: eosinophilic esophagitis, achalasia, neurodegenerative disorders, Sjögren syndrome

Systematic DDX

- Vascular
    - Acute or prior stroke, aortic aneurysm causing compression (dysphagia aortica)
- Infectious/inflammatory
    - **Infectious esophagitis**
        - **Fungal:** Candida
        - **Viral:** CMV, HSV-1
        - **Bacterial:** Actinomyces, Mycobacteria
        - **Parasites:** Chagas disease (Trypanosoma cruzi), Toxoplasma gondii
    - **Autoimmune and connective tissue disorders:** scleroderma (CREST syndrome), Sjögren syndrome, eosinophilic esophagitis

- **Neoplastic**
  - Primary head and neck malignancy (pharyngeal, tongue, esophageal, thyroid), mediastinal masses, metastases (from lung or breast)
- **Dysfunction**
  - **Neurodegenerative:** Alzheimer disease, Parkinson disease, amyotrophic lateral sclerosis
  - **Demyelinating/neuromuscular disorders:** multiple sclerosis, Lambert-Eaton myasthenic syndrome, myasthenia gravis
  - **Myopathic disorders:** inflammatory myopathies (polymyositis, dermatomyositis), muscular dystrophy
  - **Peripheral/autonomic myopathies:** Guillain-Barré syndrome
  - **Motility disorders:** achalasia, GERD (Barrett esophagus), diffuse esophageal spasm
- **Injury/trauma**
  - Traumatic brain injury, caustic injury from heat or chemicals, endotracheal intubation, Boerhaave syndrome, secondary to oncologic treatment (surgery, radiation, chemotherapy)
- **Compression/obstruction**
  - Food bolus impaction, Zenker diverticulum, esophageal (Schatzki) rings, hiatal hernia
- **Anomalies of development/aging**
  - Cleft lip/palate, laryngeal/tracheoesophageal malformations, bronchopulmonary dysplasia, thyroglossal duct cyst, cerebral palsy
- **Toxic-metabolic**
  - **Medications:** pill esophagitis (antimicrobials, NSAIDs, aspirin, bisphosphonates), opioids
  - **Endocrine/metabolic disorders:** malnutrition, hypothyroidism, hyperthyroidism, diabetes mellitus, electrolyte abnormalities, Plummer-Vinson syndrome

Notes

General considerations: Evaluation for dysphagia generally begins by characterizing the symptoms based on onset, timing, progression, involvement of solids/liquids/both, and associated symptoms such as odynophagia, coughing, or regurgitation. Dysphagia to solids alone often suggests a mechanical obstruction, whereas difficulty with both solids and liquids is more associative of a motility disorder. Workup may be supported by studies such as endoscopy, barium swallow, or manometry depending on the suspected cause. Broadly, urgent assessment is warranted for suspected airway compromise, rapidly progressive symptoms, or red-flag features like hematemesis or severe weight loss. Supportive measures, such as diet modification or temporary nutritional supplementation, may be needed while diagnostic work-up proceeds, particularly in patients at risk for aspiration or malnutrition.

Red flags: unintended weight loss, decreased appetite, odynophagia, chest pain, vomiting, unexplained anemia (especially in a patient over age 50)

Special populations: In pediatric populations, congenital anomalies and foreign body aspiration are frequent considerations, with younger patients sometimes unable to articulate or indicate pain and discomfort. Older patients are more likely to have dysphagia secondary to neurodegenerative disease, malignancy, or medication-related swallowing impairment, which raises the risk of aspiration and malnutrition. The hormonal and mechanical changes of pregnancy may lead to dysphagia from GERD, as well as throat irritation from hyperemesis-related injury. Immunosuppressed patients are more susceptible to opportunistic infections such as Candida, CMV, or HSV, and symptoms may rapidly progress.

Further Reading

- Azer SA, Kanugula AK, Kshirsagar RK. Dysphagia. In: StatPearls. StatPearls Publishing; 2023. http://www.ncbi.nlm.nih.gov/books/NBK559174/
- Carucci LR, Turner MA. Dysphagia revisited: common and unusual causes. Radiographics. 2015 Jan;35(1):105-22.
- Skarbinski KF, Glennon E. Dysphagia: A review. The Nurse Practitioner. 2020;45(7):9. doi:10.1097/01.NPR.0000669120.41930.5e
- Wilkinson JM, Codipilly DC, Wilfahrt RP. Dysphagia: evaluation and collaborative management. American family physician. 2021 Jan 15;103(2):97-106.

Sore Throat (Pharyngitis)

Introduction

Sore throat, also called pharyngitis if attributed to inflammation of the pharynx, is one of the most common chief complaints. The presentation may overlap with tonsillitis, which refers to inflammation at an adjacent anatomical site. Both conditions, however, occur most often in children and young adults and can share etiologies. Patients typically present with fever, odynophagia, and can also have tonsillopharyngeal exudates. Viral infections account for more than half of acute tonsillopharyngitis cases, but bacterial causes (particularly Streptococcus pyogenes/group A Strep) are also common. Infectious and inflammatory conditions at other sites, complicated or deep infections, and rare vascular and neoplastic etiologies can present similarly.

Checklist DDX

Serious/life-threatening: epiglottitis, retropharyngeal abscess, carotid artery dissection, parapharyngeal space infection, peritonsillar abscess, submandibular space infection, Diphtheria, giant cell arteritis, leukemia/lymphoma

Common: viral pharyngitis, Group A streptococcal pharyngitis, postnasal drip from allergic rhinitis or upper respiratory infection (URI), gastroesophageal reflux disease (GERD), environmental irritants

Commonly misdiagnosed: infectious mononucleosis (Epstein-Barr virus [EBV]), acute HIV infection, peritonsillar abscess, GERD

Systematic DDX

- **Vascular**
    - Carotid artery dissection, giant cell arteritis
- **Infectious/inflammatory**
    - **Sites of infection:** epiglottitis, submandibular space infection, peritonsillar abscess, retropharyngeal abscess, parapharyngeal space infection
    - **Etiologies:**
        - **Viral:** adenovirus (most common), EBV, cytomegalovirus (CMV), herpes simplex virus (HSV), varicella zoster virus (VZV), HIV, rhinovirus, coronavirus, enterovirus (coxsackievirus A), influenza, parainfluenza

- - **Bacterial:** Streptococcus pyogenes/group A Strep (most common), Neisseria gonorrhoeae, Chlamydia trachomatis, Corynebacterium diphtheriae, Mycoplasma pneumoniae, Treponema pallidum, Bordetella pertussis
    - **Fungal:** Candida albicans, Histoplasma capsulatum
  - **Inflammatory/autoimmune:** environmental allergic reaction, allergic rhinitis with postnasal drip, SLE, Behçet Syndrome, Kawasaki Syndrome, sarcoidosis
- **Neoplastic**
  - Oropharyngeal cancers, other malignancies of the head and neck, lymphoma, leukemia
- **Dysfunction**
  - GERD, cricopharyngeal dysfunction, vocal cord dysfunction, obstructive sleep apnea
- **Injury/trauma**
  - Excessive shouting, recent intubation, direct traumatic injury, thermal burns
- **Compression/obstruction**
  - Foreign body impaction
- **Anomalies of development/aging**
  - Branchial cleft cysts, laryngomalacia, vascular rings, age-related mucosal atrophy
- **Toxic-metabolic**
  - **Irritant/toxin:** smoke/dust/fumes exposure, poorly humidified air, caustic inhalation/ingestion, chemotherapy- or radiotherapy-induced mucositis
  - **Endocrine:** thyroiditis, thyroid nodules
- **Everything else**
  - Idiopathic chronic pharyngitis, psychogenic globus sensation

Notes

General considerations: Diagnosis and evaluation are mainly clinical, with rapid strep tests, throat cultures, nucleic acid antigen testing (NAAT), and Monospot testing for confirming or excluding etiologies. Recent guidelines favor confirming infection before beginning antibiotic treatments to address over-prescription and drug resistance. Most cases self-resolve within a few days, so supportive therapy with analgesics, antipyretics, and adequate hydration is often suggested. Serious complications involving the tonsils (massive growth, suspected neoplasia, or recurrent throat infections) can be indications for tonsillectomy.

Red flags: signs of airway obstruction (difficulty breathing, noisy breathing, stridor), drooling, muffled ("hot potato") voice, asymmetric facial or neck swelling, sepsis, drooping or deviating uvula

Special populations: Young children may present with less specific symptoms, so clinicians and caregivers should be monitoring for feeding difficulties, drooling, or behavioral changes to rapidly identify pathology and prevent complications such as rheumatic fever. In adolescents and young adults, infectious mononucleosis caused by EBV is a common cause of sore throat, often accompanied by posterior cervical lymphadenopathy and fatigue. In the elderly, pharyngitis warrants careful evaluation for neoplastic causes or systemic illnesses such as giant cell arteritis.

Further Reading

- Weber R. Pharyngitis. Primary Care: Clinics in Office Practice. 2014;41(1):91-98. doi:10.1016/j.pop.2013.10.010
- Vincent MT, Celestin N, Hussain AN. Pharyngitis. afp. 2004;69(6):1465-1470.
- Harberger S, Graber M. Bacterial Pharyngitis. In: StatPearls. StatPearls Publishing; 2023. http://www.ncbi.nlm.nih.gov/books/NBK559007/
- Ashurst JV, Edgerley-Gibb L. Streptococcal Pharyngitis. In: StatPearls. StatPearls Publishing; 2023. Accessed July 3, 2023. http://www.ncbi.nlm.nih.gov/books/NBK525997/

Neck Mass

Introduction

Composing a differential for a neck mass requires consideration of the numerous anatomical structures of the neck, including the tonsils, local lymph nodes, thyroid gland, salivary glands and their associated ducts, soft tissue growths, and vasculature. Causes can be developmental, such as with cystic masses, or due to skin or subcutaneous infection, such as abscess or lymphadenitis. However, malignancy must also be ruled out, as neck masses may represent primary cancers or metastatic disease.

Checklist DDX

Serious/life-threatening: malignancy (lymphoma, metastatic head/neck cancers, thyroid carcinoma); tuberculosis, deep neck infections; carotid artery aneurysm, arteriovenous malformation, jugular vein thrombosis, traumatic hematoma

Common: reactive viral lymphadenitis, bacterial lymphadenitis, thyroid nodules/goiter, salivary gland swelling, lipoma

Commonly misdiagnosed: malignancy (HPV-associated oropharyngeal squamous cell carcinoma, lymphoma), paraganglioma, sarcoidosis

Systematic DDX

- **Vascular**
    - Carotid artery aneurysm, arteriovenous malformation, jugular vein thrombosis
- **Infectious/inflammatory**
    - **Sites of infection:** anterior cervical, parapharyngeal, retropharyngeal infection/abscess
    - **Salivary gland inflammation:** sialadenitis, Sjögren disease, sarcoidosis
    - **Organisms:**
        - **Bacterial lymphadenitis:** Staphylococcus aureus, Streptococcus pyogenes, Tuberculosis, Bartonella henselae
        - **Viral lymphadenitis:** rubella, EBV, CMV, HIV
        - **Fungal lymphadenitis:** Histoplasma, Coccidioides, Cryptococcus, Sporothrix
        - **Parasitic lymphadenitis:** Toxoplasmosis

- **Neoplastic**
  - **Benign tumors:** lipoma, thyroid adenoma, salivary gland adenoma, schwannoma, neurofibroma
  - **Malignant tumors:** thyroid carcinoma, salivary gland carcinoma, lymphoma, metastatic carcinoma (head/neck including HPV-associated, breast, lung)
  - **Vascular tumors (can be benign or malignant):** paraganglioma (carotid body, vagal tumor)
  - **Uncommon lymphoproliferative disorders:** Castleman disease, Kikuchi disease
- **Injury/trauma**
  - Traumatic hematoma, chemical burn/irritation, postoperative seroma, radiation-induced soft tissue swelling
- **Compression/obstruction**
  - Enlarged thyroid (goiter, thyroid nodule, thyroid tumor, thyroiditis), sialolithiasis
- **Anomalies of development/aging**
  - **Congenital neck cysts:** branchial cleft cyst, thyroglossal duct cyst, dermoid cyst, cystic hygroma
  - Ectopic thyroid tissue (lingual, sublingual, suprahyoid)
- **Toxic-Metabolic**
  - Thyroid enlargement from iodine imbalance, amyloidosis

Notes

General considerations: An evaluation of neck mass should assess for urgency via airway compromise, signs of infection, or rapidly progressing swelling. Additional information includes onset, growth rate, associated symptoms, as well as the mass' location, consistency/texture, mobility, and tenderness. Imaging and tissue sampling may be required if there is any concern for neoplasm.

Red flags: airway obstruction, hoarseness, dysphagia, cranial nerve deficits, signs of malignancy (weakness, fatigue, weight loss), risk factors for cancers of the head and neck

Special populations: Congenital cystic lesions and infectious lymphadenopathy are more common in children, while infectious mononucleosis from EBV is a frequent cause of posterior cervical lymphadenopathy in adolescents, which raises the risk of splenic injury/rupture. HPV-associated oropharyngeal squamous cell carcinoma is also a preventable concern that emphasizes the importance of vaccination.

Further Reading

- Almuqamam, M. (2023, August 12). Deep neck infections. StatPearls [Internet]. https://www.ncbi.nlm.nih.gov/books/NBK513262/
- Emerick, K. (2023, November 6). Differential diagnosis of a neck mass. UpToDate. https://www.uptodate.com/contents/differential-diagnosis-of-a-neck-mass
- Haynes J, Arnold KR, Aguirre-Oskins C, Chandra S. Evaluation of neck masses in adults. Am Fam Physician [Internet]. 2015 May 15 [cited 2025 Sep 14]; Available from: https://www.aafp.org/pubs/afp/issues/2015/0515/p698.html
- McDowell RH. Neck abscess. StatPearls [Internet]. 2022 Sep 19 [cited 2025 Sep 14]; Available from: https://www.ncbi.nlm.nih.gov/books/NBK459170/

Cardiovascular

Saeed Rahmani

Long H. Tu

Nicholas Cochran-Caggiano

Chest Pain

Introduction

Chest pain is one of the most frequent complaints in both primary care and emergency settings, accounting for approximately 1% of all ambulatory visits. While only 2% to 4% of these patients are found to have life-threatening conditions such as acute coronary syndrome (ACS), it remains a leading cause of death globally. It is essential to rapidly distinguish between cardiac and non-cardiac causes to initiate appropriate management. The initial evaluation should focus on determining whether immediate referral to an emergency department is necessary, particularly to rule out ACS, a life-threatening condition that encompasses unstable angina, and myocardial infarction.

Checklist DDX

Serious/life-threatening: acute coronary syndrome (ACS), aortic dissection, pulmonary embolism (PE), tension pneumothorax, esophageal rupture (Boerhaave syndrome), pericardial effusion

Common: musculoskeletal pain (e.g., costochondritis), gastroesophageal reflux disease (GERD), anxiety and panic disorders, pleuritis, pneumonia

Commonly misdiagnosed: pericarditis, herpes zoster, gallbladder disease

Systematic DDX

- **Cardiovascular/vascular**
    - **Cardiac:** acute myocardial infarction (STEMI, NSTEMI), unstable angina, coronary vasospasm (Prinzmetal's angina), spontaneous coronary artery dissection
    - **Pulmonary:** pulmonary embolism, pulmonary hypertension, sickle cell acute chest syndrome
    - **Structural:** aortic dissection, intramural hematoma, aortic stenosis, hypertrophic cardiomyopathy, congenital coronary anomalies, aortic coarctation
    - **Infectious:** pericardial/mediastinal infection, endocarditis
    - **Inflammatory:** pericarditis, Dressler's syndrome (post-MI pericarditis), myocarditis, endocarditis, takotsubo cardiomyopathy, vasculitis (Takayasu, giant cell)

- o **Arrhythmogenic:** arrhythmias causing ischemia or chest discomfort
- **Pulmonary/respiratory**
  - o **Pleural:** pneumothorax (simple, tension), pneumomediastinum, pleuritis/pleurisy, pleural effusion, pericardial fat necrosis
  - o **Parenchymal:** pneumonia (bacterial, viral, fungal, atypical), lung abscess, tuberculosis, acute asthma/COPD exacerbation, post-viral inflammation
  - o **Neoplastic:** lung cancer with chest wall or mediastinal invasion, metastatic disease, lymphoma with mediastinal involvement
- **Gastrointestinal**
  - o **Esophageal:** gastroesophageal reflux (GERD), esophagitis, esophageal spasm, Mallory-Weiss tear, esophageal rupture (Boerhaave syndrome)
  - o **Upper GI:** peptic ulcer, gastritis, gastric volvulus, hiatal hernia
  - o **Biliary/pancreatic:** cholecystitis, biliary colic, pancreatitis, hepatitis/hepatic congestion
- **Musculoskeletal/chest wall**
  - o **Neoplastic:** primary or metastatic chest wall/pleural/mediastinal malignancy, lymphoma; paraneoplastic syndrome with chest discomfort, malignant pericardial effusion
  - o **Inflammatory:** costochondritis (Tietze syndrome), fibromyalgia
  - o **Traumatic:** rib fracture, sternal fracture, chest wall contusion, muscular strain, post-traumatic neuralgia
  - o **Neuropathic:** intercostal neuralgia, herpes zoster (pre-eruption or postherpetic), cervical or thoracic radiculopathy, thoracic outlet syndrome
  - o **Structural:** osteoarthritis of the thoracic spine, connective tissue disease (Marfan syndrome, Ehlers-Danlos syndrome, osteogenesis imperfecta)
- **Trauma/iatrogenic**
  - o **Procedures:** post-cardiac intervention complications (pericarditis, coronary injury), esophageal instrument injury, chest drain/pacemaker lead pain
  - o **Radiation:** radiation-induced pericarditis/pneumonitis
- **Miscellaneous**
  - o **Autoimmune:** SLE, RA with serositis, sarcoidosis, polymyalgia rheumatica
  - o **Metabolic/endocrine:** diabetic ketoacidosis, severe electrolyte imbalance (hypocalcemia), thyrotoxicosis-induced angina

- **Psychiatric:** anxiety disorders (panic attack, generalized anxiety disorder) somatic (somatic symptom disorder, depression with somatic focus), hyperventilation syndrome
- **Drug-induced:** cocaine, amphetamines, chemotherapy-related chest pain
- **Unclassified:** precordial catch syndrome, mediastinitis, pneumomediastinum, amyloidosis, idiopathic causes

Notes

General considerations: Chest pain requires rapid triage to differentiate benign from life-threatening causes. Key red flags include pain radiating to the jaw, neck, or arms, particularly when associated with shortness of breath, syncope, or diaphoresis. Immediate electrocardiography and troponin levels should be obtained to evaluate for myocardial infarction. A careful history, physical examination, and targeted imaging or laboratory tests guide further workup.

Red flags: pain radiating to the jaw, neck, or arms; associated dyspnea, sweating, or nausea; sudden tearing or ripping chest pain suggesting aortic dissection; syncope or near-syncope; palpitations or dizziness; prior history of coronary artery disease or known atherosclerosis; exertional or stress-related chest pain; hemoptysis or leg swelling suggesting pulmonary embolism

Special populations: In women and older adults, atypical presentations of ACS (such as fatigue or dyspnea without chest pain) are common. In younger patients, musculoskeletal or gastrointestinal causes predominate, but family history of sudden cardiac death should prompt evaluation for inherited disorders such as hypertrophic cardiomyopathy as well as congenital long QT, Wolf-Parkinson-White, and Brugada syndromes.

Further Reading

- Johnson K, Ghassemzadeh S. Chest Pain. [Updated 2022 Dec 14]. In: StatPearls [Internet]. Treasure Island (FL): StatPearls Publishing; 2025 Jan-. Available from: https://www.ncbi.nlm.nih.gov/books/NBK470557/ McConaghy JR, Sharma M, Patel H. Acute chest pain in adults: outpatient evaluation. Am Fam Physician. 2020 Dec 15;102(12):721-727.
- McConaghy JR, Sharma M, Patel H. Acute Chest Pain in Adults: Outpatient Evaluation. Am Fam Physician. 2020 Dec 15;102(12):721-727. PMID: 33320506.

- Wachter C, Markus B, Schieffer B. Kardiologische Ursachen fur Thoraxschmerz. Der Internist. 2017 Jan;58(1):8-21. doi: 10.1007/s00108-016-0165-0.
- Hedayati T, Yadav N, Khanagavi J. Non-ST-Segment Acute Coronary Syndromes. Cardiol Clin. 2018 Feb;36(1):37-52. doi: 10.1016/j.ccl.2017.08.003.
- Li SY, Zhou MG, Ye T, Cheng LC, Zhu F, Cui CY, et al. Frequency of ST-segment elevation myocardial infarction, non-ST-segment myocardial infarction, and unstable angina: results from a Southwest Chinese Registry. Rev Cardiovasc Med. 2021 Mar 30;22(1):239-245. doi: 10.31083/j.rcm.2021 01.103.
- Gulati M, Levy PD, Mukherjee D, Amsterdam E, Bhatt DL, Birtcher K, et al. 2021 AHA/ACC/ASE/CHEST/SAEM/SCCT/SCMR Guideline for the Evaluation and Diagnosis of Chest Pain. J Am Coll Cardiol. 2021;78(22). doi: 10.1016/j.jacc.2021.07.053. Available from: https://www.jacc.org/doi/abs/10.1016/j.jacc.2021.07.053

Tachycardia

Introduction

Tachycardia is characterized by a heart rate exceeding 100 beats per minute (bpm). It can be a normal response to stress, exercise, or fever, but persistent tachycardia at rest is often a marker of underlying heart conditions. Tachycardia is one of the most common presentations in emergency settings, particularly in the form of atrial fibrillation with rapid ventricular response. Atrial fibrillation affects 1.5% to 5% of the population. It is associated with an increased risk of stroke and sudden cardiac death, making early evaluation and management crucial.

Checklist DDX

Serious/life-threatening: ventricular tachycardia (VT), ventricular fibrillation (VF), atrial fibrillation (AFib) with rapid ventricular response (RVR)

Common: sinus tachycardia, atrial fibrillation (AFib), supraventricular tachycardia (SVT)

Commonly misdiagnosed: atrial flutter, multifocal atrial tachycardia, catecholaminergic polymorphic ventricular tachycardia, inappropriate sinus tachycardia

Systematic DDX

- **Vascular (cardiovascular)**
    - **Rhythm disturbances:** atrial fibrillation, supraventricular tachycardia (atrioventricular nodal reentrant tachycardia, atrioventricular reentrant tachycardia), ventricular tachycardia, ventricular fibrillation, atrial flutter, Wolff–Parkinson–White syndrome, multifocal atrial tachycardia, junctional tachycardia, sinus tachycardia, catecholaminergic polymorphic ventricular tachycardia (CPVT)
    - **Structural/inflammatory:** heart failure (acute or chronic), acute coronary syndrome (myocardial infarction), pericarditis, myocarditis, cardiomyopathies (dilated, hypertrophic, restrictive), valvular heart disease causing compensatory tachycardia or AFib

- **Infectious/inflammatory**
    - Sepsis, systemic inflammatory response syndrome (SIRS), myocarditis, infective endocarditis with systemic effects, fever from any infection causing reflex sinus tachycardia
- **Endocrine/metabolic**
    - **Electrolyte disturbances contributing to arrhythmogenesis:** hypokalemia, hypomagnesemia
    - Hyperthyroidism (thyroid storm), pheochromocytoma, hypoglycemia (especially in diabetics), anemia causing compensatory tachycardia, adrenal insufficiency
- **Neurologic**
    - Autonomic dysreflexia, autonomic instability (secondary to Parkinsonian, diabetes, multiple sclerosis etc.), stroke or transient ischemic attacks with sympathetic overactivity, increased intracranial pressure or brain injury stimulating sympathetic tone, seizures with postictal tachycardia
- **Toxic-metabolic**
    - **Stimulants:** caffeine, amphetamines, cocaine, methamphetamines; beta-agonists (e.g., albuterol), theophylline toxicity
    - **Withdrawal from:** beta-blockers or sedatives, tricyclic antidepressants
    - **Miscellaneous:** alcohol intoxication or withdrawal
- **Respiratory/pulmonary**
    - **Vascular:** pulmonary embolism
    - **Respiration:** pneumonia, bronchitis, chronic obstructive pulmonary disease (COPD) exacerbation, severe asthma exacerbation, hypoxia of any cause stimulating sympathetic drive, acute respiratory distress syndrome (ARDS)

Notes

General considerations: Evaluation of tachycardia should include a review of medications, recent illnesses, and possible metabolic or endocrine triggers. An electrocardiogram (ECG) is essential to differentiate between supraventricular and ventricular rhythms and to identify features such as pre-excitation or QT prolongation.

Red flags: heart rate above 150 beats per minute at rest, associated chest pain or tightness, shortness of breath, dizziness or fainting, palpitations in the setting of known heart disease, sudden onset of rapid heart rate, syncope or near-syncope

Special populations: In children, supraventricular tachycardia and congenital arrhythmia syndromes are more common considerations. In older adults, atrial fibrillation and structural heart disease are frequent causes. In pregnancy, increased heart rate may be physiologic, but underlying arrhythmias or thyrotoxicosis should be excluded with testing if symptoms are significant.

Further Reading

- Henning A, Krawiec C. Sinus tachycardia. In: StatPearls. Treasure Island (FL): StatPearls Publishing; 2024 Jan. Available from: https://www.ncbi.nlm.nih.gov/books/NBK553128/ (accessed July 2025).
- Waldmann V, Jouven X, Narayanan K, et al. Association Between Atrial Fibrillation and Sudden Cardiac Death: Pathophysiological and Epidemiological Insights. Circ Res. 2020 Jul 3;127(2):301-309. doi: 10.1161/CIRCRESAHA.120.316756. Epub 2020 Jul 2. PMID: 32833581.
- Gopinathannair R, Olshansky B. Management of tachycardia. F1000Prime Rep. 2015 May 12;7:60. doi:10.12703/P7-60.
- Singh M, Morin DP, Link MS. Sudden cardiac death in long QT syndrome, Brugada syndrome, and catecholaminergic polymorphic ventricular tachycardia. Prog Cardiovasc Dis. 2019 May-Jun;62(3):227-234. doi:10.1016/j.pcad.2019.05.006.
- Sitorus GDS, Ragab AAY, Houck CA, Lanters EAH, Heida A, van Gastel VE, Muskens AJQM, de Groot NMS. Ventricular dysrhythmias during long-term follow-up in patients with inherited cardiac arrhythmia. Am J Cardiol. 2019 Nov 1;124(9):1436-1441. doi:10.1016/j.amjcard.2019.07.050.
- Tanaka Y, Kawabata M, Scheinman MM, Hirao K. Catecholaminergic polymorphic ventricular tachycardia with QT prolongation. Pacing Clin Electrophysiol. 2015 Dec;38(12):1499-1502. doi:10.1111/pace.12735.
- Kim JY, Oh IY, Lee H, Lee JH, Cho Y, Gil Y, Jung S, Kim DI, Shin MG, Yoo JY, Kwak JY. The efficacy of detecting arrhythmia is higher with 7-day continuous electrocardiographic patch monitoring than with 24-h Holter monitoring. J Arrhythm. 2023 Jun;39(3):422-429. doi:10.1002/joa3.12865.

Bradycardia

Introduction

Bradycardia is defined as a heart rate below 60 bpm. While it can be normal in highly trained athletes, bradycardia in the general population, particularly in symptomatic patients, is often indicative of an underlying pathological condition. It is a common finding in aging populations and those on medications such as beta-blockers or calcium channel blockers. In severe cases, bradycardia can result in syncope or even sudden death.

Checklist DDX

Serious/life-threatening: complete (third-degree) AV block, sick sinus syndrome (sinus node dysfunction, tachy-brady syndrome), Mobitz type II second-degree AV block

Common: sinus bradycardia, medication-induced bradycardia (Many drugs used to manage hypertension or heart conditions, like calcium channel blockers and beta-blockers, can result in bradycardia.), hypothyroidism, opioid overdose

Commonly misdiagnosed: sick sinus syndrome, digoxin toxicity, obstructive sleep apnea, Lyme disease.

Systematic DDX

- Vascular (cardiovascular)
  - **Conduction disorders:** complete atrioventricular block (third-degree), heart block (first- and second-degree), sick sinus syndrome, sinoatrial exit block, junctional escape rhythms
  - **Structural/ischemic:** myocardial infarction (especially inferior), aortic stenosis, congestive heart failure, cardiomyopathies, cardiac fibrosis, post-cardiac surgery or intervention effects
- Infectious/inflammatory
  - Lyme disease (causing heart block), viral myocarditis, bacterial endocarditis, Chagas disease
- Neurologic
  - Increased intracranial pressure, brainstem stroke or posterior circulation stroke, autonomic dysfunction (e.g., autonomic neuropathy), vasovagal syncope, carotid sinus hypersensitivity

- **Respiratory**
  - Obstructive sleep apnea causing cyclic bradycardia, respiratory acidosis, severe hypoxia, chronic lung disease with hypoxemia
- **Toxic-metabolic**
  - **Medications:** beta-blockers, calcium channel blockers, digoxin toxicity, opioids, sedatives, tranquilizers, lithium, antiarrhythmics (e.g., amiodarone), clonidine
  - **Metabolic:** hypoglycemia, electrolyte disturbances (e.g., hyponatremia, hyperkalemia, hypercalcemia)
  - **Endocrine:** hypothyroidism (myxedema coma), Addison's disease (adrenal insufficiency)
- **Everything else**
  - Hypothermia

Notes

General considerations: Bradycardia may be physiologic or secondary to systemic illness, medications, or structural heart disease. Evaluation should include review of medications, thyroid function, and ECG to identify conduction blocks. Management includes addressing reversible causes. Common reversible causes according to advanced cardiac life support (ACLS) include hypoxia, hypothermia, hydrogen ion (acidosis), and toxicology such as overdose of drugs like digoxin. Management focuses on identifying and correcting these reversible causes and, in some cases, may require pacing.

Red flags: heart rate below 40 beats per minute, syncope or fainting episodes, dizziness or lightheadedness, chest pain, shortness of breath, confusion or altered mental status, signs of shock (pallor, sweating, hypotension), history of heart block or pacemaker dependence

Special populations: In children, congenital heart block and metabolic abnormalities are more common. In older adults, degenerative conduction disease, polypharmacy, and hypothyroidism are frequent causes. In pregnancy, bradycardia is rare and should prompt evaluation for medication effects or underlying systemic illness. In areas where Lyme disease is endemic acute onset of heart block, particularly in younger individuals, should prompt testing for tickborne illness.

Further Reading

- Sidhu S, Marine JE. Evaluating and managing bradycardia. Trends Cardiovasc Med. 2020 Jul;30(5):265-272. doi: 10.1016/j.tcm.2019.07.001. Epub 2019 Jul 9.
- Hafeez Y, Grossman SA. Sinus Bradycardia. In: StatPearls. Treasure Island (FL): StatPearls Publishing; 2024 Jan.
- Barstow C, McDivitt JD. Cardiovascular Disease Update: Bradyarrhythmias. FP Essent. 2017 Mar;454:18-23. PMID: 28266824.
- Olshansky B, Sullivan RM. Inappropriate sinus tachycardia. Europace. 2019 Feb 1;21(2):194-207. doi: 10.1093/europace/euy128. PMID: 29931244.
- Hawks MK, Paul MLB, Malu OO. Sinus Node Dysfunction. Am Fam Physician. 2021 Aug 1;104(2):179-185. PMID: 34383451.
- Wung SF. Bradyarrhythmias: Clinical Presentation, Diagnosis, and Management. Crit Care Nurs Clin North Am. 2016 Sep;28(3):297-308. doi: 10.1016/j.cnc.2016.04.003. PMID: 27484658.
- da Silva RMFL, Borges ASR, Silva NP, Resende ES, Tse G, Liu T, Roever L, Biondi-Zoccai G. How Heart Rate Should Be Controlled in Patients with Atherosclerosis and Heart Failure. Curr Atheroscler Rep. 2018 Sep 17;20(11):54. doi: 10.1007/s11883-018-0757-3. PMID: 30225613.
- Palatnick W, Jelic T. Calcium channel blocker and beta blocker overdose, and digoxin toxicity management. [Internet]. 2020 Sep 15;22(Suppl 9):1-42. Available from: https://www.ncbi.nlm.nih.gov/pubmed/33136356.

Arrhythmia

Introduction

Arrhythmia refers to any disturbance in the normal rhythm of the heart, ranging from benign premature beats to life-threatening conditions like ventricular fibrillation. Globally, arrhythmias are a significant public health concern, especially as populations age. Atrial fibrillation (AFib), the most common arrhythmia, affects an estimated 12 million people in the United States and more than 60 million people worldwide. Its prevalence is expected to rise due to aging populations and the increasing burden of cardiovascular risk factors such as hypertension, diabetes, and obesity. AFib is associated with a five-fold increased risk of stroke and a three-fold increased risk of heart failure. Other arrhythmias, such as ventricular tachycardia (VT) and ventricular fibrillation (VF), are significant causes of sudden cardiac death, responsible for more than 300,000 deaths annually in the United States alone. These numbers underscore the critical need for early detection, appropriate management, and preventive strategies in high-risk populations.

Checklist DDX

Serious/life-threatening: ventricular fibrillation (VF), ventricular tachycardia (VT), torsades de pointes, atrial fibrillation (AFib) with rapid ventricular response

Common: atrial fibrillation (AFib), atrial flutter, premature ventricular contractions (PVCs)

Commonly misdiagnosed: supraventricular tachycardia, Wolff–Parkinson–White syndrome, electrolyte-induced arrhythmias, compensatory sinus tachycardia

Systematic DDX

- **Vascular (cardiovascular)**
    - **Rhythm disturbances:** atrial fibrillation, ventricular tachycardia, ventricular fibrillation, supraventricular tachycardia (atrioventricular nodal reentrant tachycardia, atrioventricular reentrant tachycardia), atrial flutter, Wolff–Parkinson–White syndrome, multifocal atrial tachycardia, junctional tachycardia, sinus tachycardia, torsades de pointes, catecholaminergic polymorphic ventricular tachycardia
    - **Structural/ischemic:** heart failure, myocardial infarction (acute and chronic ischemic injury), dilated cardiomyopathy,

    hypertrophic cardiomyopathy, restrictive cardiomyopathy, valvular heart disease (mitral stenosis, aortic stenosis, mitral regurgitation), ischemic scar causing reentrant arrhythmias, cardiac sarcoidosis or amyloidosis, arrhythmogenic right ventricular cardiomyopathy
- **Infectious/inflammatory**
    - Myocarditis (viral, bacterial, autoimmune), infective endocarditis, pericarditis, Chagas disease, Lyme carditis, HIV-associated cardiomyopathy with arrhythmias
- **Neurologic**
    - Stroke (including brainstem), autonomic dysfunction (dysautonomia), seizures with postictal arrhythmia, increased intracranial pressure, vasovagal syncope leading to transient arrhythmias
- **Toxic-metabolic**
    - **Electrolyte imbalances:** hypokalemia, hyperkalemia, hypomagnesemia, hypocalcemia
    - **Medications/toxins:** beta-agonists, digitalis toxicity, cocaine, amphetamines, caffeine, alcohol intoxication and withdrawal, antiarrhythmic drugs (amiodarone, sotalol), tricyclic antidepressants, lithium toxicity, chemotherapeutic agents (doxorubicin)
    - **Endocrine:** hyperthyroidism, hypothyroidism, pheochromocytoma, diabetes-related autonomic neuropathy

Notes

General considerations: Arrhythmias can range from benign to life-threatening. Identification involves detailed history, ECG interpretation, and often additional testing such as Holter monitoring or electrophysiological studies. Catheter ablation is increasingly used in refractory cases.

Red flags: sudden onset of rapid or irregular heartbeat, chest pain or tightness, syncope or loss of consciousness, shortness of breath, dizziness or lightheadedness, rapid heart rate above 200 beats per minute, history of heart disease, recent myocardial infarction, heart failure, palpitations with hypotension, sweating, or nausea

Special populations: In children, congenital conduction disorders and inherited arrhythmia syndromes are more prevalent. In older adults, atrial fibrillation and structural heart disease predominate. In pregnancy, arrhythmias may be triggered by volume changes, thyroid dysfunction, or medication effects.

Further Reading

- Desai DS, Hajouli S. Arrhythmias. In: StatPearls. Treasure Island (FL): StatPearls Publishing; 2024 Jan.
- Fu DG. Cardiac arrhythmias: diagnosis, symptoms, and treatments. Cell Biochem Biophys. 2015 Nov;73(2):291-296. doi: 10.1007/s12013-015-0626-4.
- Lin Y, Wu HK, Wang TH, Chen TH, Lin YS. Trend and risk factors of recurrence and complications after arrhythmias radiofrequency catheter ablation: a nation-wide observational study in Taiwan. BMJ Open. 2019 May 30;9(5). doi: 10.1136/bmjopen-2018-023487. PMID: 31152025.
- Alblaihed L, Al-Salamah T. Wide Complex Tachycardias. Emerg Med Clin North Am. 2022 Nov;40(4):733-753. doi: 10.1016/j.emc.2022.06.010. PMID: 36396219.
- Link MS, Bockstall K, Weinstock J, Alsheikh-Ali AA, Semsarian C, Estes NAM 3rd, et al. Ventricular tachyarrhythmias in patients with hypertrophic cardiomyopathy and defibrillators: triggers, treatment, and implications. J Cardiovasc Electrophysiol. 2017 May;28(5):531-537. doi: 10.1111/jce.13194.

Murmur

Introduction

Cardiac murmurs are abnormal heart sounds caused by turbulent blood flow through the heart's chambers or valves, or through abnormal passages in the heart. They are crucial clinical indicators for diagnosing underlying cardiovascular conditions, ranging from benign to life-threatening. Murmurs are detected through auscultation, an essential part of the physical examination. Sensitivity and specificity of identifying murmurs through auscultation can be as high as 70% and 98%, respectively. Due to imperfect sensitivity, auscultation is typically used for screening, with echocardiography used for confirmation and further characterization. Murmurs may result from valvular pathologies (e.g., aortic stenosis or mitral regurgitation), congenital heart defects (e.g., atrial or ventricular septal defects, patent ductus arteriosus, or tetralogy of Fallot), or increased blood flow states (e.g., anemia, hyperthyroidism, or pregnancy). Murmurs are graded by intensity, timing, and quality, and may be systolic, diastolic, or continuous. Their pitch, location, and radiation (such as to the neck or axilla) help characterize the etiology. Selected notes on differentiating murmurs are included in this section.

Checklist DDX

Serious/life-threatening: aortic stenosis, mitral regurgitation, ventricular septal defect (VSD), hypertrophic obstructive cardiomyopathy (HOCM), aortic regurgitation

Common: innocent/flow murmurs, aortic stenosis, mitral valve prolapse, pulmonary stenosis, atrial septal defect (ASD)

Commonly misdiagnosed: small ventricular septal defects, mild mitral regurgitation, high-output murmurs (e.g., in anemia or hyperthyroidism)

Systematic DDX

By murmur site and characteristics
- **Right 2nd intercostal space (aortic area)**
    - Harsh, crescendo-decrescendo systolic ejection murmur, radiates to carotids: aortic stenosis
- **Left 2nd intercostal space (pulmonic area)**
    - Harsh, crescendo-decrescendo systolic ejection murmur: pulmonary stenosis

- o Early to mid-systolic ejection, crescendo-decrescendo, usually softer: innocent/physiologic flow murmurs (e.g., anemia, pregnancy, thyrotoxicosis)
- **Left upper sternal border (including 2nd-3rd intercostal spaces)**
    - o High-pitched, crescendo-decrescendo systolic ejection murmur: coarctation of the aorta (may radiate to back/scapula)
    - o Grade 2-5 systolic ejection murmur possibly radiating to neck: aortic valve stenosis
    - o Systolic ejection murmur with radiation to infraclavicular areas, axilla, and back: pulmonary valve stenosis
    - o Early diastolic decrescendo murmur (Graham Steell murmur): pulmonary regurgitation (pulmonary hypertension)
    - o Continuous "machinery-like" murmur: patent ductus arteriosus
- **Left lower sternal border (including 3rd-4th intercostal spaces)**
    - o Holosystolic murmur louder with inspiration: tricuspid regurgitation
    - o Holosystolic murmur, often with a palpable thrill: ventricular septal defect (especially congenital)
    - o Harsh crescendo-decrescendo systolic murmur increasing with Valsalva or standing, decreases with squatting: hypertrophic obstructive cardiomyopathy
    - o Mid-diastolic rumbling murmur with opening snap: tricuspid stenosis
    - o Systolic murmur with wide fixed split S2: atrial septal defect
    - o High-pitched early diastolic decrescendo murmur, best heard sitting and leaning forward: aortic regurgitation
- **Apex (5th intercostal space, midclavicular line)**
    - o Blowing holosystolic (pansystolic) murmur, radiates to axilla, S4: mitral regurgitation
    - o Mid-systolic click followed by a late systolic murmur: mitral valve prolapse
    - o Low-pitched, mid-to-late diastolic rumbling murmur with opening snap, best heard with bell: mitral stenosis
    - o Harsh systolic murmur with palpable thrill (mid to lower left sternal border or apex): tetralogy of Fallot
- **Supraclavicular/neck area**
    - o Harsh crescendo-decrescendo systolic murmur radiating to neck: aortic stenosis
    - o Continuous murmur with whirring quality: venous hum (usually innocent in children)

- **Notes on murmur characteristics**
    - **Innocent/physiologic murmurs:** Typically systolic, short duration, soft, musical or vibratory, limited to a small area, intensity varies with position or respiration. Commonly heard at left lower sternal border or pulmonic area in children and young adults.
    - **Maneuvers modifying murmurs:**
        - Valsalva/standing increases HOCM murmur and mitral valve prolapse, decreases most others
        - Squatting increases blood return, decreases HOCM and MVP, increases AS and MR
        - Sustained handgrip increases afterload, decreases MR, AS, and HOCM murmurs
        - Inspiration increases right heart murmurs (tricuspid, pulmonary)
        - Expiration enhances left heart murmurs (mitral, aortic)

Pathophysiologic approach
- **Vascular (cardiovascular)**
    - **Valvular pathologies:** aortic stenosis, aortic regurgitation, mitral stenosis, mitral regurgitation, tricuspid stenosis, tricuspid regurgitation, pulmonary stenosis, pulmonary regurgitation, bicuspid aortic valve, prosthetic valve dysfunction
    - **Congenital heart defects:** atrial septal defect (ASD), ventricular septal defect (VSD), patent ductus arteriosus (PDA), tetralogy of Fallot, coarctation of the aorta, Ebstein anomaly
    - **Cardiomyopathies:** hypertrophic obstructive cardiomyopathy (HOCM), dilated cardiomyopathy
    - **Other structural:** left ventricular outflow tract obstruction, papillary muscle dysfunction or rupture, subaortic membrane, cardiac tumors (e.g., myxoma)
- **Respiratory**
    - Pulmonary hypertension, high-output states (e.g., anemia, hyperthyroidism), chronic obstructive pulmonary disease (COPD), severe asthma
- **Endocrine/metabolic**
    - Hyperthyroidism, pregnancy (increased cardiac output leading to flow murmurs), anemia, fever, high flow from Paget's disease of bone
- **Neurologic**
    - Neurogenic causes (e.g., neurogenic shock leading to altered hemodynamics)

Notes

General considerations: Echocardiography is the preferred diagnostic tool to evaluate murmur etiology and assess valve structure and function. Transesophageal echocardiography may be necessary if transthoracic imaging is insufficient. Chest radiograph can evaluate heart size and pulmonary congestion, particularly in heart failure due to valvular disease. Cardiac catheterization is indicated for cases requiring precise pressure measurements, surgical planning, or for intervention such as transcatheter aortic valve replacement (TAVR) in cases of severe aortic stenosis.

Red flags: loud murmur (grade 4 or higher), murmur associated with syncope or dizziness, chest pain or shortness of breath, cyanosis or peripheral edema, history of rheumatic fever or endocarditis, family history of sudden cardiac death, murmur in a patient with a known congenital heart defect

Special populations: In children, innocent murmurs are common but structural heart defects must be excluded. In older adults, degenerative valve disease predominates. In pregnancy, increased flow may produce benign flow murmurs, but careful evaluation is warranted if symptoms are present.

Further Reading

- Landefeld J, Tran-Reina M, Henderson M. Approach to the patient with a murmur. Med Clin North Am. 2022 May;106(3):545-555. doi: 10.1016/j.mcna.2021.12.011. Epub 2022 Apr 4.
- Thomas SL, Heaton J, Makaryus AN. Physiology, cardiovascular murmurs. In: StatPearls. Treasure Island (FL): StatPearls Publishing; 2024 Jan.
- Reyna MA, Kiarashi Y, Elola A, Oliveira J, Renna F, Gu A, et al. Heart murmur detection from phonocardiogram recordings: The George B. Moody PhysioNet Challenge 2022. PLOS Digit Health. 2023 Sep;2(9). doi: 10.1371/journal.pdig.0000324.
- Lim GB. AI used to detect cardiac murmurs. Nat Rev Cardiol. 2021 Jul;18(7):460. doi: 10.1038/s41569-021-00567-8.
- Huq A, Rahman A. Cardiac murmurs in children. Aust J Gen Pract. 2024;53(7):453-62. doi: 10.3316/informit.T2024071000013490315256417.

Hypotension

Introduction

Hypotension is a clinical condition characterized by low blood pressure, defined as systolic blood pressure below 90 mmHg, diastolic pressure below 60 mmHg, or a mean arterial pressure below 65 mmHg. It can be benign in healthy individuals, such as athletes, but it is often a sign of an underlying problem when accompanied by symptoms like dizziness, fainting, or shock. In emergency settings, hypotension is a critical marker of severe illness, such as sepsis, hemorrhage, or cardiogenic shock. Immediate evaluation and treatment are vital, as sustained hypotension can result in inadequate perfusion of organs, leading to multi-organ failure. The underlying cause must be identified and corrected rapidly, often requiring fluid resuscitation, vasopressors, or other interventions. Tools like bedside ultrasound, laboratory markers, and cross-sectional imaging may help guide the diagnosis and management of hypotension, especially when associated with shock.

Checklist DDX

Serious/life-threatening: myocardial infarction, pulmonary embolism, aortic dissection, hypovolemia, sepsis, pericardial tamponade, tension pneumothorax, cardiomyopathy, tachyarrhythmia

Common: dehydration (due to vomiting, diarrhea), medications (antihypertensives, beta-blockers, or calcium channel blockers), cardiac conditions (arrhythmias, valvular heart disease, heart failure affecting stroke volume or heart rate), sepsis

Commonly misdiagnosed: adrenal insufficiency, autonomic dysfunction, medication side effects.

Systematic DDX

- Vascular (cardiovascular)
  - **Ischemic/structural:** myocardial infarction, heart failure, valvular heart disease, aortic dissection, cardiomyopathy
  - **Shock/flow issues:** cardiogenic shock, hypovolemic shock (e.g., hemorrhage, dehydration), distributive shock (sepsis, anaphylaxis), pericardial effusion with tamponade, massive pulmonary embolism, tension pneumothorax
  - **Arrhythmias:** bradyarrhythmias (heart block), tachyarrhythmias causing poor cardiac output

- **Infectious/inflammatory**
    - Sepsis/septic shock, toxic shock syndrome, other systemic inflammatory states causing distributive shock
- **Endocrine/metabolic**
    - Addison's disease, adrenal crisis, hypothyroidism (myxedema), hyperthyroidism
- **Neurologic**
    - Autonomic dysfunction (diabetic autonomic neuropathy, Parkinson's disease, multiple system atrophy), stroke (especially brainstem infarction); spinal cord injury or lesions causing neurogenic shock
- **Toxic-metabolic**
    - **Medications causing hypotension:** antihypertensives (ACE inhibitors, ARBs, beta blockers, calcium channel blockers, diuretics), sedatives, narcotics (opioids), alcohol, vasodilators, anesthetics
    - Overdose of vasodilatory drugs or beta blockers, drug-induced adrenal suppression
- **Respiratory**
    - Massive pulmonary embolism, severe chronic obstructive pulmonary disease (COPD) exacerbation, severe asthma exacerbation, tension pneumothorax
- **Hypovolemia**
    - **Dehydration:** vomiting, diarrhea, or inadequate intake; severe malnutrition or cachexia
    - **Hemorrhage:** gastrointestinal bleeding, trauma, ruptured aneurysm (e.g., ruptured abdominal aortic aneurysm or splenic artery aneurysm)
    - **Third spacing:** anaphylaxis, pancreatitis, burns, severe sepsis

Notes

General considerations: Hypotension should be evaluated in the context of symptoms and clinical setting. It may reflect hypovolemia, decreased cardiac output, peripheral vasodilation, or obstruction. Management depends on identifying and treating the underlying cause, such as fluid resuscitation for hypovolemia, vasopressors for distributive shock, or emergent intervention for obstructive etiologies like tamponade or pulmonary embolism. Early detection and classification of shock (hypovolemic, cardiogenic, distributive, or obstructive) are crucial to guide therapy.

Red flags: persistent mean arterial pressure below 65 mmHg with symptoms; sudden drop in blood pressure associated with chest pain or dyspnea; cold clammy skin, weak pulse, confusion, or lethargy; decreased urine output; altered mental status or loss of consciousness; recent trauma or significant blood loss; evidence of sepsis such as fever, chills, or rapid heart and respiratory rates; history of heart disease, recent myocardial infarction, or arrhythmia

Special populations: In older adults, polypharmacy and autonomic dysfunction are frequent contributors. In pregnancy, hypotension may be physiologic but should prompt evaluation for hemorrhage or sepsis if symptomatic. In patients with endocrine disorders such as Addison's disease, adrenal insufficiency must be considered.

Further Reading

- Owens PE, Lyons SP, O'Brien ET. Arterial hypotension: prevalence of low blood pressure in the general population using ambulatory blood pressure monitoring. J Hum Hypertens. 2000 Apr;14(4):243-7. doi: 10.1038/sj.jhh.1000973.
- Sharma S, Hashmi MF, Bhattacharya PT. Hypotension. In: StatPearls. Treasure Island (FL): StatPearls Publishing; 2024 Jan. Available from: https://www.ncbi.nlm.nih.gov/books/NBK499961. [PMID: 29763136].
- Egi M, Ogura H, Yatabe T, Atagi K, Inoue S, Iba T, et al. The Japanese Clinical Practice Guidelines for Management of Sepsis and Septic Shock 2020 (J-SSCG 2020). J Intensive Care. 2021 Aug 25;9(1):53. Available from: https://doi.org/10.1186/s40560-021-00555-7.
- Tehrani BN, Truesdell AG, Psotka MA, Rosner C, Singh R, Sinha SS, et al. A Standardized and Comprehensive Approach to the Management of Cardiogenic Shock. JACC Heart Fail. 2020 Nov;8(11):879-91. Available from: https://doi.org/10.1016/j.jchf.2020.09.005.
- Samsky MD, Morrow DA, Proudfoot AG, Hochman JS, Thiele H, Rao SV. Cardiogenic Shock After Acute Myocardial Infarction: A Review. JAMA. 2021;326(18):1840-50. Available from: https://doi.org/10.1001/jama.2021.18323.
- Yang X, Liu Z, Hu C, Li Y, Zhang X, Wei L. Incidence and risk factors for hypotension after carotid artery stenting: Systematic review and meta-analysis. Int J Stroke. 2024;19(1):40-9. Available from: https://doi.org/10.1177/17474930231190837.

Cardiac Arrest

Introduction

Cardiac arrest is a sudden and severe medical emergency marked by the abrupt cessation of heart function, resultant lack of circulation, loss of consciousness, and absent breathing. It is a critical condition with a high mortality rate, requiring immediate intervention to prevent irreversible damage or death. Each year, more than 350,000 individuals experience out-of-hospital cardiac arrest in the United States alone, with survival rates below 10% despite cardiopulmonary resuscitation (CPR), defibrillation, and other interventions. Cardiac arrest can occur without warning, often in individuals with no prior history of heart disease. Its leading cause is ischemic heart disease, particularly coronary artery disease (up to 70%), although other cardiac and non-cardiac factors may contribute.

Checklist DDX

Common (all serious/life-threatening): arrhythmia (such as ventricular fibrillation [VF] or pulseless ventricular tachycardia [VT]), severe electrolyte imbalances (e.g., hyperkalemia), massive pulmonary embolism, acute myocardial infarction (AMI), cardiac tamponade, tension pneumothorax, intracranial hemorrhage, toxic overdoses (e.g., tricyclic antidepressants, beta-blockers, calcium channel blockers), respiratory failure (e.g., due to chronic obstructive pulmonary disease [COPD] or acute respiratory distress syndrome [ARDS]), sepsis, severe trauma (causing hypovolemia or blunt trauma)

Commonly misdiagnosed: pulmonary embolism, myocarditis, pericardial tamponade, drug-induced cardiac toxicity, inherited arrhythmogenic syndromes (e.g., long QT syndrome, Brugada syndrome)

Systematic DDX

- **Vascular (cardiovascular)**
    - **Ischemic:** myocardial infarction (STEMI, NSTEMI), coronary artery disease, coronary artery dissection
    - **Structural/valvular:** dilated cardiomyopathy, hypertrophic cardiomyopathy, aortic stenosis, aortic dissection, congenital heart disease
    - **Failure/flow:** congestive heart failure with low output, massive pulmonary embolism causing obstructive shock, pericardial effusion (tamponade)

- **Infectious/inflammatory**
    - Sepsis-induced cardiac dysfunction, severe pneumonia with hypoxia, infective endocarditis with embolic complications, myocarditis due to viral/bacterial/fungal agents
- **Neurologic**
    - Massive stroke (ischemic or hemorrhagic), especially brainstem strokes, increased intracranial pressure causing Cushing response, seizures with hypoxia or apnea, central nervous system trauma with autonomic dysfunction
- **Respiratory**
    - Massive pulmonary embolism, tension pneumothorax, severe asthma, acute exacerbations of chronic obstructive pulmonary disease (COPD), acute respiratory distress syndrome (ARDS)
- **Toxic-metabolic**
    - **Endocrine crises:** thyroid storm (severe hyperthyroidism), myxedema coma (severe hypothyroidism), Addisonian crisis (adrenal insufficiency)
    - **Electrolyte disturbances:** hyperkalemia, hypokalemia, hypocalcemia, magnesium abnormalities
    - **Metabolic:** severe hypoglycemia, diabetic ketoacidosis, severe acidosis or alkalosis
    - **Drug overdose:** opioids (respiratory depression), tricyclic antidepressants (arrhythmogenic), beta-blockers, calcium channel blockers
    - **Poisoning:** carbon monoxide, cyanide, other chemical or environmental toxins
    - **Others:** cocaine-induced arrhythmias or myocardial ischemia, amphetamines causing vasospasm or cardiomyopathy, alcohol intoxication causing arrhythmias or severe electrolyte abnormalities
- **Other**
    - **Trauma:** blunt or penetrating cardiac injury, cardiac tamponade
    - **Hypovolemia:** significant bleeding or dehydration causing shock
    - **Primary arrhythmia disorders:** long QT syndrome, Brugada syndrome, catecholaminergic polymorphic ventricular tachycardia, electrical abnormalities (e.g., Wolff-Parkinson-White syndrome with tachyarrhythmias)
    - Hypothermia causing arrhythmias and cardiac instability

Notes

General considerations: The rapid identification of reversible causes is central to management. Advanced cardiac life support (ACLS) guidelines emphasize the "H's and T's" as a framework for potentially reversible causes: hypoxia, hypovolemia, hydrogen ion (acidosis), hypo- or hyperkalemia, hypothermia, toxins, tamponade, tension pneumothorax, and thrombosis (coronary or pulmonary). Continuous high-quality CPR, early defibrillation when indicated, and prompt identification of underlying etiologies are essential for survival.

Red flags: not applicable (all etiologies of cardiac arrest are serious, regardless of associated symptoms)

Special populations: In children, cardiac arrest often results from respiratory failure, congenital heart disease, or severe sepsis. In older adults, underlying coronary artery disease, heart failure, and polypharmacy are frequent contributors. In pregnancy, additional considerations include amniotic fluid embolism, pulmonary embolism, cardiomyopathy, and complications of hypertensive disorders such as eclampsia.

Further Reading

- Allencherril J, Lee PYK, Khan K, Loya A, Pally A. Etiologies of in-hospital cardiac arrest: a systematic review and meta-analysis. Resuscitation. 2022 Jun;175:88-95. doi:10.1016/j.resuscitation.2022.03.005.
- Teeter W, Haase D. Updates in traumatic cardiac arrest. Emerg Med Clin North Am. 2020 Nov;38(4):891-901. doi:10.1016/j.emc.2020.06.009.
- Sumer RW, Woods WA. Cardiac arrest in special populations. Cardiol Clin. 2024 May;42(2):289-306. doi:10.1016/j.ccl.2024.02.013.
- Beun L, Yersin B, Osterwalder J, Carron PN. Pulseless electrical activity cardiac arrest: time to amend the mnemonic "4H&4T"? Swiss Med Wkly. 2015 Jul 31;145:w14178. doi:10.4414/smw.2015.14178.
- Imazio M, De Ferrari GM. Cardiac tamponade: an educational review. Eur Heart J Acute Cardiovasc Care. 2021 Mar 5;10(1):102-109. doi:10.1177/2048872620939341.
- Jung J. Optimizing survival outcomes for adult patients with nontraumatic cardiac arrest. Emerg Med Pract. 2016 Oct;18(10):1-24.

Pulmonary

Omar Zaree

Long H. Tu

Zachary Boivin

Shortness of Breath (Dyspnea)

Introduction

Shortness of breath, or dyspnea, is a frequent clinical symptom that can be challenging to assess due to its broad range of underlying causes, spanning cardiopulmonary, metabolic, neuromuscular, and psychological disorders. Symptoms can develop suddenly over hours to days (acute) or persist for more than 4 to 8 weeks (chronic). Key history elements include onset, duration, and whether dyspnea occurs at rest or during exertion. Key physical examination components are vital signs, mental status, breathing effort, use of accessory muscles, and signs of hypoxia or hemodynamic instability. Distinct findings on examination, such as jugular venous distention, wheezing, rales, or peripheral edema, can help guide clinicians toward specific diagnoses.

Checklist DDX

Serious/life-threatening: severe asthma exacerbation, severe chronic obstructive pulmonary disease (COPD) exacerbation, congestive heart failure (CHF), pulmonary embolism, pneumothorax, acute respiratory distress syndrome (ARDS), anaphylaxis, cardiac tamponade, myocardial ischemia

Common: asthma, COPD, anxiety, panic attack, pneumonia, CHF

Commonly misdiagnosed: anemia, thyroid disease, toxic-metabolic disorders, sepsis, medication-induced dyspnea, and neuromuscular disorders

Systematic DDX

Pathophysiologic approach
- **Pulmonary**
    - Asthma, acute exacerbation of COPD, pneumonia, pulmonary embolism, lung malignancy, pneumothorax, aspiration, foreign body aspiration
- **Cardiovascular**
    - CHF, pulmonary edema, acute coronary syndrome, pericardial tamponade, valvular heart defect, pulmonary hypertension, cardiac arrhythmia, or intracardiac shunting

- **Infection**
    - **Viral:** RSV, CMV pneumonia (transplant patients), COVID-19, influenza
    - **Bacterial:** epiglottitis, empyema, legionnaires' disease, lung abscess, TB
    - **Fungal:** aspergillosis, histoplasmosis, coccidioidomycosis
- **Autoimmune and inflammatory**
    - **Allergy:** anaphylaxis, angioedema, asthma
    - **Granulomatous inflammation:** eosinophilic granulomatosis with polyangiitis (EGPA), granulomatosis with polyangiitis (GPA), sarcoidosis
    - **Connective tissue disease:** rheumatoid arthritis, systemic lupus erythematosus (SLE), Sjogren syndrome
    - **Other:** idiopathic pulmonary fibrosis (IPF)
- **Neuromuscular**
    - **Mechanical restriction:** severe obesity, kyphoscoliosis, chest trauma with fracture or flail chest
    - **Others:** central nervous system or spinal cord dysfunction, phrenic nerve paralysis, myopathy, neuropathy
- **Toxic-metabolic**
    - **Inhaled irritants:** chlorine, cyanide, ammonia, sulfur dioxide, nitrogen oxide, carbon monoxide, smoke
    - **Chemical warfare agents:** phosgene, mustard gas, sarin
    - **Heavy metal poisoning:** mercury, lead, arsenic
    - **Alkaline/acidic substance/ hydrocarbons:** gasoline, kerosene, diesel (chemical pneumonitis)
    - **Met-hemoglobin inducing agents:** benzocaine, nitrites, dapsone
    - **Other:** organophosphate poisoning, salicylate overdose, metabolic acidosis
- **Psychogenic**
    - Hyperventilation syndrome, psychogenic dyspnea, vocal cord dysfunction syndrome
- **Others**
    - **Hematologic:** anemia
    - **Renal:** acute renal failure, metabolic acidosis
    - **Endocrinology:** thyrotoxicosis, diabetic ketoacidosis (DKA)
    - **Gastroenterology:** liver cirrhosis, ascites
    - **Miscellaneous:** sepsis, obesity hypoventilation syndrome

- **Acute vs. chronic**
  - **Acute**
    - **Pulmonary/chest wall:** flail chest, bronchospasm, pulmonary embolism, pneumothorax, pulmonary (bronchitis or pneumonia), asthma exacerbation, COPD exacerbation, hemorrhage, trauma, aspiration
    - **Cardiovascular:** acute myocardial ischemia, acute CHF exacerbation, hypertensive emergency, cardiac tamponade, pericarditis
    - **Head/neck:** angioedema, anaphylaxis, foreign body, infection
    - **Gastrointestinal:** ascites, intra-abdominal process
    - **CNS/neuromuscular:** stroke, myasthenic crisis, encephalitis
    - **Psychiatric:** anxiety, panic disorder
    - **Toxic-metabolic:** salicylate poisoning, carbon monoxide poisoning, diabetic ketoacidosis, fever, sepsis
  - **Chronic**
    - **Pulmonary**
      - **Alveolar:** bronchoalveolar carcinoma, chronic pneumonia
      - **Interstitial:** medications (methotrexate, bleomycin, amiodarone, busulfan, etc..), radiation, lymphangitic spread of malignancy, passive congestion, idiopathic pulmonary fibrosis
      - **Obstructive:** asthma, bronchitis, bronchiectasis, bronchiolitis obliterans, COPD, intrabronchial neoplasm, tracheomalacia
      - **Restrictive (extrinsic):** kyphoscoliosis, obesity, pleural disease (effusion), pneumothorax
      - **Vascular:** pulmonary emboli, idiopathic pulmonary hypertension
    - **Cardiac**
      - **Arrhythmia:** atrial fibrillation, inappropriate sinus tachycardia, sick sinus syndrome/bradycardia
      - **Myocardial:** cardiomyopathy, coronary ischemia
      - **Restrictive:** constrictive pericarditis, pericardial effusion/tamponade
      - **Valvular/septal:** congenital heart disease/intracardiac shunt, aortic regurgitation/stenosis, mitral regurgitation/stenosis
    - **Gastrointestinal**
      - GERD/aspiration, neoplasia, abdominal wall hernia, ascites

- Neuromuscular
  - **Metabolic:** acidosis (e.g., renal failure), glycogen storage disease, mitochondrial disease, thyroid disease
  - **Neurogenic:** amyotrophic lateral sclerosis (ALS), muscular dystrophies, phrenic nerve palsy, poliomyelitis
- Upper airway
  - Head/neck tumor, vocal cord paralysis/dysfunction, goiter
- Others
  - **Anemia:** iron deficiency anemia, hemolysis
  - **Deconditioning/obesity:** sedentary lifestyle, obesity hypoventilation syndrome
  - **Pain/splinting:** pleural-based malignancy
  - **Psychological/functional:** anxiety/hyperventilation, panic disorder, depression
  - Pregnancy

Notes

General considerations: The evaluation of dyspnea begins with identification and stabilization of any life-threatening conditions. Diagnostic investigations play a crucial role in the further evaluation of dyspnea. Initial tests may include chest radiography to identify pulmonary or cardiac etiologies. Blood biomarkers, such as B-type natriuretic peptide (BNP) and high-sensitivity troponin (hs-trop), can help differentiate cardiac from pulmonary causes, and pulmonary function tests—including spirometry and lung volume measurements—can further clarify obstructive versus restrictive disease patterns. Arterial blood gas analysis can be helpful assess gas exchange and acid-base status. In recent years, bedside point-of-care lung ultrasound (POCUS) and echocardiography have become valuable tools for the rapid assessment of acute dyspnea in emergency settings.

Red flags: accessory muscles use, inability to speak full sentences, stridor, hemoptysis, chest pain, sudden onset or severe dyspnea, altered mental status

Special populations: In children, dyspnea most frequently results from acute respiratory tract infections, asthma exacerbations (often viral-triggered), allergic rhinitis, or airway obstruction. Early recognition is essential to avoid life-threatening cases. Dyspnea in pregnancy is mostly physiologic; however, severe or sudden onset dyspnea can be a sign of preeclampsia, CHF, or pulmonary embolism. In older adults, symptoms may be underreported or attributed to aging, so thorough evaluation is critical.

Further Reading

- Santus P, Radovanovic D, Saad M, Zilianti C, Coppola S, Chiumello DA, Pecchiari M. Acute dyspnea in the emergency department: a clinical review. Internal and Emergency Medicine. 2023 Aug;18(5):1491-507.
- Berliner D, Schneider N, Welte T, Bauersachs J. The differential diagnosis of dyspnea. Deutsches Ärzteblatt International. 2016 Dec 9;113(49):834.
- Wahls SA. Causes and evaluation of chronic dyspnea. American family physician. 2012 Jul 15;86(2):173-80.
- Sharma S, Hashmi MF, Badireddy M. Dyspnea on Exertion. StatPearls. Treasure Island (FL).
- Soni, Nilam J., Robert Arntfield, and Pierre Kory, eds. Point-of-Care Ultrasound. Philadelphia, PA: Elsevier/Saunders, 2015. Print. p50-83

Dyspnea on Exertion

Introduction

Dyspnea on exertion is shortness of breath triggered by physical activity and relieved by rest. It is a symptom of a disease and not a disease on its own. It usually arises from disorders in the respiratory and the cardiac systems with the most common cause being congestive heart failure (CHF). To a lesser extent, however, other systemic disorders can result in dyspnea on exertion, and diagnostic approach and treatment are typically tailored according to etiology.

Checklist DDX

Serious/life-threatening: pulmonary edema, pneumonia, acute myocardial ischemia, anaphylaxis, cardiac tamponade, pulmonary embolism, pulmonary arterial hypertension, intracardiac shunting, cardiac arrhythmia, lung cancer, angioedema

Common: asthma, COPD, CHF, obesity, anemia

Commonly misdiagnosed: exercise-induced bronchoconstriction, exercise-induced laryngeal obstruction, deconditioning, pulmonary arterial hypertension, mitochondrial myopathies, muscle dystrophies

Systematic DDX

- Pulmonary
    - **Obstructive airway disease:** acute exacerbation of COPD, asthma
    - **Restrictive lung disease:** interstitial lung disease, sarcoidosis
    - **Infectious and inflammatory:** pneumonia, aspiration, pleurisy
    - **Structural:** pneumothorax, idiopathic subglottic tracheal stenosis
    - **Neoplasia:** lung cancer
    - **Other:** exercise induced laryngeal obstruction, post-pneumonectomy, congenital bronchial atresia, idiopathic pulmonary arteriovenous malformation
- Cardiovascular
    - **Ischemic/embolic:** acute myocardial ischemia, pulmonary embolism
    - **Functional:** CHF, pulmonary edema, myocardial dysfunction, pulmonary arterial hypertension

- - Structural: valvular heart defect, intracardiac shunting, cardiac tamponade, aortopulmonary window
  - Others: arrhythmia, cardiac preload failure, carcinoid heart disease
- Others
  - Immunologic and inflammatory: sepsis, anaphylaxis, angiooedema
  - Gastrointestinal: liver cirrhosis, hiatal hernia
  - Endocrinology and metabolic: obesity, thyrotoxicosis, metabolic acidosis
  - Nephrology: acute renal failure
  - Toxic (if inhaled during exertion): smoke, pollen, mold spores, dust, chemical fumes, air pollution
  - Miscellaneous: psychogenic (i.e. anxiety), deconditioning, muscle dystrophies, mitochondrial myopathies, chest wall pain

Notes

General considerations: Since CHF is the most common cause of dyspnea on exertion, point-of-care or comprehensive echocardiogram is crucial to look for any cardiac abnormalities, with less common causes having other distinct features. For instance, long term smoking with prolonged cough might suggest COPD; a history of smoking and diabetes mellitus can contribute to acute coronary syndrome. Thus, history plays a critical role in diagnosing dyspnea on exertion.

Red flags: dyspnea at rest or rapidly worsening dyspnea, chest pain, pressure or tightness, syncope or presyncope, palpitations with exertional dyspnea, hemoptysis, orthopnea or paroxysmal nocturnal dyspnea, marked hypoxemia or cyanosis, signs of right or left heart failure (e.g., jugular venous distention, peripheral edema, S3 gallop, ascites), unexplained tachycardia, hypotension, new ECG changes, evidence of severe anemia (e.g., pallor, tachycardia, hypotension), neurological symptoms (e.g., confusion, agitation, or altered mental status)

Special populations: In children and adolescents, dyspnea on exertion is more commonly caused by exercise-induced bronchoconstriction and physiologic deconditioning, and less commonly caused by congenital heart disease. Hypertrophic cardiomyopathy and arrhythmias must be considered in young athletes with exertional symptoms. In older patients, dyspnea on exertion might be challenging due to atypical presentations and underreporting of symptoms. Diagnostic yield is lower, and red flag symptoms such as syncope or acute decompensation may be subtle or absent. Physiologic dyspnea is common in pregnancy, but red flags such as hypoxemia, chest pain, or syncope should prompt urgent evaluation for other causes. In obese patients, restrictive lung mechanics or sleep-disordered breathing should be considered since obesity can mask or mimic other causes of dyspnea on exertion.

Further Reading

- Durbin W, Hardie W. Unexplained dyspnea on exertion: cardiopulmonary exercise testing as a diagnostic tool. Physiology. 2025 May 12;40(S1):2016.
- Rao VN, Kelsey MD, Blazing MA, Pagidipati NJ, Fortin TA, Fudim M. Unexplained dyspnea on exertion: the difference the right test can make. Circulation: Heart Failure. 2022 Feb;15(2):e008982.
- Morgan WC, Hodge HL. Diagnostic evaluation of dyspnea. American family physician. 1998 Feb 15;57(4):711-6.
- Paunikar S, Chakole V. Pulmonary shunt in critical care: a comprehensive review of pathophysiology, diagnosis, and management strategies. Cureus. 2024 Sep 3;16(9).
- Vézina FA, Milad D, Godbout K, Bernier M, Maltais F, Nadreau É, Sénéchal M. An unusual cause of exertional dyspnea in a 55 years old man. Respiratory Medicine Case Reports. 2020 Jan 1;29:101004.

Wheezing

Introduction

Wheezing is a high-pitched, whistling sound heard during breathing, caused by the narrowing or blockage of airways from the larynx to the distal bronchioles. Although it's commonly associated with asthma and COPD, wheezing can also occur with foreign body aspiration, congestive heart failure (CHF), airway tumors, or any condition that causes the airways to narrow. Wheezing can be divided according to systemic causes and type "expiratory vs inspiratory," anatomical distribution "unilateral vs widespread," and "functional vs structural."

Checklist DDX

Serious/life-threatening: status asthmaticus, anaphylaxis, foreign body aspiration, acute CHF, pulmonary embolism

Common: asthma, COPD, infection, allergic reaction

Commonly misdiagnosed: gastroesophageal reflux disease (GERD), vocal fold dysfunction, pulmonary edema (cardiac asthma), large mass (ex: thyroid nodule, enlarged lymph node) causing airway obstruction, pulmonary embolism

Systematic DDX

Pathophysiologic approach
- **Inflammatory and immunologic**
    o **Airway disease:** COPD, asthma, allergic reaction (up to anaphylaxis)
    o **Pulmonary parenchyma:** sarcoidosis, ARDS, hypersensitivity pneumonitis
    o **Immunodeficiencies:** IgG/IgA deficiencies, AIDS, B-cell deficiency
- **Infectious**
    o **Bacterial:** pneumonia, tuberculosis, pertussis.
    o **Viral:** RSV, rhinovirus, influenza, croup
    o **Fungal:** histoplasmosis, aspergillosis, coccidioidomycoses (esp. in immunocompromised patients)
    o **Parasitic:** echinococcosis, ascariasis, schistosomiasis
- **Cardiovascular**
    o Pulmonary embolism, CHF

- Toxic
    - **Illicit drugs:** cocaine, heroin
    - **Environmental and occupational pollutants:** volatile organ compounds (paints, solvents, cleaning agents), irritant gases (chlorine, ammonia, smoke, carbon monoxide, chemical fumes)
- Neoplasia
    - Lung cancer, bronchial carcinoid tumor, carcinoid syndrome, systemic mastocytosis
- Miscellaneous
    - Foreign body aspiration, GERD, bronchiectasis
- Special scenarios
    - **Medications:** ACE inhibitors, beta blockers, aspirin, NSAIDs
    - **Congenital:** vascular ring, laryngeal web, tracheoesophageal fistula, tracheomalacia, laryngomalacia
    - **Genetic:** cystic fibrosis (CF), primary ciliary dyskinesia
    - **Rare:** vocal cord dysfunction, alpha-1 antitrypsin deficiency, tracheobronchomalacia, Churg-Strauss syndrome, sarcoidosis, relapsing polychondritis, bronchial stenosis, pulmonary Langerhans cell histiocytosis
    - **Others:** vocal cord dysfunction, pulmonary infiltrate and blood eosinophilia (Loeffler's syndrome, chronic eosinophilic pneumonia, tropical eosinophilia, hypereosinophilic syndrome, various vasculitides, and allergic bronchopulmonary aspergillosis)

Diffuse vs. unilateral
- Diffuse wheeze
    - **Extrathoracic:** anaphylaxis, angioedema, vocal cord paralysis, laryngeal stenosis, goiter with thoracic inlet obstruction, anxiety with hyperventilation, lymphoma
    - **Intrathoracic central airway:** Tracheal stenosis, mediastinal tumors, hyperdynamic airway collapse due to tracheomalacia, mucus plugs, thoracic aortic aneurysm, foreign body inhalation
    - **Intrathoracic lower airway:** bronchitis/bronchiolitis, COPD, pulmonary edema (cardiac asthma), bronchial mass, bronchiectasis, pneumothorax, inhaled irritant or corrosive agent exposure
- Unilateral wheeze
    - **Intraluminal obstruction:** endotracheal tube malposition, aspiration (foreign body or mucus plug)
    - **Intrinsic airway disease:** bronchogenic carcinoma, bronchial stenosis, bronchiectasis

- o Extrinsic compression
  - Neoplasia: bronchogenic carcinoma, thymic carcinoma, lymphoma
  - Benign mass effect: retrosternal goiter, aortic aneurysm
- o Infection: pneumonia

Inspiratory vs. expiratory vs. mixed
- Inspiratory wheeze
  - o Laryngeal/tracheal stenosis, vocal cord dysfunction, epiglottitis, laryngomalacia, laryngotracheitis
- Expiratory wheeze
  - o Asthma, COPD, bronchiolitis (esp. in infants), foreign body aspiration, CHF with pulmonary edema, bronchiectasis, infections (RSV, pneumonia, bronchitis), anaphylaxis, tracheomalacia, GERD, cystic fibrosis
- Mixed
  - o Severe asthma, advanced COPD

Structural vs. functional approach
- Structural
  - o Tumors, foreign body, bronchial stricture, goiter, vocal cord dysfunction, tracheomalacia, bronchomalacia, vascular ring, bronchogenic cyst, aortic aneurysm, lymphadenopathy, bronchiectasis, mediastinal mass
- Functional
  - o Asthma, anaphylaxis, angioedema, allergens, cold air, exercise, irritants, GERD, psychogenic wheezing, pulmonary edema (cardiac asthma)

Notes

General considerations: Inspiratory wheezes are mostly associated with upper airway obstruction whereas expiratory wheezes are associated with lower airway obstruction or constriction. Focal lung diseases such as pneumonia and foreign body aspiration are more likely to produce unilateral wheezes unlike ARDS and other systemic lung disorders, which cause diffuse wheezes. History and physical exam can help uncover the cause of wheezing. A silent chest, or the absence of wheezing, in an asthma patient can either indicate improvement of bronchoconstriction or severe airway obstruction. In the latter case, the airflow is so restricted that no wheezing is produced. If a silent chest is accompanied by exhaustion, it suggests respiratory muscle fatigue and need for either noninvasive positive pressure ventilation or invasive mechanical ventilation with endotracheal intubation.

Red flags: sudden onset with allergy symptoms (hives or swelling of the lips or face, etc.), severe difficulty breathing, bluish lip color, occurs after choking on a small object or food, recurrent symptoms

Special populations: In infants and young children, wheezing most likely results from low birth weight, prematurity, or a history of recurrent respiratory infections (such as bronchiolitis). Children with atopy or a family history of allergy are at higher risk for recurrent wheezing and later development of asthma. In elderly adults, wheezing might be a sign of serious/life-threatening conditions such as CHF and should be followed by detailed clinical assessment.

Further Reading

- Irwin RS, Barnes PJ, Hollingsworth H. Evaluation of wheezing illnesses other than asthma in adults. UpToDate. Waltham: UpToDate. 2013.
- Gong H. Wheezing and asthma. Clinical Methods: The History, Physical, and Laboratory Examinations. 3rd edition. 1990.
- Pasterkamp H. The highs and lows of wheezing: a review of the most popular adventitious lung sound. Pediatric pulmonology. 2018 Feb;53(2):243-54.

Cough

Introduction

Cough is a natural, primitive reflex that functions as part of the body's immune defense to guard against foreign substances. It is linked to a wide range of clinical conditions and causes. Due to the ambiguous nature of this symptom, its potential for a hidden underlying cause, its significant impact on quality of life, and the absence of objective evaluation tools, cough should be considered a serious concern until a harmless cause is identified. Patient's age and characteristics of cough might give a clue about the etiology. It can be classified based on duration, with acute cough lasting less than 3 weeks, subacute lasting 3 to 8 weeks, and chronic cough lasting more than 8 weeks; or based on mucus production, where a productive cough contains mucus and a dry cough does not. Treatment of cough varies based on the cause.

Checklist DDX

Serious/life-threatening: severe asthma exacerbation, COPD exacerbation, pneumonia, congestive heart failure (CHF), pulmonary embolism, lung cancer, anaphylaxis, tuberculosis, aspiration

Common: post-viral cough, upper airway cough syndrome, common cold, influenza, COVID-19, asthma, COPD, acute bronchitis, pneumonia, GERD

Commonly misdiagnosed: protracted bacterial bronchitis, somatic cough syndrome, diffuse panbronchiolitis, GERD, lung cancer

Systematic DDX

Pathophysiologic approach
- **Pulmonary**
    - **Upper respiratory tract:** upper respiratory infection, upper airway cough syndrome, sinusitis, laryngitis, pertussis, laryngotracheiitis
    - **Lower respiratory tract:** asthma, COPD, acute bronchitis, pneumonia, interstitial lung disease, tuberculosis, lung carcinoma, bronchiectasis
- **Cardiovascular**
    - CHF, pulmonary edema, pulmonary embolism, pericarditis

- **Infectious**
    - **Viral:** upper respiratory infection, influenza, COVID-19, RSV, parainfluenza, influenza
    - **Bacterial:** pertussis, tuberculosis, bacterial pneumonia (streptococcal pneumonia, H. influenzae, Moraxella catarrhalis, staph aureus, gram negative bacilli, etc.)
    - **Fungal:** histoplasmosis, coccidioidomycosis, blastomycosis (fungal infection is more common in immunocompromised patients)
- **Immunologic/allergic**
    - Allergic rhinitis/sinusitis, anaphylaxis, nonasthmatic eosinophilic bronchitis, immunodeficiencies (chronic granulomatous disease, Bruton agammaglobulinemia, severe combined immunodeficiency, etc.)
- **Environmental/occupational**
    - Inhaled irritants (smoke, chemical, dust, pollutants, carbon monoxide), pneumoconiosis, asbestosis, silicosis
- **Others**
    - **Medications:** ace inhibitors, beta blockers, NSAIDs, aspirin, methacholine
    - **Genetic:** cystic fibrosis (CF), primary ciliary dyskinesia
    - **Miscellaneous:** sarcoidosis, foreign body aspiration, vagal nerve stimulation, psychogenic, GERD
    - **Rare:** cerumen impaction, esophageal achalasia, tracheoesophageal fistula, Zenker diverticulum, Ortner syndrome, peritoneal dialysis, pneumonitis, tracheobronchial collapse, esophageal tracheobronchial reflex

Considerations by chronicity

- **Acute**
    - **Infections:** upper respiratory tract disease (pharyngitis, sinusitis, tracheitis, rhinitis, otitis, laryngotracheitis "Croup"), lower respiratory tract disease (pneumonia, abscess, empyema, bronchiolitis "RSV")
    - **Other:** aspiration, foreign body, pulmonary embolism, inhaled irritant
- **Subacute**
    - Postinfectious cough, eosinophilic bronchitis, pertussis, cough variant asthma
- **Recurrent**
    - Asthma, CF, GERD, aspiration, anatomic abnormalities (tracheobronchomalacia, tracheoesophageal fistula, vascular ring, abnormal position or origin of large bronchi), passive smoking

- **Chronic**
    - Asthma, CF, GERD, aspiration, pertussis, anatomic abnormality, passive smoking, mycoplasma, psychogenic, tuberculosis, tumor, upper airway cough syndrome, nonasthmatic eosinophilic bronchitis, medications (ace inhibitors, beta blockers, aspirin, NSAIDs, etc.), protracted bacterial bronchitis

Dry vs. wet
- **Dry**
    - Laryngitis, sore throat, tonsillitis, croup, sinusitis, asthma, allergies, GERD, inhaled irritants (air pollution, dust, smoke), ace inhibitors
- **Wet**
    - Asthma, acute bronchitis, common cold, pneumonia, COPD (chronic bronchitis or emphysema)

Notes

General considerations: The diagnostic approach varies according to the duration of cough. Certain cough characteristics can aid in diagnosis such as whooping cough in pertussis, hoarseness or stridor in croup/laryngeal involvement, sudden onset in foreign body aspiration, and environmental exposure in psittacosis/histoplasmosis/coccidioidomycosis. The initial step in managing acute cough is to determine whether the cause is a life-threatening condition or not. The treatment is based on the etiology.

Red flags: unintentional weight loss, fever, cough lasting more than three weeks, hemoptysis, choking, shortness of breath, chest pain, unexplained tiredness, swelling of legs/face, history of smoking, persistent wheezing, hoarseness

Special populations: In immunocompromised patients, causes of cough can be broader, including fungal and opportunistic bacterial/viral infections, medication-induced pulmonary toxicity, or neoplasms. Cough that worsens when lying down may signal CHF. Persistent or severe coughs in pregnancy require medical evaluation and treatment to prevent maternal discomfort and potential risks such as preterm labor or fetal growth abnormalities.

Further Reading

- Michaudet C, Malaty J. Chronic cough: evaluation and management. American family physician. 2017 Nov 1;96(9):575-80.

- Amos LB. Cough. Nelson pediatric symptom-based diagnosis. 2017 May 12:15.
- Coughlin L. Cough: Diagnosis and M management. American Family Physician. 2007 Feb 15;75(4).

Hemoptysis

Introduction

Hemoptysis is the coughing up blood from the lower respiratory tract (i.e., from below the vocal cords), typically originating from the bronchial arteries; whereas massive hemoptysis is a life-threatening volume of blood (ranging from 100 mL/24 hrs to more than 1,000 mL/24 hrs) and can cause airway obstruction or blood loss. Pseudohemoptysis, expectoration of blood that comes from the upper respiratory tract and/or the upper gastrointestinal tract, can mimic hemoptysis and can be differentiated by the characteristics of blood and the associated symptoms. True hemoptysis is marked by frothy sputum, bright red blood, and possibly a choking sensation if the bleeding is massive.

Checklist DDX

Serious/life-threatening: pulmonary embolism, lung cancer, tuberculosis, trauma, coagulopathy.

Common: respiratory infections, COPD, cancer, and bronchiectasis (developed countries); TB (worldwide); lower respiratory tract infection and foreign body aspiration (children)

Commonly misdiagnosed: granulomatosis with polyangiitis (GPA), SLE, Goodpasture's syndrome, idiopathic pulmonary hemosiderosis, pulmonary arteriovenous malformations, intercostal-to-pulmonary arterial fistula.

Systematic DDX

- **Pulmonary**
    - **Airway/tracheobronchial:** bronchial tumors, bronchiectasis, bronchitis, foreign body, trauma
    - **Parenchymal**
        - **Infectious:** fungal (aspergillosis, paragonimiasis), leptospirosis, lung abscess, parasitic diseases, pneumonia, TB and non-TB mycobacteria
        - **Rheumatologic:** Goodpasture syndrome, Behcet syndrome, GPA, Henoch Schonlein purpura, microscopic polyangiitis, sarcoidosis, lupus, mixed cryoglobulinemia
        - **Others:** cystic fibrosis (CF), cocaine, diffuse alveolar damage, acute lung allograft rejection, idiopathic pulmonary hemosiderosis, lung contusion

- **Vascular**
  - Pulmonary embolism/infarction, arteriovenous malformation, bronchovascular fistula, pulmonary hypertension, aneurysm/pseudoaneurysm, dieulafoy lesion (of airway), bronchial telangectasia
- **Cardiac**
  - Right sided endocarditis, pulmonary edema (congestive heart failure, mitral stenosis, congenital heart disease)
- **Iatrogenic**
  - **Medications:** anticoagulants, thrombolytic/fibrinolytic, anti-angiogenics (bevacizumab)
  - **Post procedural:** lung biopsy, heart/pulmonary artery catheterization, bronchoscopy, endotracheal tube erosion, airway stent
- **Miscellaneous**
  - Coagulopathy, thoracic/pulmonary endometriosis, thrombocytopenia
- **Pseudohemoptysis**
  - **Gastrointestinal (hematemesis):** ulcer, gastritis, esophageal variceal bleed
  - **Upper respiratory airway source:** epistaxis, ulcers, telangectasias
  - Serratia marcescens (gram negative bacteria producing red pigment)

Notes

Notes: Between 20% to 50% of cases may ultimately not receive a definitive diagnosis or are idiopathic. Chest radiographs can initially help, though have limited sensitivity in detecting the bleeding source. CT angiography with contrast is more sensitive for identifying bleeding sources. Effective management involves treating the underlying cause to prevent recurrence, which varies depending on the predisposing factor. Bronchial artery embolization can address many cases of massive bleeding. Surgery is generally considered for patients who do not respond to medical treatment or embolization. Endotracheal intubation can be difficult, and massive hemoptysis may require selective mainstem intubation of the non-affected lung.

Red flags: massive hemoptysis, back pain, presence of a pulmonary artery catheter or tracheostomy, malaise, weight loss, fatigue, extensive smoking history, dyspnea at rest during examination, absent or decreased breath sounds

Special populations: In children, congenital heart disease, CF, and idiopathic pulmonary hemosiderosis are notable causes of hemoptysis, while infections remain the most common etiology in those without pre-existing structural lung or cardiac disease. Children with tracheostomies or immunosuppression (e.g., post-transplant) are also at increased risk for recurrent or severe hemoptysis. In regions with high tuberculosis prevalence, tuberculosis remains a leading cause, particularly among young adults and recent immigrants. Older adults, esp. in those with a history of smoking, are at increased risk for hemoptysis secondary to malignancy or chronic pulmonary disease. Patients with structural lung disease (e.g., bronchiectasis, prior pulmonary infections, or sequelae of pulmonary embolism) and those on anticoagulant therapy are consistently identified as high-risk groups for both initial and recurrent hemoptysis.

Further Reading

- Godfrey S. Pulmonary hemorrhage/hemoptysis in children. Pediatric pulmonology. 2004 Jun;37(6):476-84.
- Ittrich H, Bockhorn M, Klose H, Simon M. The diagnosis and treatment of hemoptysis. Deutsches Ärzteblatt international. 2017 Jun 5;114(21):371.
- Gagnon S, Quigley N, Dutau H, Delage A, Fortin M. Approach to hemoptysis in the modern era. Canadian respiratory journal. 2017;2017(1):1565030.
- Larici AR, Franchi P, Occhipinti M, Contegiacomo A, del Ciello A, Calandriello L, Storto ML, Marano R, Bonomo L. Diagnosis and management of hemoptysis. Diagnostic and interventional radiology. 2014 Apr 30;20(4):299.
- Earwood JS, Thompson TD. Hemoptysis: evaluation and management. American family physician. 2015 Feb 15;91(4):243-
- O'Gurek D, Choi HY. Hemoptysis: evaluation and management. American family physician. 2022 Feb;105(2):144-51.

Snoring

Introduction

Snoring is the sound that occurs when the tissues in the throat vibrate against each other. During sleep, the throat's "upper airway dilator" muscles relax, leading to a narrow upper airway that increases airflow, causing soft tissue vibration. History and physical examination form the basis of snoring evaluation, with additional studies conducted according to specific findings. Since snoring isn't considered a disease but a (potentially bothersome) symptom, it is typically treated based on the patient's preference, except in certain cases where conservative, instrumental, or surgical approaches are required.

Checklist DDX

Serious/life-threatening: obstructive sleep apnea (OSA), central sleep apnea, airway neoplasia

Common: OSA, smoking, alcohol use, supine sleeping position, obesity, advanced age, alcohol, central fat distribution, adenoid and tonsillar hypertrophy, male sex, pregnancy, chronic nasal congestion (e.g. allergic rhinitis), deviated nasal septum, nasal polyps

Commonly misdiagnosed: hypothyroidism, oropharyngeal or laryngeal tumors, acromegaly (esp. in absence of characteristic features), central sleep apnea, upper airway resistance syndrome

Systematic DDX

Pathophysiologic approach
- Pulmonary
    - **Obstructive disorders of upper/lower airway:** OSA, COPD, asthma
    - **Upper respiratory infections** (common cold "viral rhinitis," sinusitis, or bronchitis)
    - **Chronic nasal congestion:** allergic rhinitis, structural causes (deviated nasal septum or nasal polyp), infectious (influenza "flu," tonsillitis and pharyngitis, adenoiditis "esp. in children")
- Neurological
    - Central sleep apnea, amyotrophic lateral sclerosis, muscle dystrophies

- **Gastrointestinal**
  - GERD
- **Cardiovascular**
  - Heart failure (if complicated by central sleep apnea)
- **Endocrinal/metabolic**
  - Hypothyroidism, acromegaly, obesity
- **Others**
  - **Medications/substances:** alcohol, sedatives, muscle relaxants, and hypnotics
  - Pregnancy

Structural vs non-structural
- **Structural/anatomic**
  - **Craniofacial skeletal abnormalities:** facial elongation, posterior facial compression, retrognathia, micrognathia, mandibular hypoplasia, brachycephalic head form
  - **Oral cavity/oropharyngeal structures:** macroglossia, long uvula, high-arched palate (esp. in women/Turner syndrome)
  - **Upper airway soft tissue hypertrophy:** adenotonsillar hypertrophy (especially in children), inferior displacement of hyoid bone
  - **Nasal cavity abnormalities:** nasal polyps, deviated nasal septum, chronic nasal congestion (e.g. allergic rhinitis), inferior turbinate hypertrophy, nasal valve collapse
  - **Genetic disorders:** Prader-Willi, Down, Marfan and Pierre Robin syndromes
- **Non-structural**
  - Obesity, central fat distribution, male sex, advanced age, alcohol use, sedative and hypnotic use, smoking, supine sleep position, pregnancy

Notes

General considerations: Primary snoring is snoring that doesn't cause awakenings, restricted airflow, frequent arousals, drops in oxygen levels, or arrhythmia. It happens in individuals who don't experience excessive daytime drowsiness, and it is not accompanied by OSA. History can be important as it provides insight into what may be triggering snoring, when it occurs during the day, and the presence of relevant comorbidities. The STOP-BANG questionnaire is a test used to screen for OSA. It has a total score of 8, with 0-2 classified as low risk, 3-4 as intermediate risk, and 5 and above as high risk. Primary snoring isn't usually treated except if it bothers the patients or their partners. Lifestyle modifications such as weight loss, avoiding alcohol and sedating medications before bedtime, or avoiding back sleeping, can be helpful in reducing snoring. CPAP is very effective in treating OSA as well as in primary snoring. Surgery can be an option to reconstruct normal anatomy if anatomical abnormalities are the cause of snoring.

Red flags: witnessed apnea, choking during sleep, morning headaches, loud and constant snoring, hypertension, BMI ≥ 35 kg/m^2, Epworth sleepiness score ≥ 10, insomnia, history of drowsiness or falling asleep while driving; ADHD-like symptoms/poor concentration and bed wetting (in children)

Special populations: OSA is more common in men, but the risk in women increases after menopause, likely due to hormonal changes affecting upper airway tone. Patients with comorbid cardiovascular or metabolic disease are at increased risk for OSA-related complications.

Further Reading

- Chen L, Pivetta B, Nagappa M, Saripella A, Islam S, Englesakis M, Chung F. Validation of the STOP-Bang questionnaire for screening of obstructive sleep apnea in the general population and commercial drivers: a systematic review and meta-analysis. Sleep Breath. 2021 Dec;25(4):1741-1751.
- Huyett P. What is snoring?. JAMA Otolaryngology–Head & Neck Surgery. 2023 Mar 1;149(3):286-.
- Stuck BA, Hofauer B. The diagnosis and treatment of snoring in adults. Deutsches Ärzteblatt International. 2019 Nov 29;116(48):817.
- Slowik JM, Sankari A, Collen JF. Obstructive sleep apnea. InStatPearls [Internet] 2024 Mar 21. StatPearls Publishing.

Abdominal and Gastrointestinal

Saeed Rahmani

Long H. Tu

Ashley A. Jacobson

Abdominal Pain

Introduction

Abdominal pain and tenderness are among the most frequent complaints in emergency and outpatient settings, accounting for a significant proportion of visits across all age groups. The clinical presentation may be acute or chronic, diffuse or localized. It is often accompanied by other symptoms such as nausea, vomiting, fever, or changes in bowel habits. Differential considerations overlap with presentations such as nausea/vomiting, gastrointestinal bleeding, and urinary or gynecologic symptoms. Major diagnostic considerations include distinguishing surgical emergencies (e.g., perforation, ischemia, obstruction) from medical and functional causes.

Abdominal pain can be subdivided by site or distribution (generalized/diffuse, right upper quadrant, left upper quadrant, right lower quadrant, left lower quadrant, epigastric, periumbilical, suprapubic, and flank pain). Location of pain is statistically associated with specific underlying etiologies (e.g., right upper quadrant with hepatobiliary disease); however, it is insufficiently reliable to rule in or rule out specific etiologies. Pain location must be considered with other history, exam, lab, and imaging findings to guide diagnosis. Where potentially helpful, we provide differential considerations by location, with the caveat that these represent associations – underlying pathology can present atypically or with variable pain distribution.

Checklist DDX

Serious/life-threatening (most common serious): mesenteric ischemia, ruptured abdominal aortic aneurysm, perforated viscus, bowel obstruction, acute appendicitis, acute cholecystitis, pancreatitis, intraabdominal hemorrhage, volvulus, testicular torsion, and tubo-ovarian abscess

> By location (note: location alone is insufficient to rule in or rule out pathology)
> - **Right upper quadrant (RUQ):** acute cholecystitis/cholangitis, hepatic abscess or rupture, perforated duodenal ulcer, pneumonia
> - **Left upper quadrant (LUQ):** splenic rupture or infarct, gastric perforation, myocardial infarction, acute pancreatitis, pneumonia
> - **Epigastric/upper central:** myocardial infarction, perforated peptic ulcer, aortic dissection or ruptured abdominal aortic aneurysm (AAA), acute pancreatitis

- **Periumbilical:** mesenteric ischemia, ruptured AAA, early appendicitis, small bowel obstruction,
- **Right lower quadrant (RLQ):** appendicitis, cecal volvulus or ischemia, ectopic pregnancy
- **Left lower quadrant (LLQ):** ectopic pregnancy, diverticulitis, ischemic colitis
- **Suprapubic/lower central:** ruptured ectopic pregnancy, acute urinary retention or bladder rupture, acute pelvic inflammatory disease
- **Diffuse/generalized:** peritonitis (from any perforated viscus), mesenteric ischemia, ruptured AAA, diabetic ketoacidosis
- **Flank:** renal colic from obstructing kidney stone, pyelonephritis with sepsis

Common: gastroenteritis, constipation, irritable bowel syndrome, peptic ulcer disease, biliary colic, urinary tract infection, diverticulitis, functional abdominal pain, gastroesophageal reflux disease, functional dyspepsia, chronic pancreatitis

Commonly misdiagnosed: functional disorders (e.g., irritable bowel syndrome, functional dyspepsia), small bowel obstruction, chronic pancreatitis, inflammatory bowel diseases (e.g., Crohn's disease), abdominal wall pain, porphyria, familial Mediterranean fever

Systematic DDX

Pathophysiologic approach
- **Vascular**
    - **Arterial/venous occlusion (and low flow states):** mesenteric ischemia, ischemic colitis, renal vein thrombosis, portal vein thrombosis, splenic infarct
    - **Aneurysm/dissection:** abdominal aortic aneurysm (AAA) rupture, aortic dissection
    - **Venous outflow obstruction:** Budd-Chiari syndrome
- **Infectious/inflammatory**
    - **Gastrointestinal:** appendicitis, diverticulitis, gastroenteritis, typhlitis, colitis (including from Clostridioides difficile), peritonitis, epiploic appendagitis, omental infarction, H. pylori gastritis
    - **Hepatobiliary:** cholecystitis, cholangitis, hepatitis
    - **Pancreatic:** pancreatitis
    - **Genitourinary:** urinary tract infection, pyelonephritis, salpingitis, pelvic inflammatory disease, tubo-ovarian abscess, Fournier's gangrene
    - **Other abdominal infections:** splenic abscess, hepatic abscess

- Neoplastic
    - **Gastrointestinal tract:** colorectal carcinoma, gastric carcinoma, small bowel adenocarcinoma, gastrointestinal stromal tumor (GIST)
    - **Hepatobiliary:** hepatocellular carcinoma, cholangiocarcinoma
    - **Pancreatic:** pancreatic cancer
    - **Renal:** renal cell carcinoma
    - **Gynecologic:** ovarian cancer
    - **Diffuse/multifocal:** lymphoma, peritoneal carcinomatosis, pseudomyxoma peritonei
- Dysfunction
    - **Functional bowel disorders:** irritable bowel syndrome, functional abdominal pain syndrome
    - **Upper GI disorders:** achalasia, functional dyspepsia, gastroparesis, gastric or duodenal ulcer
    - **Pancreatic:** chronic pancreatitis
    - **Endocrine/metabolic functional pain:** diabetic ketoacidosis, diabetic gastropathy
    - **Biliary:** sphincter of Oddi dysfunction
    - **Other functional syndromes:** cyclic vomiting syndrome, chronic intestinal pseudo-obstruction
- Injury/trauma
    - **Blunt trauma:** splenic rupture, liver laceration, traumatic pancreatic injury, bowel injury
    - **Penetrating trauma:** stab wounds, gunshot wounds
    - **Post-surgical:** postoperative pain, post-laparoscopic referred shoulder pain
    - **Wall/musculoskeletal:** abdominal wall hematoma, rectus sheath hematoma
    - **Diaphragmatic/structural:** diaphragmatic rupture
- Compression/obstruction
    - **Small bowel:** adhesive bowel obstruction, hernia, intussusception, superior mesenteric artery syndrome, bezoar
    - **Large bowel:** volvulus, colorectal tumor obstruction, fecal impaction, sigmoid elongation/redundancy
    - **Biliary:** gallstone ileus, biliary obstruction from stone or tumor
    - **Ureteric/urinary:** ureteric obstruction from calculus or mass
    - **Gastric:** gastric outlet obstruction
- Anomalies of development/aging
    - **Congenital:** pyloric stenosis, congenital malrotation, annular pancreas, Meckel diverticulum, Hirschsprung disease, intestinal duplication cyst, persistent vitelline duct

- ○ **Age-related/degenerative:** diverticulosis, sigmoid redundancy
- **Toxic-metabolic**
  - ○ **Drug-induced:** medication-induced pain (NSAIDs, opioids), iron overdose
  - ○ **Alcohol-related:** alcohol-induced gastritis, alcohol-induced pancreatitis
  - ○ **Metabolic/renal:** uremia, hypercalcemia, diabetic gastropathy
  - ○ **Toxins/poisons:** lead poisoning, mushroom poisoning (Amanita phalloides), organophosphate toxicity
  - ○ **Metabolic disorders:** porphyria
- **Everything else**
  - ○ **Abdominal wall/somatic:** abdominal wall pain, hernia without obstruction
  - ○ **Autoinflammatory/hereditary:** familial Mediterranean fever, hereditary angioedema
  - ○ **Hematologic/systemic:** sickle cell crisis, vasculitis (e.g., polyarteritis nodosa)
  - ○ **Referred pain:** thoracic causes (pneumonia, myocardial infarction, pericarditis)
  - ○ **Dermatologic/neurologic:** herpes zoster
  - ○ **Psychological:** depression, somatization disorder

By location (note: location alone is insufficient to rule in or rule out pathology)
- **Right upper quadrant (RUQ)**
  - ○ **Vascular:** Budd-Chiari syndrome (hepatic vein thrombosis)
  - ○ **Infectious/inflammatory:** acute cholecystitis, cholangitis, hepatitis, hepatic abscess
  - ○ **Neoplastic:** hepatocellular carcinoma, cholangiocarcinoma, metastatic liver lesions
  - ○ **Dysfunction:** biliary dyskinesia, chronic cholecystitis
  - ○ **Injury/trauma:** liver laceration, blunt trauma to right upper abdomen
  - ○ **Compression/obstruction:** gallstone disease with or without biliary obstruction
  - ○ **Anomalies/aging:** large liver cysts, biliary atresia (congenital)
  - ○ **Toxic-metabolic:** alcohol-induced hepatitis, drug-induced liver injury (e.g., acetaminophen toxicity)
  - ○ **Everything else:** abdominal wall strain or herpes zoster (early)
- **Left upper quadrant (LUQ)**
  - ○ **Vascular:** splenic infarct or rupture, rare mesenteric ischemia affecting splenic flexure

- o **Infectious/inflammatory:** pancreatitis (tail), gastritis, gastric ulcer, splenic abscess
- o **Neoplastic:** pancreatic tail cancer, gastric carcinoma, splenic lymphoma
- o **Dysfunction:** chronic pancreatitis, functional dyspepsia
- o **Injury/trauma:** splenic rupture, blunt trauma
- o **Compression/obstruction:** gastric outlet obstruction (due to tumor or scarring)
- o **Anomalies/aging:** wandering spleen (rare), age-related gastric mucosal changes
- o **Toxic-metabolic:** alcohol-induced pancreatitis or gastritis, medication-induced gastritis (NSAIDs)
- o **Everything else:** abdominal wall pain, referred pain from cardiac ischemia/myocardial infarction
- **Epigastric**
  - o **Vascular:** abdominal aortic aneurysm (AAA) rupture, mesenteric ischemia
  - o **Infectious/inflammatory:** acute pancreatitis (head), gastritis, peptic ulcer disease (gastric or duodenal), hepatitis
  - o **Neoplastic:** pancreatic head carcinoma, gastric cancer, esophageal cancer
  - o **Dysfunction:** gastroparesis, achalasia, functional dyspepsia, diabetic ketoacidosis
  - o **Injury/trauma:** pancreatic trauma, esophageal rupture
  - o **Compression/obstruction:** gastric outlet obstruction, pancreatic pseudocyst compressing adjacent organs
  - o **Anomalies/aging:** congenital anomalies of pancreas or stomach
  - o **Toxic-metabolic:** pancreatitis, medication-induced gastritis
  - o **Everything else:** abdominal wall pain, referred pain from cardiac ischemia/myocardial infarction, psychological causes
- **Periumbilical**
  - o **Vascular:** early mesenteric ischemia, early small bowel ischemia
  - o **Infectious/inflammatory:** early appendicitis, enteritis, small bowel obstruction
  - o **Neoplastic:** small bowel tumors, lymphoma
  - o **Dysfunction:** irritable bowel syndrome
  - o **Injury/trauma:** trauma to small bowel or mesentery
  - o **Compression/obstruction:** small bowel obstruction, hernias (umbilical or incisional)
  - o **Anomalies/aging:** Meckel's diverticulum, congenital malrotation
  - o **Toxic-metabolic:** medication-induced enteritis

- o **Everything else:** abdominal wall pain, psychological causes
- **Right lower quadrant (RLQ):**
  - o **Vascular:** mesenteric ischemia involving terminal ileum or cecum
  - o **Infectious/inflammatory:** appendicitis, Crohn's disease, pelvic inflammatory disease (female), tubo-ovarian abscess, urinary tract infection
  - o **Neoplastic:** cecal carcinoma, lymphoma
  - o **Dysfunction:** irritable bowel syndrome, chronic inflammatory bowel disease
  - o **Injury/trauma:** trauma to ileum or cecum
  - o **Compression/obstruction:** inguinal hernia, ileocecal intussusception, bowel obstruction
  - o **Anomalies/aging:** Meckel's diverticulum
  - o **Toxic-metabolic:** medication-induced colitis
  - o **Everything else:** abdominal wall pain, testicular torsion (referred pain), psychological causes
- **Left lower quadrant (LLQ):**
  - o **Vascular:** ischemic colitis (watershed areas)
  - o **Infectious/inflammatory:** diverticulitis, ulcerative colitis, pelvic inflammatory disease (female), tubo-ovarian abscess, urinary tract infection
  - o **Neoplastic:** sigmoid colon carcinoma, lymphoma
  - o **Dysfunction:** irritable bowel syndrome
  - o **Injury/trauma:** trauma to sigmoid colon
  - o **Compression/obstruction:** inguinal hernia, bowel obstruction, volvulus of sigmoid colon
  - o **Anomalies/aging:** diverticulosis
  - o **Toxic-metabolic:** medication-induced colitis
  - o **Everything else:** abdominal wall pain, psychological causes
- **Suprapubic/lower central abdomen:**
  - o **Vascular:** rarely pelvic vascular thrombosis
  - o **Infectious/inflammatory:** Fournier's gangrene, urinary tract infection, cystitis, acute pelvic inflammatory disease, prostatitis (male)
  - o **Neoplastic:** bladder carcinoma, gynecologic cancers (e.g., cervical, uterine)
  - o **Dysfunction:** chronic pelvic pain syndrome, bladder dysfunction
  - o **Injury/trauma:** bladder rupture, pelvic trauma
  - o **Compression/obstruction:** urinary retention, bladder outlet obstruction

- o **Anomalies/aging:** congenital anomalies of urinary tract or reproductive organs
- o **Toxic-metabolic:** medication-induced cystitis
- o **Everything else:** abdominal wall somatic pain, psychological causes
- **Flank pain**
  - o **Vascular:** renal vein thrombosis (less common)
  - o **Infectious/Inflammatory:** pyelitis/pyelonephritis, perinephric abscess
  - o **Neoplastic:** renal cell carcinoma, other urinary tract neoplasia
  - o **Dysfunction:** chronic kidney disease pain (rarely painful)
  - o **Injury/trauma:** renal trauma, rib fractures
  - o **Compression/obstruction:** nephrolithiasis (kidney stones), ureteric obstruction
  - o **Anomalies/aging:** congenital renal anomalies
  - o **Toxic-metabolic:** uremic pain
  - o **Everything else:** musculoskeletal pain, herpes zoster
- **Diffuse/generalized abdominal pain**
  - o **Vascular:** mesenteric ischemia, ruptured abdominal aortic aneurysm (AAA)
  - o **Infectious/inflammatory:** generalized peritonitis, severe gastroenteritis, diabetic ketoacidosis-related visceral pain
  - o **Neoplastic:** peritoneal carcinomatosis
  - o **Dysfunction:** severe irritable bowel syndrome or functional gastrointestinal disorders
  - o **Injury/trauma:** perforated viscus, abdominal trauma
  - o **Compression/obstruction:** diffuse bowel obstruction, paralytic ileus
  - o **Anomalies/aging:** widespread age-related changes in bowel motility
  - o **Toxic-metabolic:** severe electrolyte imbalances causing ileus or pain
  - o **Everything else:** abdominal wall pain, familial Mediterranean fever, psychological causes

Notes

General considerations: A thorough history and physical examination remain central to diagnosis with imaging (preferably contrast-enhanced CT in nonpregnant adults) and laboratory studies tailored to clinical suspicion. In children and pregnant patients, ultrasonography is preferred for initial imaging.

Red flags: sudden or severe pain, persistent vomiting or inability to tolerate liquids, bloody vomit or stool, high fever, signs of shock, severe abdominal tenderness or rigidity (peritonitis), unexplained weight loss, jaundice, difficulty breathing or chest pain, new or worsening pain in patients with a history of abdominal surgery or cancer, dizziness, confusion, altered consciousness

Special populations: In children, common causes include constipation, gastroenteritis, urinary tract infections, and appendicitis, while congenital anomalies such as pyloric stenosis, Meckel diverticulum, or malrotation, and emergencies like intussusception or incarcerated hernia, must also be considered. In older adults, malignancy, mesenteric ischemia, abdominal aortic aneurysm, medication side effects, and conditions such as diverticulosis, cholelithiasis, and constipation are more prevalent. Pregnant women may experience pain from obstetric causes like ectopic pregnancy, placental abruption, or round ligament pain, but gastrointestinal, urinary, and vascular pathologies must not be overlooked as pregnancy can mask or alter presentations. Patients with immunocompromise have higher risk for atypical infections.

Further Reading

- Yew KS, George MK, Allred HB. Acute abdominal pain in adults: evaluation and diagnosis. American family physician. 2023 Jun;107(6):585-96.
- Rogers SO, Kirton OC. Acute abdomen in the modern era. N Engl J Med. 2024;391(1):60-67. doi:10.1056/NEJMra2304821.
- Yamashita S, Tago M, Katsuki NE, Nishi TM, Yamashita SI. Relationships between sites of abdominal pain and the organs involved: a prospective observational study. BMJ open. 2020 Jun 1;10(6):e034446.
- Buel KL, Wilcox J, Mingo PT. Acute abdominal pain in children: evaluation and management. Am Fam Physician. 2024;110(6):621-631.
- Börner N, Kappenberger AS, Weber S, et al. The acute abdomen: structured diagnosis and treatment. Dtsch Arztebl Int. 2025;122(5):137-144. doi:10.3238/arztebl.m2025.0019.
- Pichetshote N, Pimentel M. An approach to the patient with chronic undiagnosed abdominal pain. Am J Gastroenterol. 2019;114(5):726-732. doi:10.14309/ajg.0000000000000130.
- Lukic S, Mijac D, Filipovic B, et al. Chronic abdominal pain: gastroenterologist approach. Dig Dis. 2022;40(2):181-186. doi:10.1159/000516977.

Abdominal Swelling or Distention

Introduction

Abdominal swelling or distention refers to a visible or palpable increase in abdominal girth, often accompanied by subjective bloating or fullness. The presentation may be acute or chronic and can be associated with pain, altered bowel habits, or systemic symptoms. The primary diagnostic task is to distinguish benign functional disorders from serious pathology such as bowel obstruction, malignancy, or organ failure. Overlap exists with related presentations including abdominal pain, ascites, abdominal masses, and genitourinary concerns.

Checklist DDX

Serious/life-threatening: acute bowel obstruction, perforated viscus, intra-abdominal hemorrhage, abdominal compartment syndrome, severe ascites (e.g., from liver failure or rapidly progressive malignancy)

Common: constipation, irritable bowel syndrome, small intestinal bacterial overgrowth, functional bloating and distention (including disorders of gut–brain interaction), dietary factors, chronic liver disease with ascites, obesity, pregnancy

Commonly misdiagnosed: ovarian cancer (especially in women over 50), chronic pancreatitis, slow transit constipation, pelvic floor dysfunction

Systematic DDX

- Vascular
    - Portal hypertension (ascites), mesenteric ischemia (bowel wall edema), Budd–Chiari syndrome
- Infectious/inflammatory
    - Peritonitis, infectious gastroenteritis, inflammatory bowel disease, chronic pancreatitis
- Neoplastic
    - **Solid tumors:** ovarian carcinoma, colorectal carcinoma, gastrointestinal stromal tumor
    - **Other:** lymphoma, lymphoproliferative disorders

- **Dysfunction**
  - **Major organ failure:** hepatic cirrhosis with ascites, renal nephrotic syndrome, cardiac heart failure, abdominal compartment syndrome
  - **Functional disorders:** functional abdominal bloating and distention (disorders of gut–brain interaction), irritable bowel syndrome, motility disorders, slow transit constipation, pelvic floor dysfunction
- **Injury/trauma**
  - Postoperative ileus, intra-abdominal hematoma
- **Compression/obstruction**
  - Small or large bowel obstruction, hernia, intra-abdominal mass, prostatic hyperplasia causing urinary retention, fecal impaction
- **Anomalies of development/aging**
  - **Congenital malformations:** malrotation, duplication cysts
  - **Physiologic:** pregnancy
  - Age-related decreased intestinal motility
- **Toxic–metabolic**
  - **Drug-related:** medication-induced constipation (opioids), medication-induced urinary retention (anticholinergics)
- **Everything else**
  - Obesity, pseudo-obstruction, psychological causes (somatization)

Notes

General considerations: Most cases of bloating and distention are functional and do not require extensive testing unless alarm features or abnormal examination findings are present. Physical examination should assess for masses, ascites, and signs of obstruction. Imaging is indicated with abnormal findings or red flag symptoms. Functional disorders may be diagnosed using the Rome IV criteria, and management typically involves a multidisciplinary approach addressing diet, motility, visceral sensitivity, and psychosocial factors.

Red flags: recent onset or worsening symptoms, severe or persistent pain, vomiting, gastrointestinal bleeding, unintentional weight loss, palpable mass, inability to urinate, defecate, or pass flatus, family history of gastrointestinal malignancy or inflammatory bowel disease

Special populations: In women over 50, persistent bloating or distention should prompt evaluation for ovarian cancer. In children, congenital anomalies, constipation, and celiac disease are common considerations. In the elderly, malignancy, heart failure, and medication side effects are more prevalent. Pregnancy and obesity are frequent benign causes, but do not exclude other pathology.

Further Reading

- Moshiree B, Drossman DA, Shaukat A. AGA clinical practice update on evaluation and management of belching, abdominal bloating, and distention: expert review. Gastroenterology. 2023;165(3):791-800.e3. doi:10.1053/j.gastro 2023.04.039.
- Byale A, Palsson OS, Simrén M, et al. Bloating and distention patients form six distinct latent clusters based on symptoms, diet, psychosocial and quality of life parameters. Am J Gastroenterol. 2025;[Epub ahead of print]. doi:10.14309/ajg.0000000000003622.
- Rogers SO, Kirton OC. Acute abdomen in the modern era. N Engl J Med. 2024;391(1):60-67. doi:10.1056/NEJMra2304821.
- Börner N, Kappenberger AS, Weber S, et al. The acute abdomen: structured diagnosis and treatment. Dtsch Arztebl Int. 2025;122(5):137-144. doi:10.3238/arztebl.m2025.0019.
- Saul H, Gursul D, Lyratzopoulos G. When do people with abdominal symptoms need a fast track referral? BMJ. 2022;377:o1198. Accessed 2025 Aug 8. doi:10.1136/bmj.o1198.

Nausea/Vomiting

Introduction

Nausea and vomiting are common symptoms encountered in both outpatient and inpatient settings. Presentations range from self-limited, benign conditions to manifestations of life-threatening disease. Acute symptoms (less than 7 days) are most often due to infections, medications, or toxins, while chronic symptoms (4 weeks or longer) require evaluation for gastrointestinal, neurologic, metabolic, endocrine, and psychiatric causes. Symptom duration between these timeframes may be considered either subacute or episodic with differential considerations drawn from both the acute and chronic designations. Underlying etiologies for nausea and vomiting overlap with that of other presentations such as abdominal pain, diarrhea, and weight loss.

Checklist DDX

Serious/life-threatening: acute gastrointestinal obstruction, bowel ischemia, acute myocardial infarction, increased intracranial pressure (e.g. bleed, mass), adrenal crisis, diabetic ketoacidosis, and severe infections (e.g., sepsis, meningitis)

Common: viral gastroenteritis, medication side effects (opioids, antibiotics, chemotherapeutics), pregnancy (especially first trimester), vestibular disorders (e.g., labyrinthitis, benign paroxysmal positional vertigo), migraine, and functional gastrointestinal disorders (e.g., gastroparesis, functional dyspepsia)

Commonly misdiagnosed: cyclic vomiting syndrome, cannabinoid hyperemesis syndrome, gastroparesis, small bowel obstruction, psychiatric causes (e.g., anxiety, eating disorders), and metabolic or endocrine disorders such as Addison's disease and hyperthyroidism

Systematic DDX

Acute (<7 days)
- **Vascular**
  - Mesenteric ischemia, acute myocardial infarction, Budd-Chiari syndrome
- **Infectious/inflammatory**
  - **Gastrointestinal:** infectious gastroenteritis (norovirus, Staphylococcus aureus enterotoxin, Bacillus cereus), bacterial food poisoning, hepatitis, pancreatitis, appendicitis, cholecystitis, cholangitis, colitis, inflammatory bowel disease (acute flare)

- o **Neurologic:** meningitis, encephalitis, labyrinthitis, vestibular neuritis, Ménière disease, otitis media
- o **Systemic:** sepsis, pelvic inflammatory disease, urinary tract infection, prostatitis, ovarian torsion, testicular torsion
- **Dysfunction**
  - o Acute episode of cyclic vomiting syndrome, cannabinoid hyperemesis syndrome, hyperemesis gravidarum
- **Injury/trauma**
  - o Concussion, increased intracranial pressure (acute), intracranial hemorrhage, postoperative nausea/vomiting (anesthesia)
- **Compression/obstruction**
  - o Small or large bowel obstruction, acute gastric outlet obstruction, superior mesenteric artery syndrome, intracranial mass effect (acute)
- **Toxic-metabolic**
  - o Acute medication or toxin exposure, acute alcohol intoxication, toxin ingestion (cyanide, carbon monoxide, ricin), adrenal crisis, diabetic ketoacidosis, acute metabolic derangements (uremia, hypercalcemia, hyponatremia)
- **Everything else**
  - o Motion sickness

Chronic (>4 weeks)
- **Vascular**
  - o Chronic mesenteric ischemia, Chronic Budd-Chiari syndrome (subacute presentation possible)
- **Infectious/inflammatory**
  - o Chronic inflammatory bowel disease, chronic prostatitis
- **Neoplastic**
  - o Gastric carcinoma (or other neoplasia), small bowel tumors, intracranial neoplasms, vestibular schwannoma
- **Dysfunction**
  - o Gastroparesis (diabetic, postsurgical, post-infectious), functional dyspepsia, achalasia, chronic cyclic vomiting syndrome, chronic cannabinoid hyperemesis syndrome, chronic gastroesophageal reflux disease (GERD)
- **Compression/obstruction:**
  - o Chronic partial gastric outlet obstruction, chronic superior mesenteric artery syndrome, chronic intracranial mass effect
- **Anomalies of development/aging**
  - o Congenital malrotation, age-related delayed gastric emptying

- **Toxic-metabolic**
    - Chronic medication side effects, chronic alcohol use, endocrine causes (Addison's disease, pregnancy-related hyperemesis), chronic metabolic derangements (uremia, hypercalcemia, hyponatremia)
- **Everything else**
    - Psychiatric disorders (anxiety, depression, eating disorders), rumination syndrome, chronic motion sickness

Notes

General considerations: A careful history and physical examination are essential to guide the diagnostic approach, with attention to onset, duration, associated symptoms, medication and substance use, and alarm features. Initial workup typically includes laboratory testing (CBC, electrolytes, pancreatic and liver enzymes, thyroid-stimulating hormone, toxin screen, pregnancy test) and may also involve upper endoscopy and radiographic imaging. Acute, self-limited cases may be managed symptomatically, while chronic or severe cases require targeted evaluation for underlying causes.

Red flags: severe abdominal pain, hematemesis, melena, weight loss, neurologic deficits, dehydration, hypotension, altered mental status

Special populations: In pregnancy, hyperemesis gravidarum and other pregnancy-related causes must be distinguished from gastrointestinal and systemic diseases. In children, infectious, anatomic, and metabolic causes predominate, while in the elderly, medication side effects, malignancy, and metabolic derangements are more common. Cannabinoid hyperemesis syndrome and cyclic vomiting syndrome are increasingly recognized in adolescents and young adults.

Further Reading

- Tome J, Kamboj AK, Sweetser S. A practical 5-step approach to nausea and vomiting. Mayo Clin Proc. 2022;97(3):600-608. doi:10.1016/j.mayocp.2021.10.030
- Johns T, Lawrence E. Evaluation and treatment of nausea and vomiting in adults. Am Fam Physician. 2024;109(5):417-425
- Lacy BE, Parkman HP, Camilleri M. Chronic nausea and vomiting: evaluation and treatment. Am J Gastroenterol. 2018;113(5):647-659. doi:10.1038/s41395-018-0039-2
- Scorza K, Williams A, Phillips JD, Shaw J. Evaluation of nausea and vomiting. Am Fam Physician. 2007;76(1):76-84

- Anderson WD, Strayer SM. Evaluation of nausea and vomiting: a case-based approach. Am Fam Physician. 2013;88(6):371-379
- Rubio-Tapia A, McCallum R, Camilleri M. AGA clinical practice update on diagnosis and management of cannabinoid hyperemesis syndrome: commentary. Gastroenterology. 2024;166(5):930-934.e1. doi:10.1053/j.gastro.2024.01.040
- Levinthal DJ, Staller K, Venkatesan T. AGA clinical practice update on diagnosis and management of cyclic vomiting syndrome: commentary. Gastroenterology. 2024;167(4):804-811.e1. doi:10.1053/j.gastro.2024.05.031

Diarrhea

Introduction

Diarrhea is a common gastrointestinal complaint characterized by the passage of loose or watery stools, often with increased frequency or volume. It can be classified by duration as acute (<14 days), persistent (14–30 days), or chronic (>4 weeks). Etiologies are broadly categorized as infectious or non-infectious, and as watery, fatty, or inflammatory. Overlap exists with other presentations such as irritable bowel syndrome, malabsorption syndromes, and gastrointestinal bleeding. Clinical assessment should be guided by onset, duration, associated symptoms, and patient risk factors to direct appropriate diagnostic evaluation and management.

Checklist DDX

Serious/life-threatening: mesenteric ischemia, sepsis, bowel obstruction, toxic megacolon, ischemic colitis, acute severe diarrhea due to invasive bacterial infection, Clostridioides difficile colitis, severe dehydration, lymphoma, colorectal cancer, VIPoma, adrenal crisis, cystic fibrosis

Common: viral gastroenteritis (norovirus, rotavirus), bacterial food poisoning (Salmonella, Shigella, Campylobacter, Escherichia coli), medication-induced diarrhea (antibiotics, laxatives), irritable bowel syndrome, lactose intolerance, celiac disease, bile acid diarrhea, microscopic colitis, inflammatory bowel disease, small intestinal bacterial overgrowth, post-surgical syndromes (short bowel, dumping)

Commonly misdiagnosed: exocrine pancreatic insufficiency, bile acid diarrhea, microscopic colitis, celiac disease, chronic parasitic infections (Giardia), functional diarrhea misattributed to organic disease or vice versa

Systematic DDX

Acute (<14 days)
- **Vascular**
    - Ischemic colitis, mesenteric ischemia
- **Infectious/inflammatory**
    - Viral gastroenteritis (norovirus, rotavirus), bacterial gastroenteritis (Salmonella, Shigella, Campylobacter, enterotoxigenic E. coli, STEC [Shiga toxin-producing Escherichia coli]), toxin-mediated gastroenteritis (Staphylococcus aureus, Bacillus cereus, Clostridium perfringens), Clostridioides difficile

- o Inflammatory bowel disease, other inflammatory colitis, appendicitis
- **Neoplastic**
  - o Rare acute presentation from obstructive colorectal carcinoma
- **Injury/trauma**
  - o Postoperative diarrhea (post-anesthesia or bowel resection), abdominal trauma
- **Compression/obstruction**
  - o Partial small bowel obstruction, encopresis, intussusception, gastric outlet obstruction
- **Toxic-metabolic**
  - o Medication-induced diarrhea (antibiotics, magnesium antacids), alcohol intoxication, toxin ingestion (cyanide, carbon monoxide), endocrine (thyrotoxicosis), metabolic derangements (uremia, hypercalcemia, hyponatremia)

Persistent (14–30 days)
- **Infectious/inflammatory**
  - o **Protozoal infections:** Giardia lamblia, Cryptosporidium spp., Cyclospora cayetanensis, Entamoeba histolytica
  - o **Other:** post-infectious irritable bowel syndrome, microscopic colitis, inflammatory bowel disease (milder or subacute flare), small intestinal bacterial overgrowth, radiation colitis, eosinophilic gastroenteritis
- **Toxic-metabolic**
  - o Medication-induced diarrhea (antibiotics, laxatives, metformin), bile acid diarrhea
- **Everything else**
  - o Irritable bowel syndrome, factitious diarrhea (laxative abuse)

Chronic (>4 weeks)
- **Vascular**
  - o Chronic mesenteric ischemia, vasculitis (Behçet syndrome)
- **Infectious/inflammatory**
  - o **Chronic parasitic infections:** Giardia, Entamoeba, Cryptosporidium, Cyclospora
  - o **Other:** inflammatory bowel disease (Crohn's disease, ulcerative colitis), microscopic colitis, radiation colitis, eosinophilic gastroenteritis, chronic small intestinal bacterial overgrowth
- **Neoplastic**
  - o Colorectal carcinoma, lymphoma, villous adenoma, Kaposi sarcoma, carcinoid tumor, gastrinoma

- - **Endocrine tumors:** VIPoma, medullary thyroid cancer, pheochromocytoma, carcinoid
- **Dysfunction**
  - IBS-D (irritable bowel syndrome with diarrhea), functional diarrhea, bile acid diarrhea, exocrine pancreatic insufficiency, celiac disease, lactose intolerance
- **Injury/trauma**
  - Radiation enteritis, post-surgical changes (bowel resection, cholecystectomy, gastric surgery)
- **Metabolic/endocrine:**
  - Hyperthyroidism, diabetic autonomic neuropathy
- **Compression/obstruction**
  - Partial small bowel obstruction, strictures
- **Anomalies of development/aging**
  - Congenital enzyme deficiencies (sucrase-isomaltase), congenital chloride diarrhea, age-related motility disorders
- **Toxic-metabolic**
  - Chronic medication-induced diarrhea (colchicine, metformin, magnesium antacids)
  - Heavy metal toxicity
- **Everything else**
  - Factitious diarrhea, psychological causes (somatization), endometriosis involving bowel

Notes

General considerations: Evaluation should distinguish acute from chronic diarrhea, infectious from non-infectious etiologies, and watery, fatty, or inflammatory subtypes. Travel history, dietary exposures, recent antibiotic use, and comorbid conditions guide diagnosis. Management prioritizes fluid and electrolyte replacement, with further evaluation based on risk factors and alarm features.

Red flags: high fever, bloody stools, severe abdominal pain, unintentional weight loss, anemia, persistent symptoms beyond several weeks, hypotension, tachycardia, oliguria, signs of hypovolemia

Special populations: Pediatric, elderly, and immunocompromised patients may have atypical presentations. They are more prone to rapid dehydration and have higher risk of severe complications. In pregnant patients, dehydration may compromise fetal perfusion. Infectious etiologies such as listeriosis require prompt recognition.

Further Reading

- Riddle MS, DuPont HL, Connor BA. ACG Clinical Guideline: Diagnosis, treatment, and prevention of acute diarrheal infections in adults. Am J Gastroenterol. 2016;111(5):602-22. doi:10.1038/ajg.2016.126
- Sokic-Milutinovic A, Pavlovic-Markovic A, Tomasevic RS, Lukic S. Diarrhea as a clinical challenge: General practitioner approach. Dig Dis. 2022;40(3):282-289. doi:10.1159/000517111
- DuPont HL. Persistent diarrhea: A clinical review. JAMA. 2016;315(24):2712-23. doi:10.1001/jama.2016.7833
- Hammer HF. Management of chronic diarrhea in primary care: The gastroenterologists' advice. Dig Dis. 2021;39(6):615-621. doi:10.1159/000515219
- Schiller LR, Pardi DS, Sellin JH. Chronic diarrhea: Diagnosis and management. Clin Gastroenterol Hepatol. 2017;15(2):182-193.e3. doi:10.1016/j.cgh.2016.07.028
- Shane AL, Mody RK, Crump JA, et al. 2017 Infectious Diseases Society of America clinical practice guidelines for the diagnosis and management of infectious diarrhea. Clin Infect Dis. 2017;65(12):e45-e80. doi:10.1093/cid/cix569
- Brenner DM, Domínguez-Muñoz JE. Differential diagnosis of chronic diarrhea: An algorithm to distinguish irritable bowel syndrome with diarrhea from other organic gastrointestinal diseases. J Clin Gastroenterol. 2023;57(7):663-670. doi:10.1097/MCG.0000000000001855
- Burgers K, Lindberg B, Bevis ZJ. Chronic diarrhea in adults: Evaluation and differential diagnosis. Am Fam Physician. 2020;101(8):472-480
- Hiner GE, Walters JR. A practical approach to the patient with chronic diarrhoea. Clin Med (Lond). 2021;21(2):124-126. doi:10.7861/clinmed.2021-0028

Constipation

Introduction

Constipation is a common gastrointestinal disorder affecting approximately 15% of the global population and occurring across all ages, characterized by infrequent bowel movements, straining, hard or lumpy stools, incomplete evacuation, and a sensation of anorectal blockage. Acute constipation (days to <2 weeks) is most often related to sudden dietary changes, dehydration, immobility, acute illness, or new medication use such as opioids, anticholinergics, calcium channel blockers, iron, and antidepressants. Acute obstruction such as colorectal cancer or volvulus must be excluded if alarm features are present. Persistent constipation (2–4 weeks) may result from ongoing medication effects, subacute metabolic or endocrine disorders such as hypothyroidism and hypercalcemia, or evolving pelvic floor dysfunction. Chronic constipation (>4 weeks) is most often idiopathic, normal transit constipation, slow transit constipation, or outlet dysfunction (dyssynergic defecation), or secondary to chronic medications, metabolic or endocrine disease, neurologic disorders such as Parkinson's disease, multiple sclerosis, or spinal cord injury, or psychosocial factors. Chronic constipation is defined by the Rome IV criteria as symptoms persisting for at least 3 months (with onset at least 6 months prior) and including at least two features in at least 25% of defecations, fewer than three spontaneous bowel movements per week, straining, hard stools, incomplete evacuation, anorectal blockage, or manual maneuvers, in the absence of diarrhea.

Checklist DDX

Serious/life-threatening: colorectal malignancy, bowel obstruction, toxic megacolon, cauda equina syndrome, stroke, botulism, hypercalcemia, myxedema coma

Common: functional constipation (normal or slow transit), IBS-C (with constipation), low fiber/low water diet, hypothyroidism, medication-induced constipation (opioids, anticholinergics, calcium channel blockers, antidepressants), pelvic floor dysfunction, electrolyte imbalances, diabetic neuropathy, spinal cord lesions

Commonly misdiagnosed: dyssynergic defecation, slow transit constipation, medication-induced constipation, secondary causes such as hypothyroidism, diabetes, neurologic disorders, and pelvic floor dysfunction

Systematic DDX

Acute (<2 weeks)
- **Vascular**
    - Acute mesenteric ischemia, ischemic colitis
- **Infectious/inflammatory**
    - Diverticulitis, stercoral colitis
- **Neoplastic**
    - Acute presentation of obstructing colorectal carcinoma
- **Dysfunction**
    - **Medication-induced**: opioids, anticholinergics, calcium channel blockers, iron, calcium supplements, certain antidepressants
    - **Other**: acute functional constipation, acute hypothyroid crisis, ileus
- **Injury/trauma**
    - Postoperative states, acute spinal cord injury
- **Compression/obstruction**
    - Large-bowel obstruction (colorectal carcinoma, sigmoid volvulus, cecal volvulus, severe diverticular stricture), fecal impaction
- **Toxic-metabolic**
    - Acute dehydration, acute hypercalcemia, hypokalemia
- **Everything else**
    - Acute pain syndromes limiting mobility, acute functional constipation after travel ("vacation constipation")

Persistent (2–4 weeks)
- **Vascular**
    - Subacute ischemic colitis
- **Infectious/inflammatory**
    - Subacute diverticulitis, subacute colitis
- **Neoplastic**
    - Evolving partial obstruction from colorectal carcinoma
- **Dysfunction**
    - Early functional constipation, early IBS-C, evolving pelvic floor dysfunction, subacute medication effect, pregnancy-associated constipation
- **Compression/obstruction**
    - Subacute large-bowel obstruction (stricture, mass)
- **Toxic-metabolic**
    - Early hypothyroidism, subacute hypercalcemia, evolving diabetic autonomic neuropathy

- **Chronic (>4 weeks)**
  - **Vascular**
    - Chronic mesenteric ischemia (rare), portal hypertension with hemorrhoidal congestion
  - **Infectious/inflammatory:**
    - **Parasitic/bacterial:** Chagas disease
    - **Inflammatory/other:** chronic proctitis, chronic radiation proctitis, chronic colitis, stercoral colitis
  - **Neoplastic**
    - Colorectal carcinoma, rectal or pelvic mass, lymphoma, pelvic malignancies causing obstruction
  - **Dysfunction**
    - **Primary:** functional constipation (normal transit, slow transit), IBS-C, dyssynergic defecation, pelvic floor dysfunction
    - **Secondary:** hypothyroidism, diabetes mellitus, Parkinson's disease, multiple sclerosis, spinal cord injury, celiac disease, chronic diabetic autonomic neuropathy, chronic medication effect
  - **Injury/trauma**
    - Chronic postoperative changes, pelvic or spinal cord injury, radiation injury
  - **Compression/obstruction**
    - Chronic partial obstruction (stricture, mass), rectocele, extrinsic compression from pelvic mass, fecal impaction
  - **Anomalies of development/aging**
    - Hirschsprung disease (in children), congenital megacolon, age-related decreased motility
  - **Toxic-metabolic:**
    - **Medication-induced:** opioids, anticholinergics, calcium channel blockers, iron, calcium supplements
    - **Metabolic:** chronic hypercalcemia, chronic hypothyroidism, chronic hypokalemia
  - **Everything else**
    - Eating disorders, psychological factors, chronic dehydration

Notes

General considerations: Dietary habits, medication use, medical and surgical histories, and targeted laboratory testing (complete blood count, electrolyte levels, thyroid function tests) alongside digital rectal examination and selective imaging or colonoscopy can help identify underlying causes and guide management. Management in benign/self-limited cases begins with lifestyle modifications including increased fiber intake, hydration, and physical activity. Pharmacologic options such as osmotic or stimulant laxatives, and in selected cases secretagogues, are considered for refractory symptoms. Biofeedback therapy is indicated for pelvic floor dysfunction.

Red flags: signs of obstruction, rectal bleeding, significant unintentional weight loss, bloody bowel movements, abdominal distension, failure to thrive, neurological abnormalities

Special populations: In children, congenital anomalies and functional constipation are common considerations. In older adults, decreased mobility, comorbidities, and polypharmacy increase risk. In pregnancy, hormonal and mechanical factors contribute to constipation and should be addressed conservatively when possible.

Further Reading

- Alavi K, Thorsen AJ, Fang SH, et al. The American Society of Colon and Rectal Surgeons Clinical Practice Guidelines for the Evaluation and Management of Chronic Constipation. Dis Colon Rectum. 2024;67(10):1244-1257. doi:10.1097/DCR.0000000000003430.
- Bharucha AE, Lacy BE. Mechanisms, evaluation, and management of chronic constipation. Gastroenterology. 2020;158(5):1232-1249.e3. doi:10.1053/j.gastro.2019.12.034.
- Wald A. Constipation: advances in diagnosis and treatment. JAMA. 2016;315(2):185-191 doi:10.1001/jama.2015.16994.
- Hungin AP. Chronic constipation in adults: the primary care approach. Dig Dis. 2022;40(2):142-146. doi:10.1159/000516489.
- Sharma A, Rao SSC, Kearns K, et al. Diagnosis, management and patient perspectives of the spectrum of constipation disorders. Aliment Pharmacol Ther. 2021;53(12):1250-1267. doi:10.1111/apt.16369.
- Pannemans J, Masuy I, Tack J. Functional constipation: individualising assessment and treatment. Drugs. 2020;80(10):947-963. doi:10.1007/s40265-020-01305-z.
- Bharucha AE, Dorn SD, Lembo A, Pressman A. American Gastroenterological Association medical position statement on constipation. Gastroenterology. 2013;144(1):211-217. doi:10.1053/j.gastro.2012.10.029.

Hematemesis

Introduction

Hematemesis, defined as the vomiting of fresh blood or coffee-ground material. It is a hallmark sign of acute upper gastrointestinal bleeding, commonly from the esophagus, stomach, or duodenum. A critical initial step is to distinguish hematemesis from hemoptysis (coughing up blood) or nasopharyngeal bleeding, both of which can mimic vomiting blood, but arise from respiratory or nasal sources rather than the gastrointestinal tract. The vomited blood may appear as bright red if fresh bleeding is ongoing, or as dark, granular "coffee-ground" material representing older, partially digested blood, which can help localize and time the bleeding event.

Checklist DDX

Serious/life-threatening: acute esophageal or gastric variceal hemorrhage, aortoenteric fistula, Boerhaave syndrome, massive bleeding from peptic ulcer disease, Dieulafoy lesion

Common: peptic ulcer disease, erosive gastritis or gastropathy, Mallory-Weiss tear, erosive esophagitis, gastric carcinoma, early-onset esophagogastric cancers

Commonly misdiagnosed: Dieulafoy lesion, gastric MALT lymphoma, atypical Mallory-Weiss tear, erosive esophagitis, hemoptysis, nasopharyngeal bleeding

Systematic DDX

- **Vascular**
  - **Portal hypertensive sources:** esophageal varices, gastric varices, portal hypertensive gastropathy
  - **Arterial sources:** Dieulafoy lesion, ruptured visceral artery aneurysm (splenic, gastroduodenal, gastric, gastroepiploic), aortoenteric fistula
  - **Other vascular malformations:** angiodysplasia, hereditary hemorrhagic telangiectasia (Osler-Weber-Rendu syndrome), arteriovenous malformations of the upper GI tract
- **Infectious/inflammatory**
  - **Gastric/duodenal:** erosive gastritis (NSAID-induced, alcohol-related, stress-related), duodenitis (NSAID-induced, infectious)
  - **Esophageal:** erosive esophagitis (reflux, pill-induced, infectious: Candida, HSV, CMV)
  - **Other inflammatory:** portal hypertensive gastropathy

- **Neoplastic**
    - **Gastric:** gastric carcinoma, gastric MALT lymphoma
    - **Esophageal:** esophageal carcinoma
- **Dysfunction**
    - **Vascular:** portal hypertension
    - **Hematologic:** coagulopathy (anticoagulant use, thrombocytopenia, clotting factor deficiencies)
- **Injury/trauma**
    - **Mucosal injury:** Mallory-Weiss tear, nasogastric tube trauma
    - **Full-thickness injury:** Boerhaave syndrome (esophageal perforation)
    - **Iatrogenic:** post-surgical bleeding, post-endoscopic bleeding (e.g., after sphincterotomy)
- **Compression/obstruction**
    - **Benign:** peptic stricture with ulceration
    - **Malignant:** tumor-related obstruction with mucosal injury
- **Anomalies of development/aging**
    - Angiodysplasia, hereditary hemorrhagic telangiectasia
- **Toxic-metabolic**
    - **Medication-induced:** NSAIDs, corticosteroids, anticoagulants, chemotherapeutic agents
    - **Chemical/alcohol-related:** alcohol-induced mucosal injury, caustic ingestion (rare)
- **Everything else**
    - Hematobilia (e.g., after liver biopsy, hepatic trauma), pancreaticobiliary fistula, swallowed blood from severe epistaxis or oral/nasal trauma

Notes

General considerations: Hematemesis mandates prompt airway, breathing, and circulation assessment with early intravenous access and resuscitation. Type and screen should be obtained. Endoscopic evaluation is essential for diagnosis and management. Patients with cirrhosis should be treated as variceal bleeders until proven otherwise.

Red flags: hemodynamic instability, altered mental status, massive hematemesis, history of aortic surgery, severe chest pain after vomiting, recent instrumentation, signs of chronic liver disease

Special populations: In children, most cases are due to accidental ingestion, gastritis. In the elderly, malignancy and drug-induced ulcers predominate. Patients with alcohol use disorders are at high risk for esophageal variceal bleeding requiring acute intervention. Pregnant patients may have Mallory-Weiss tears due to hyperemesis gravidarum.

Further Reading

- Kaplan DE, Ripoll C, Thiele M, et al. AASLD practice guidance on risk stratification and management of portal hypertension and varices in cirrhosis. Hepatology. 2024;79(5):1180-1211. doi:10.1097/HEP.0000000000000647.
- Vu QD, Menias CO, Bhalla S, et al. Aortoenteric fistulas: CT features and potential mimics. Radiographics. 2009;29(1):197-209. doi:10.1148/rg.291075185.
- Vakil N. Peptic ulcer disease: a review. JAMA. 2024;332(21):1832-1842. doi:10.1001/jama.2024.19094.
- Zeng Q, Dai JF, Cao H, Zhang S. Dieulafoy disease with gastric MALT lymphoma: a case report. Medicine (Baltimore). 2020;99(41):e22651. doi:10.1097/MD.0000000000022651.

Hematochezia

Introduction

Hematochezia is the passage of fresh blood or clots per rectum, most often indicating acute lower gastrointestinal bleeding. The clinical presentation ranges from scant blood on toilet paper to massive, life-threatening hemorrhage. While hematochezia typically reflects bleeding from the colon or rectum, rapid upper gastrointestinal bleeding can also present as hematochezia, especially in cases of hemodynamic instability or large-volume blood loss. Overlap exists with melena (black, tarry stools) and occult gastrointestinal bleeding. Distinguishing the source is critical for management.

Checklist DDX

Serious/life-threatening: massive diverticular bleeding, colonic angiodysplasia, brisk upper gastrointestinal bleeding (e.g., peptic ulcer, varices), ischemic colitis with transmural necrosis, rectal ulcer in critically ill patients, colorectal malignancy, post-polypectomy bleeding

Common: diverticulosis, external and internal hemorrhoids, anal fissures, colorectal polyps, angiodysplasia, ischemic or infectious colitis

Commonly misdiagnosed: small bowel bleeding, upper gastrointestinal bleeding presenting as hematochezia, solitary rectal ulcer, radiation proctitis, early colorectal cancer

Systematic DDX

- Vascular
    - **Arterial sources:** diverticular bleeding, colonic angiodysplasia (arteriovenous malformations), ischemic colitis
    - **Venous sources:** hemorrhoids (internal/external), rectal varices (portal hypertension-related)
    - **Other vascular lesions:** Dieulafoy's lesion (colon/rectum), aortoenteric fistula, hereditary hemorrhagic telangiectasia (Osler-Weber-Rendu), post-polypectomy bleeding
- Infectious/inflammatory
    - **Infectious colitis:** bacterial (Shigella, Salmonella, Campylobacter, Escherichia coli O157:H7, C. difficile), viral (CMV), parasitic (Entamoeba histolytica, Schistosoma)

- o **Inflammatory bowel disease:** ulcerative colitis, Crohn's disease (colonic involvement)
- o **Radiation-induced:** radiation proctitis, post-radiation mucosal injury
- o **Other:** stercoral ulceration, solitary rectal ulcer syndrome
- **Neoplastic**
    - o **Malignant:** colorectal carcinoma, rectal carcinoma, anal carcinoma
    - o **Benign:** colorectal polyps (adenomatous, villous), colonic villous adenomas
- **Dysfunction**
    - o **Coagulopathy:** anticoagulant therapy, antiplatelet therapy, thrombocytopenia, clotting factor deficiencies
- **Injury/trauma**
    - o **Anorectal trauma:** anal fissure, hemorrhoids (bleeding component), rectal ulcer
    - o **Iatrogenic:** post-endoscopy bleeding, post-surgical anastomotic bleeding
    - o **Direct trauma:** foreign body insertion, anal intercourse–related injury
- **Compression/obstruction**
    - o **Mass-related:** obstructing colorectal tumor with mucosal ulceration
    - o **Stricture-related:** inflammatory or ischemic stricture ulceration
    - o **Other:** intussusception
- **Anomalies of development/aging**
    - o **Congenital:** Meckel diverticulum (consider in children), congenital AVM
    - o **Other:** age-related mucosal vessel fragility, anorectal malformations
- **Toxic-metabolic**
    - o **Medication-induced:** NSAIDs, aspirin, chemotherapeutic agents (mucosal injury), potassium chloride tablets
    - o **Chemical injury:** alcohol-induced mucosal injury, caustic enemas or irritants
- **Everything else**
    - o Solitary rectal ulcer syndrome, small bowel bleeding with rapid transit, massive upper GI bleed presenting as hematochezia

Notes

General considerations: Initial management focuses on hemodynamic stabilization, exclusion of an upper gastrointestinal source, and risk stratification. Most cases are self-limited, but severe bleeding requires urgent intervention. Further evaluation includes complete blood count, coagulation profile, liver function tests, type and screen, fecal occult blood tests, sigmoidoscopy, and colonoscopy.

Red flags: hemodynamic instability, ongoing brisk bleeding, age over 60, history of colorectal cancer or polyps, associated severe abdominal pain

Special populations: In children, hematochezia is most often due to anal fissures, polyps, or infectious colitis. In young adults, benign anorectal disease predominates, but early-onset colorectal cancer must be considered. In the elderly, diverticulosis, angiodysplasia, and malignancy are more common.

Further Reading

- Nagata N, Kobayashi K, Yamauchi A, et al. Identifying bleeding etiologies by endoscopy affected outcomes in 10,342 cases with hematochezia: CODE BLUE-J study. Am J Gastroenterol. 2021;116(11):2222-2234.
- Gralnek IM, Neeman Z, Strate LL. Acute lower gastrointestinal bleeding. N Engl J Med. 2017;376(11):1054-1063.
- Eckmann JD, Chedid VG, Loftus CG. A rational approach to the patient with hematochezia. Curr Opin Gastroenterol. 2018;34(1):38-45.
- Aaron AE, Amabile A, Andolfi C, et al. Gastrointestinal surgical emergencies textbook. Chicago (IL): American College of Surgeons; 2021.
- Sengupta N, Feuerstein JD, Jairath V, et al. Management of patients with acute lower gastrointestinal bleeding: an updated ACG guideline. Am J Gastroenterol. 2023;118(2):208-231.
- Demb J, Liu L, Murphy CC, et al. Time to endoscopy or colonoscopy among adults younger than 50 years with iron-deficiency anemia and/or hematochezia in the VHA. JAMA Netw Open. 2023;6(11):e2341516.
- Khan R, Hyman D. Hematochezia in the young patient: a review of health-seeking behavior, physician attitudes, and controversies in management. Dig Dis Sci. 2010;55(2):233-239.

Melena

Introduction

Melena is characterized by black, tarry, and often foul-smelling stools, typically resulting from the digestion of blood as it transits the gastrointestinal tract. Melena typically suggests bleeding proximal to the ligament of Treitz, but small bowel and right-sided colonic sources are also possible. Major diagnostic considerations include distinguishing melena from dark stools due to iron, bismuth, or certain foods, and differentiating it from hematochezia, which may occur with brisk upper gastrointestinal bleeding or distal sources. Melena may overlap with hematemesis in severe upper gastrointestinal bleeding and can persist for days after bleeding has ceased due to gastrointestinal transit time.

Checklist DDX

Serious/life-threatening: massive upper gastrointestinal bleeding from peptic ulcer disease, esophageal or gastric varices, aortoenteric fistula, malignancy, angiodysplasia

Common: peptic ulcer disease, erosive gastritis, esophagitis, Mallory-Weiss tear, small bowel angiodysplasia

Commonly misdiagnosed: confusion with iron or bismuth ingestion, overlooked melena in patients with slow colonic transit; small bowel bleeding, right-sided colonic bleeding, nasopharyngeal and oropharyngeal sources

Systematic DDX

- **Vascular**
    - **Varices:** esophageal, gastric (portal hypertension-related)
    - **Ruptured visceral artery aneurysm:** gastric, gastroepiploic, splenic, or gastroduodenal artery
    - **Other vascular lesions:** aortoenteric fistula, arteriovenous malformations, Dieulafoy lesion, angiodysplasia of the upper GI tract, gastric antral vascular ectasia, hereditary hemorrhagic telangiectasia

- **Infectious/inflammatory**
    - **Peptic ulcer disease:** gastric or duodenal ulcer (often due to H. Pylori or NSAIDs)

- o **Erosive/inflammatory mucosal disease:** erosive gastritis, erosive duodenitis, erosive esophagitis (reflux, pill-induced, infectious)
- o **Small bowel ulceration:** cytomegalovirus, NSAID-induced enteropathy
- o **Inflammatory bowel disease with proximal involvement:** ulcerative colitis, Crohn's disease
- o Infectious enteritis involving proximal small bowel (rare cause of melena)
- **Neoplastic**
  - o **Upper gastrointestinal malignancies:** gastric carcinoma, esophageal carcinoma, duodenal carcinoma; gastric lymphoma (including MALT lymphoma), ampullary or periampullary carcinoma
  - o **Small bowel tumors:** gastrointestinal stromal tumor, lymphoma, metastatic lesions
- **Dysfunction**
  - o **Portal hypertension:** varices, portal hypertensive gastropathy
  - o **Coagulopathy:** anticoagulant or antiplatelet use, thrombocytopenia, clotting factor deficiencies
- **Injury/trauma**
  - o **Mucosal tears:** Mallory-Weiss tear
  - o **Boerhaave syndrome:** esophageal perforation with bleeding
  - o **Iatrogenic:** post-endoscopic procedures, post-surgery, post-sphincterotomy, nasogastric tube–induced mucosal injury
- **Compression/obstruction**
  - o Obstructing tumors or strictures with ulceration, peptic stricture with ulceration
- **Anomalies of development/aging**
  - o **Vascular malformations and fragility:** congenital vascular malformations, age-related mucosal fragility
  - o Meckel diverticulum
- **Toxic-metabolic**
  - o **Drug/alcohol related:** NSAID-induced ulceration, aspirin-induced gastritis, corticosteroid-induced mucosal injury, alcohol-induced mucosal injury
  - o Chemotherapy-related mucosal ulceration
- **Everything else**
  - o **Swallowed blood:** epistaxis, oral surgery
  - o **Biliopancreatic sources:** bleeding from the biliary tree (e.g., after liver biopsy, trauma, tumor), pancreaticobiliary fistula,

> hemosuccus pancreaticus (bleeding from the pancreatic duct, often due to splenic artery aneurysm)
> - **Other:** massive lower GI bleeding with slow transit, post-radiation mucosal injury

Notes

General considerations: Initial management should include labs (complete blood count, coagulation studies, type and screen) with consideration of imaging and/or endoscopy. Even small-volume bleeding (>50 mL) can cause melena, and stool color may persist after bleeding has stopped. If initial evaluation is unrevealing, second-look endoscopy and small bowel assessment can be considered.

Red flags: hemodynamic instability, syncope, ongoing melena with iron deficiency anemia, history of liver disease or portal hypertension, recent aortic surgery, constitutional/systemic symptoms suggesting malignancy

Special populations: In children, consider peptic ulcer disease, Meckel diverticulum, or varices. In older adults, malignancy, angiodysplasia, and nonsteroidal anti-inflammatory drug-induced ulcers are common. In pregnancy, variceal hemorrhage risk increases with portal hypertension.

Further Reading

- Aaron AE, Amabile A, Andolfi C, et al. Gastrointestinal surgical emergencies textbook. Chicago (IL): American College of Surgeons; 2021.
- Laine L, Laursen SB, Zakko L, et al. Severity and outcomes of upper gastrointestinal bleeding with bloody vs coffee-grounds hematemesis. Am J Gastroenterol. 2018;113(3):358-366. doi:10.1038/ajg.2018.5.
- Gerson LB, Fidler JL, Cave DR, Leighton JA. ACG clinical guideline: diagnosis and management of small bowel bleeding. Am J Gastroenterol. 2015;110(9):1265-1287. doi:10.1038/ajg.2015.246.
- Dina I, Nedelcu M, Iacobescu CG, Baboi ID, Bălăceanu AL. Rare etiologies of upper gastrointestinal bleeding: a narrative review. J Clin Med. 2025;14(14):4972. doi:10.3390/jcm14144972.
- Shung DL, Laine L. Upper gastrointestinal bleeding: review of current evidence and implications for management. Aliment Pharmacol Ther. 2024;59(9):1062-1081. doi:10.1111/apt.17949.

Pelvic and Genitourinary

Saeed Rahmani

Long H. Tu

Curtis Xu

Primary and Secondary Amenorrhea

Introduction

Amenorrhea is the absence of menses in a female of reproductive age. Primary amenorrhea is when a girl has never menstruated by 15 years of age or >3 years after thelarche. Secondary amenorrhea is when menses stops for ≥3 months in a woman with previously regular cycles or ≥6 months in a woman with irregular cycles. Although pregnancy, breastfeeding and menopause are normal reasons for absent periods, amenorrhea can also signify disruption anywhere along the hypothalamic–pituitary–ovarian–uterine axis. Important etiologic groups include outflow-tract obstruction, primary ovarian insufficiency, hypothalamic or pituitary disorders, other endocrine disorders, and physiologic or medication-induced conditions.

The International Federation of Gynecology and Obstetrics (FIGO) provides an approach called HyPO-P, which is acronym that can be used to categorize ovulatory disorders into etiologies related to the hypothalamus, pituitary, ovary, and polycystic ovary syndrome (PCOS). Causes may be further stratified using the "GAIN-FIT-PIE" mnemonic: genetic, autoimmune, iatrogenic, neoplasm (GAIN); functional, infectious/inflammatory, trauma/vascular (FIT); and physiological, idiopathic, endocrine (PIE). We will detail both this approach and a primary pathophysiologic approach; there is no need to memorize the all details of either – getting a sense of the framework is most important.

Checklist DDX

Serious/life-threatening: intracranial tumors (pituitary adenoma, craniopharyngioma), Sheehan syndrome or pituitary apoplexy, adrenal or ovarian neoplasms with androgen or estrogen secretion, ectopic pregnancy, ovarian torsion, severe eating disorders, chronic systemic illnesses that predispose to electrolyte disturbances, cardiac arrhythmia, Asherman syndrome

Common: pregnancy, functional hypothalamic amenorrhea (due to stress, weight loss, or excessive exercise), polycystic ovary syndrome (PCOS), primary ovarian insufficiency, hyperprolactinemia, thyroid dysfunction (hypothyroidism or hyperthyroidism), congenital anatomic abnormalities (Müllerian agenesis, imperforate hymen, transverse vaginal septum), gonadal dysgenesis (e.g., Turner syndrome), obesity and metabolic syndrome, menopause, medication effects (hormonal contraception, antipsychotics, glucocorticoids, chemotherapy)

Commonly misdiagnosed: functional hypothalamic amenorrhea (often mistaken for PCOS), mild hyperprolactinemia, subtle thyroid dysfunction, constitutional delay of puberty, outflow-tract anomalies such as transverse vaginal septum or Asherman syndrome

Systematic DDX

HyPO-P system

- Hypothalamus
    - **Genetic:** congenital gonadotropin-releasing hormone deficiency (Kallmann syndrome, Prader–Willi syndrome)
    - **Autoimmune:** neurosarcoidosis
    - **Iatrogenic:** head trauma affecting hypothalamic–pituitary axis
    - **Neoplasm:** hypothalamic hamartoma, craniopharyngioma, lymphoma, gliomas, Langerhans cell histiocytosis, metastatic mass
    - **Functional:** functional hypothalamic amenorrhea due to stress, weight loss, or excessive exercise; constitutional delay of puberty
    - **Infectious/inflammatory:** tuberculous or granulomatous hypophysitis
    - **Trauma/vascular:** head trauma affecting hypothalamic function
    - **Physiological:** constitutional delay of puberty
    - **Idiopathic:** idiopathic hypothalamic dysfunction
    - **Endocrine:** disruptions secondary to endocrine abnormalities (thyroid disorders)
- Pituitary
    - **Genetic:** congenital pituitary hormone deficiencies
    - **Autoimmune:** autoimmune hypophysitis
    - **Iatrogenic:** pituitary surgery or radiation (implied)
    - **Neoplasm:** craniopharyngioma, germinoma, lymphoma, germ cell tumors, meningioma, Langerhans cell histiocytosis, prolactin-secreting pituitary adenoma (prolactinoma), non-functioning pituitary adenoma, metastatic mass
    - **Functional:** hyperprolactinemia due to medications or hypothyroidism; hypopituitarism
    - **Infectious/inflammatory:** tuberculous or granulomatous hypophysitis
    - **Trauma/vascular:** pituitary infarction or hemorrhage (Sheehan syndrome), pituitary apoplexy
    - **Physiological:** pituitary changes in pregnancy
    - **Idiopathic:** idiopathic pituitary dysfunction

- o **Endocrine:** hyperprolactinemia secondary to hypothyroidism or drugs
- **Ovary**
  - o **Genetic:** gonadal dysgenesis (Turner syndrome, Swyer syndrome)
  - o **Autoimmune:** autoimmune oophoritis
  - o **Iatrogenic:** salpingectomy, chemotherapy, radiation-induced ovarian failure, intrauterine curettage or other instrumentation causing Asherman syndrome
  - o **Neoplasm:** granulosa cell tumor, dysgerminoma, Sertoli–Leydig cell tumor, thecoma
  - o **Functional:** primary ovarian insufficiency
  - o **Infectious/inflammatory:** pelvic inflammatory disease with intrauterine adhesions (Asherman syndrome)
  - o **Trauma/vascular:** ovarian torsion leading to ischemic injury
  - o **Physiological:** natural menopause and perimenopause, pregnancy, ectopic pregnancy
  - o **Idiopathic:** idiopathic ovarian insufficiency
  - o **Endocrine:** androgen-secreting ovarian tumors
- **Polycystic ovary syndrome (PCOS)**
  - o **Genetic:** familial predisposition and genetic variants
  - o **Iatrogenic:** medications exacerbating hyperandrogenism or ovulatory dysfunction
  - o **Functional:** insulin resistance, metabolic syndrome, hormonal feedback alterations
  - o **Endocrine:** hyperandrogenism, LH/FSH imbalance
- **Other anatomical categories (not a part of HyPO-P but clinically relevant)**
  - o **Outflow tract/uterine anomalies**
    - **Congenital/anomalies of development:** imperforate hymen, transverse vaginal septum, vaginal atresia, cervical stenosis, Müllerian agenesis (Mayer–Rokitansky–Küster–Hauser syndrome), intrauterine adhesions (Asherman syndrome)
    - **Compression/obstruction:** large pituitary adenomas compressing pituitary stalk
  - o **Adrenal/other endocrine disorders**
    - **Neoplasm:** virilizing adrenal tumors, androgen-secreting neoplasms
      Endocrine: Cushing syndrome, congenital adrenal hyperplasia (including 17-α-hydroxylase deficiency), 5-α-reductase deficiency, aromatase deficiency, complete androgen insensitivity syndrome

- Systemic/toxic-metabolic/nutritional causes
    - **Functional:** eating disorders (anorexia nervosa, bulimia), excessive exercise, obesity, metabolic syndrome
    - **Iatrogenic:** antipsychotics (dopamine antagonists), chemotherapeutic agents, radiation therapy, glucocorticoids, opioids, hormonal contraceptives, spironolactone
    - **Other:** diabetes mellitus, celiac disease, chronic kidney disease, inflammatory bowel disease, cirrhosis, severe systemic illness
- Miscellaneous / psychological causes
    - Psychogenic causes (depression, anxiety, chronic stress, severe psychological stress), postpartum lactation or prolonged breastfeeding, other rare endocrine disorders

Pathophysiologic approach
- **Vascular**
    - Pituitary infarction or hemorrhage (Sheehan syndrome) and pituitary apoplexy
- **Infectious/inflammatory**
    - Tuberculous or granulomatous hypophysitis; neurosarcoidosis; pelvic inflammatory disease with intra-uterine adhesions (Asherman syndrome)
- **Neoplastic**
    - **Pituitary/hypothalamic tumors:** prolactin-secreting pituitary adenoma, non-functioning pituitary adenoma, craniopharyngioma, hypothalamic hamartoma, germinoma, lymphoma, germ cell tumors, meningioma, Langerhans cell histiocytosis, gliomas, metastatic masses
    - **Ovarian tumors:** granulosa cell tumor, dysgerminoma, Sertoli–Leydig cell tumor, thecoma
    - **Other endocrine or adrenal tumors:** virilizing adrenal tumors, androgen-secreting neoplasms
- **Dysfunction**
    - **Hypothalamic:** functional hypothalamic amenorrhea due to stress, weight loss or excessive exercise; congenital gonadotropin-releasing hormone deficiency (Kallmann syndrome, Prader–Willi syndrome); constitutional delay of puberty
    - **Pituitary:** hyperprolactinemia (prolactinoma, medications, hypothyroidism); hypopituitarism (empty sella syndrome, Sheehan syndrome); other pituitary hormone deficiencies

- Ovarian: primary ovarian insufficiency; polycystic ovary syndrome; gonadal dysgenesis (Turner syndrome, Swyer syndrome); autoimmune oophoritis.
- Thyroid: hypothyroidism, hyperthyroidism
- Adrenal/androgen disorders: Cushing syndrome, congenital adrenal hyperplasia (including 17-α-hydroxylase deficiency), 5-α-reductase deficiency, aromatase deficiency, complete androgen insensitivity syndrome

- **Injury/trauma**
  - Head trauma affecting the hypothalamic–pituitary axis; postpartum hemorrhage with subsequent pituitary ischemia; ovarian torsion; intra-uterine curettage or other instrumentation causing Asherman syndrome
- **Compression/obstruction**
  - Outflow-tract obstruction (imperforate hymen, transverse vaginal septum, vaginal atresia, cervical stenosis); intra-uterine adhesions; large pituitary adenomas compressing the pituitary stalk
- **Anomalies of development/aging**
  - Chromosomal or genetic anomalies: Turner syndrome, Swyer syndrome, Kallmann syndrome, Prader–Willi syndrome, androgen insensitivity syndrome, 5-α-reductase deficiency, 17-α-hydroxylase deficiency, aromatase deficiency
  - Congenital anatomic anomalies: Müllerian agenesis (Mayer–Rokitansky–Küster–Hauser syndrome), vaginal atresia
  - Developmental delay/aging: constitutional delay of puberty; natural menopause and perimenopause
- **Toxic-metabolic**
  - Chronic systemic diseases: diabetes mellitus, celiac disease, chronic kidney disease, inflammatory bowel disease, cirrhosis, severe systemic illness.
  - Medications and toxic exposures: Antipsychotics (dopamine antagonists), chemotherapeutic agents and radiation therapy, glucocorticoids, opioids, hormonal contraceptives, spironolactone
- **Nutritional/metabolic**
  - Eating disorders (anorexia nervosa, bulimia), malnutrition, excessive exercise, severe psychological stress, obesity and metabolic syndrome
- **Everything else**
  - Idiopathic amenorrhea, psychogenic causes (depression, anxiety, chronic stress), postpartum lactation or prolonged breastfeeding, other rare endocrine disorders

Notes

General considerations: Amenorrhea is a symptom rather than a disease; evaluation should first rule out pregnancy. Detailed menstrual and medical histories, including age of menarche, weight changes, exercise patterns, psychosocial stressors and medication use can help to prioritize etiologies. Physical examination should assess pubertal development, body mass index, signs of androgen excess and genital tract patency. Targeted laboratory tests include serum β-human chorionic gonadotropin, prolactin, thyroid-stimulating hormone, follicle-stimulating hormone, luteinizing hormone, estradiol and, when appropriate, androgens; pelvic ultrasonography and, in selected cases, cross-sectional imaging of the brain to assess for sellar or hypothalamic masses.

Red flags: sudden severe pelvic, headache, visual changes, rapid personality changes, galactorrhea, rapid virilization, severe weight loss, electrolyte abnormalities, bradyarrhythmias

Special populations: In adolescents, consider genetic disorders and constitutional delay of puberty. In reproductive-age women, pregnancy and functional hypothalamic amenorrhea are frequent causes; clinicians should ask about stress, exercise and eating patterns, and counsel about bone health. Amenorrhea is physiologic in pregnancy and lactation; however, postpartum pituitary hemorrhage can result in hypopituitarism and persistent amenorrhea (Sheehan syndrome). In perimenopausal and older women, it is critical to differentiate physiologic menopause from pathologic amenorrhea, i.e., related to systemic conditions.

Further Reading

- Klein DA, Paradise SL, Reeder RM. Amenorrhea: a systematic approach to diagnosis and management. American Family Physician. 2019;100(1):39-48.
- Munro MG, Balen AH, Cho S, et al. The FIGO ovulatory disorders classification system. Fertility and Sterility. 2022;118(4):768-786.
- Munro MG, Balen AH, Cho S, et al. The FIGO ovulatory disorders classification system. International Journal of Gynecology and Obstetrics. 2022;159(1):1-20.
- Saadedine M, Kapoor E, Shufelt C. Functional hypothalamic amenorrhea: recognition and management of a challenging diagnosis. Mayo Clinic Proceedings. 2023;98(9):1376-1385.
- Amenorrhea: absence of periods. American College of Obstetricians and Gynecologists (ACOG) Patient FAQ. Accessed July 30 2025.

Vaginal Discharge

Introduction

Vaginal discharge is a common gynecologic symptom characterized by fluid secreted from the vaginal and cervical glands. Its causes range widely from normal physiological changes related to hormonal fluctuations and menstruation to infections, inflammation, and rarely, neoplastic conditions. The most frequent pathological causes are infectious vaginitis, including bacterial vaginosis, vulvovaginal candidiasis, and trichomoniasis, which often alter the color, consistency, and odor of the discharge. Other causes include cervicitis, pelvic inflammatory disease (PID), atrophic vaginitis (particularly in postmenopausal women), and less commonly malignancies such as cervical or vaginal cancer. Accurate diagnosis is essential since the underlying etiology guides specific management and has varying implications for reproductive health and overall well-being.

Checklist DDX

Serious/life-threatening: pelvic inflammatory disease (PID), retained foreign body (with resulting toxic shock syndrome), cervicitis due to Neisseria gonorrhoeae or Chlamydia trachomatis, vaginal or cervical malignancy

Common: bacterial vaginosis, vulvovaginal candidiasis, trichomoniasis, physiologic discharge (e.g., ovulatory, pregnancy-related), atrophic vaginitis (postmenopausal), non-infectious irritant or allergic vaginitis

Commonly misdiagnosed: desquamative inflammatory vaginitis, aerobic vaginitis, atrophic vaginitis, cervicitis (especially chlamydia/gonorrhea), physiologic discharge mistaken for infection

Systematic DDX

- **Vascular**
    - Vaginal or cervical neoplasms with necrosis or bleeding
- **Infectious/inflammatory**
    - Bacterial vaginosis (overgrowth of anaerobes), vulvovaginal candidiasis (Candida spp.), trichomoniasis (Trichomonas vaginalis), aerobic vaginitis, desquamative inflammatory vaginitis, cervicitis (Chlamydia trachomatis, Neisseria gonorrhoeae, HSV), PID
- **Neoplastic**
    - Vaginal or cervical cancer, especially if discharge is bloody, malodorous, or persistent

- **Dysfunction**
    - Atrophic vaginitis (postmenopausal estrogen deficiency), lichen planus, lichen sclerosus
- **Injury/trauma**
    - Foreign body (e.g., retained tampon), sexual trauma, chemical or irritant exposure
- **Anomalies of development/aging**
    - Atrophic vaginitis, congenital outflow tract anomalies
- **Toxic-metabolic**
    - Medications (e.g., antibiotics altering flora), diabetes mellitus (predisposing to candidiasis)
- **Everything else**
    - Physiologic discharge (mid-cycle, pregnancy), allergic reactions (e.g., to hygiene products)

Notes

General considerations: Diagnosis relies on a combination of history, physical examination, and targeted testing. Professional societies have recommended pH testing, KOH whiff test, and wet mount microscopy as first-line office diagnostics, with nucleic acid amplification tests (NAATs) for trichomoniasis and cervicitis when available. Point-of-care tests have limitations however, and laboratory confirmation should be considered in recurrent or atypical cases. Empiric therapy without diagnosis increases the risk of inappropriate treatment and recurrent symptoms.

Red flags: concurrent pelvic or abdominal pain, pain during sex, signs of sexually transmitted infections (itches, genital sores or lesions), changes in vaginal discharge

Special populations: In postmenopausal women, estrogen deficiency predisposes to atrophic vaginitis and infections. In pediatric populations, consider foreign bodies and noninfectious irritation. In pregnant individuals, discharge may be physiologic or related to infections that can impact pregnancy outcomes.

Further Reading

- Shroff S. Infectious Vaginitis, Cervicitis, and Pelvic Inflammatory Disease. Med Clin North Am. 2023;107(2):299-315. doi:10.1016/j.mcna.2022.10.009.
- Workowski KA, Bachmann LH, Chan PA, et al. Sexually Transmitted Infections Treatment Guidelines, 2021. MMWR Recomm Rep. 2021;70(4):1-187. doi:10.15585/mmwr.rr7004a1.

- Miller JM, Binnicker MJ, Campbell S, et al. Guide to Utilization of the Microbiology Laboratory for Diagnosis of Infectious Diseases: 2024 Update. Clin Infect Dis. 2024. doi:10.1093/cid/ciae104.
- Anderson MR, Klink K, Cohrssen A. Evaluation of Vaginal Complaints. JAMA. 2004;291(11):1368-1379. doi:10.1001/jama.291.11.1368.
- Neal CM, Kus LH, Eckert LO, Peipert JF. Noncandidal Vaginitis: A Comprehensive Approach to Diagnosis and Management. Am J Obstet Gynecol. 2020;222(2):114-122. doi:10.1016/j.ajog.2019.09.001.
- Paavonen J, Brunham RC. Bacterial Vaginosis and Desquamative Inflammatory Vaginitis. N Engl J Med. 2018;379(23):2246-2254. doi:10.1056/NEJMra1808418.
- Hillier SL, Austin M, Macio I, et al. Diagnosis and Treatment of Vaginal Discharge Syndromes in Community Practice Settings. Clin Infect Dis. 2021;72(9):1538-1543. doi:10.1093/cid/ciaa260.

Vaginal Bleeding

Vaginal bleeding encompasses any bleeding from the vagina, including normal menstruation, but is most clinically relevant when abnormal in timing, volume, or context. Abnormal uterine bleeding (AUB) is a common presentation in reproductive-aged women and adolescents, and may signal structural, hormonal, systemic, or malignant processes. The International Federation of Gynecology and Obstetrics (FIGO) has standardized the nomenclature and classification of AUB using the PALM-COEIN system. This acronym helps organize structural and nonstructural etiologies of vaginal bleeding

Checklist DDX

Serious/life-threatening: ectopic pregnancy, retained products of conception, gestational trophoblastic disease, uterine or cervical malignancy, severe coagulopathy (e.g., von Willebrand disease), acute hemorrhage from uterine rupture or trauma

Common: anovulatory cycles (especially in adolescents and perimenopausal women), uterine fibroids (leiomyoma), endometrial polyps, adenomyosis, ovulatory dysfunction, endometrial hyperplasia, endometrial/vaginal atrophy in postmenopausal women, iatrogenic causes (anticoagulants, hormonal therapy), pregnancy-related complications (miscarriage)

Commonly misdiagnosed: coagulopathies (especially in adolescents), endometrial or cervical polyps, ovulatory dysfunction, endometrial hyperplasia

Systematic DDX

PALM-COEIN system
- **Structural causes**
  - **Polyp**
    - Includes benign growths like endometrial or cervical polyps
  - **Adenomyosis**
    - Abnormal presence of endometrial glands and stroma in the myometrium
  - **Leiomyoma (fibroids)**
    - Benign smooth muscle tumors of the uterus

- - o **Malignancy and hyperplasia**
      - Endometrial, cervical, vaginal, or vulvar cancer; endometrial hyperplasia, rare ovarian tumors (e.g., granulosa cell tumor)
- **Nonstructural causes**
  - o **Coagulopathy**
      - Systemic coagulopathies (e.g., von Willebrand disease, platelet disorders), medications impacting coagulation such as anticoagulants
  - o **Ovulatory dysfunction**
      - Ovulatory dysfunction (anovulation, polycystic ovary syndrome), other hormonal abnormalities (thyroid disease, hyperprolactinemia)
  - o **Endometrial causes**
      - Pelvic inflammatory disease, sexually transmitted infections causing endometrial friability, endometritis, cervicitis, endometrial/vaginal atrophy (postmenopausal bleeding)
  - o **Iatrogenic**
      - Iatrogenic trauma (e.g., post-procedural), medications (hormonal agents)
  - o **Not yet classified**
      - **Vascular causes:** uterine arteriovenous malformations, gestational trophoblastic disease, rare vascular tumors
      - **Injury/trauma causes:** vaginal or cervical lacerations, sexual assault, retained foreign body

Pathophysiologic approach
- **Vascular**
  - o Uterine arteriovenous malformations, gestational trophoblastic disease, and rare vascular tumors
- **Infectious/inflammatory**
  - o Endometritis, cervicitis, pelvic inflammatory disease, and sexually transmitted infections causing endometrial friability
- **Neoplastic**
  - o Endometrial, cervical, vaginal, or vulvar cancer; endometrial hyperplasia; and rare ovarian tumors (e.g., granulosa cell tumor)
- **Dysfunction**
  - o Ovulatory dysfunction (anovulation, polycystic ovary syndrome), thyroid dysfunction, hyperprolactinemia, and chronic liver or renal disease

- **Injury/trauma**
    - Vaginal or cervical lacerations, sexual assault, retained foreign body, and iatrogenic trauma (e.g., post-procedural)
- **Compression/obstruction**
    - Cervical stenosis (post-surgical or congenital), intrauterine adhesions (Asherman syndrome)
- **Anomalies of development/aging**
    - Congenital uterine anomalies, endometrial/vaginal atrophy (postmenopausal bleeding)
- **Toxic-metabolic**
    - Medications (anticoagulants, hormonal agents), systemic coagulopathies (e.g., von Willebrand disease, platelet disorders), and severe hepatic dysfunction
- **Everything else**
    - Physiologic bleeding (menarche, perimenopause), idiopathic AUB

Notes

General considerations: Initial evaluation must exclude pregnancy and assess hemodynamic stability. Adolescents with heavy bleeding should be evaluated for coagulopathies, and postmenopausal bleeding warrants prompt assessment for malignancy. Laboratory and imaging studies are tailored to clinical suspicion. A thorough history should address bleeding pattern, associated symptoms, and risk factors for malignancy or systemic disease. Quality-of-life impact and psychosocial context should also be assessed, especially in adolescents.

Red flags: hemodynamic instability (tachycardia, hypotension, syncope), heavy bleeding (soaking through greater than one pad per hour), severe anemia, systemic symptoms (e.g., poor growth, fatigue), abnormal genital examination (e.g., mass, trauma, skin changes), suspicion of sexual abuse or neoplasm; in reproductive-aged women, suspected or confirmed pregnancy with bleeding

Special populations: In adolescents, heavy menstrual bleeding (HMB) is often due to anovulatory cycles but may signal an underlying bleeding disorder. In pregnant women, any vaginal bleeding is a red flag for ectopic pregnancy, miscarriage, or placental pathology. In the second and third trimesters, placental abruption, previa, and vasa previa must be considered. In postmenopausal women, any vaginal bleeding is a red flag for endometrial or cervical malignancy.

Further Reading

- Jain V, Munro MG, Critchley HOD. Contemporary Evaluation of Women and Girls With Abnormal Uterine Bleeding: FIGO Systems 1 and 2. Int J Gynaecol Obstet. 2023;162 Suppl 2:29-42. doi:10.1002/ijgo.14946.
- Marnach ML, Laughlin-Tommaso SK. Evaluation and Management of Abnormal Uterine Bleeding. Mayo Clin Proc. 2019;94(2):326-335. doi:10.1016/j.mayocp.2018.12.012.
- Borzutzky C, Jaffray J. Diagnosis and Management of Heavy Menstrual Bleeding and Bleeding Disorders in Adolescents. JAMA Pediatr. 2020;174(2):186-194. doi:10.1001/jamapediatrics.2019.5040.
- Munro MG. Classification of Menstrual Bleeding Disorders. Rev Endocr Metab Disord. 2012;13(4):225-234. doi:10.1007/s11154-012-9220-x.
- Lebduska E, Beshear D, Spataro BM. Abnormal Uterine Bleeding. Med Clin North Am. 2023;107(2):235-246. doi:10.1016/j.mcna.2022.10.014.
- Brenner PF. Differential Diagnosis of Abnormal Uterine Bleeding. Am J Obstet Gynecol. 1996;175(3 Pt 2):766-769. doi:10.1016/s0002-9378(96)80082-2.
- Drever N, Peek S, Moussaoui D, et al. Vaginal Bleeding in Children: A Retrospective Audit at a Tertiary Paediatric Gynaecology Service. J Paediatr Child Health. 2023;59(4):653-659. doi:10.1111/jpc.16366.
- Hernandez A, Dietrich JE. Abnormal Uterine Bleeding in the Adolescent. Obstet Gynecol. 2020;135(3):615-621. doi:10.1097/AOG.0000000000003693.

Testicular Pain

Introduction

Testicular pain is a frequently encountered urologic concern with a wide range of potential causes that can vary from benign conditions to life-threatening emergencies. Acute scrotal pain is considered a medical emergency because of the possibility of testicular torsion—a condition where the spermatic cord twists, cutting off blood supply to the testicle, leading to sudden, severe pain and swelling. Other acute causes include infections like epididymitis or trauma. Chronic testicular pain may result from infections, vascular issues such as varicocele, neoplasms, or referred pain from conditions outside the scrotum, such as nerve irritation or gastrointestinal problems.

Checklist DDX

Serious/life-threatening: testicular torsion, Fournier gangrene, incarcerated or strangulated inguinal hernia, epididymo-orchitis with abscess, testicular neoplasm, testicular trauma with rupture

Common: epididymitis (sexually and non-sexually transmitted), torsion of testicular appendage, hydrocele, varicocele, referred pain from nephrolithiasis, inguinal hernia

Commonly misdiagnosed: torsion of testicular appendage (often mistaken for torsion), epididymitis (misdiagnosed as torsion), referred pain from renal colic, chronic orchialgia, early testicular neoplasm presenting with pain

Systematic DDX

- **Vascular**
    - Testicular torsion, torsion of testicular appendage, varicocele, infarction from trauma or vasculitis
- **Infectious/inflammatory**
    - Epididymitis (Chlamydia trachomatis, Neisseria gonorrhoeae, Escherichia coli), epididymo-orchitis, viral orchitis (mumps, Coxsackie, EBV, VZV), Fournier gangrene, abscess
- **Neoplastic**
    - Testicular tumor (usually painless, but may present with pain if hemorrhage or infarction), paratesticular tumors

- **Dysfunction**
    - Hydrocele, varicocele, chronic orchialgia, post-vasectomy pain syndrome
- **Injury/trauma**
    - Testicular rupture, hematoma, contusion, or referred pain from pelvic or spinal injury
- **Compression/obstruction**
    - Incarcerated or strangulated inguinal hernia, spermatic cord compression, obstructive uropathy
- **Anomalies of development/aging**
    - Undescended testis (torsion risk), retractile testis, testicular atrophy
- **Toxic-metabolic**
    - Drug-induced epididymitis
- **Everything else**
    - Referred pain from renal colic, musculoskeletal pain, nerve entrapment syndromes

Notes

General considerations: Testicular torsion is a urologic emergency; salvage rates decline rapidly after 6 hours. The TWIST score is a validated tool for risk stratification and can guide the need for immediate surgical exploration versus imaging. Epididymitis is the most common cause of acute scrotal pain in adults and may be managed with empiric antibiotics targeting likely pathogens. Isolated orchitis is rare in adults except with mumps or other viral infections; laboratory confirmation is recommended. Fournier gangrene requires emergent surgical debridement and broad-spectrum antibiotics. Chronic pain may require multidisciplinary evaluation.

Red flags: sudden and severe pain (especially with nausea or vomiting), fever, scrotal erythema/swelling, crepitus, hard testicle on exam

Special populations: In neonates and infants, torsion may present subtly and requires prompt evaluation. In adolescents, testicular torsion and torsion of appendages are common; rapid diagnosis is critical. In older adults, epididymitis and referred pain from renal or spinal origins are more common. In immunocompromised patients or diabetics, Fournier gangrene must be considered.

Further Reading

- Workowski KA, Bachmann LH, Chan PA, et al. Sexually Transmitted Infections Treatment Guidelines, 2021. MMWR Recomm Rep. 2021;70(4):1-187. doi:10.15585/mmwr.rr7004a1.
- Miller JM, Binnicker MJ, Campbell S, et al. Guide to Utilization of the Microbiology Laboratory for Diagnosis of Infectious Diseases: 2024 Update. Clin Infect Dis. 2024. doi:10.1093/cid/ciae104.
- Langan RC, Puente MEE. Scrotal Masses. Am Fam Physician. 2022;106(2):184-189.
- Fitzgibbons RJ, Forse RA. Clinical Practice. Groin Hernias in Adults. N Engl J Med. 2015;372(8):756-763. doi:10.1056/NEJMcp1404068.
- Kang C, Punjani N, Lee RK, et al. Effect of Varicoceles on Spermatogenesis. Semin Cell Dev Biol. 2022;121:114-124. doi:10.1016/j.semcdb.2021.04.005.
- Hoang VT, Van HAT, Hoang TH, et al. A Review of Classification, Diagnosis, and Management of Hydrocele. J Ultrasound Med. 2024;43(3):599-607. doi:10.1002/jum.16380.
- Gupta RT, Kalisz K, Khatri G, et al. ACR Appropriateness Criteria® Acute Onset Flank Pain-Suspicion of Stone Disease (Urolithiasis). J Am Coll Radiol. 2023;20(11S):S315-S328. doi:10.1016/j.jacr.2023.08.020.
- Qin KR, Qu LG. Diagnosing With a TWIST: Systematic Review and Meta-Analysis of a Testicular Torsion Risk Score. J Urol. 2022;208(1):62-70. doi:10.1097/JU.0000000000002496.
- Montrief T, Long B, Koyfman A, Auerbach J. Fournier Gangrene: A Review for Emergency Clinicians. J Emerg Med. 2019;57(4):488-500. doi:10.1016/j.jemermed.2019.06.023.

Dysuria

Introduction

Dysuria, defined as pain, burning, or discomfort during urination, is a common symptom encountered across diverse clinical settings and can result from a wide spectrum of causes affecting the urinary tract and adjacent structures. The symptom often signifies underlying infectious, inflammatory, obstructive, neoplastic, or functional processes involving either the lower or upper urinary tract, as well as related genital or pelvic organs. Etiologies vary from benign conditions like uncomplicated urinary tract infections to serious pathologies such as pyelonephritis, infection of obstructing ureteral calculi, or malignancy that require urgent evaluation and intervention.

Checklist DDX

Serious/life-threatening: pyelonephritis, urosepsis, obstructing ureteral calculi with infection, acute bacterial prostatitis

Common: acute cystitis (uncomplicated urinary tract infection), urethritis (gonococcal and nongonococcal), vulvovaginal candidiasis, bacterial vaginosis, trichomoniasis, chronic prostatitis/chronic pelvic pain syndrome, nephrolithiasis, interstitial cystitis/bladder pain syndrome, genitourinary syndrome of menopause, benign prostatic hyperplasia

Commonly misdiagnosed: urethritis mistaken for cystitis, interstitial cystitis/bladder pain syndrome, chronic prostatitis, nephrolithiasis presenting with dysuria, genital herpes without classic lesions

Systematic DDX

- **Vascular**
    - Renal infarction
- **Infectious/inflammatory**
    - **Bacterial:** acute cystitis, pyelonephritis, urethritis (Neisseria gonorrhoeae, Chlamydia trachomatis, Mycoplasma genitalium), Trichomonas vaginalis, acute and chronic prostatitis
    - **Viral:** herpes simplex virus
    - **Fungal:** vulvovaginal candidiasis
    - **Local inflammation:** interstitial cystitis/bladder pain syndrome, bacterial vaginosis, lichen sclerosus, contact dermatitis

- o **Systemic inflammatory processes:** (manifestation of) psoriasis, reactive arthritis, Behçet syndrome, Sjögren syndrome
- **Neoplastic and hematologic**
  - o Bladder cancer, urethral carcinoma, prostate cancer, vulvovaginal cancer
- **Dysfunction**
  - o Benign prostatic hyperplasia, pelvic floor dysfunction, neurogenic bladder, chronic pelvic pain syndrome
- **Injury/trauma**
  - o Urethral trauma (catheterization, instrumentation, sexual activity), chemical or radiation cystitis, trauma secondary to intercourse
- **Compression/obstruction**
  - o Ureteral calculi, bladder calculi, obstructing tumors, urethral strictures
- **Anomalies of development/aging**
  - o Atrophic vaginitis/genitourinary syndrome of menopause, congenital urinary tract anomalies, posterior urethral valves
- **Toxic-metabolic**
  - o Drug-induced cystitis (cyclophosphamide, ketamine), metabolic derangements predisposing to nephrolithiasis, dietary irritants (caffeine, spicy foods)
- **Everything else**
  - o Referred pain (gynecologic or gastrointestinal), psychogenic causes

Notes

General considerations: A thorough history including sexual exposure, symptom chronology, and associated systemic signs is critical. Urinalysis and urine culture remain cornerstone diagnostics for urinary tract infections, with pyuria and nitrites supporting diagnosis but not excluding other causes. Nucleic acid amplification testing is recommended for urethritis and sexually transmitted infections. In men, digital rectal examination and urine culture guide prostatitis diagnosis. Imaging is generally reserved for suspected obstruction or complicated infection.

Red flags: fever, flank pain, costovertebral angle tenderness, systemic toxicity, signs of sepsis, obstructing stones with infection, rapidly progressive pain

Special populations: Pregnant individuals require careful differentiation of dysuria from physiologic urinary frequency and prompt treatment of infections to prevent adverse outcomes. Postmenopausal women with dysuria should be evaluated for atrophic changes and malignancy risk. Men with chronic dysuria require assessment for chronic prostatitis and pelvic pain syndromes.

Further Reading

- Urinary Tract Infections in Pregnant Individuals. Obstetrics and Gynecology. 2023;142(2):435–445. doi:10.1097/AOG.0000000000005269.
- Sell J, Nasir M, Courchesne C. Urethritis: rapid evidence review. Am Fam Physician. 2021;103(9):553–558.
- Workowski KA, Bachmann LH, Chan PA, et al. Sexually transmitted infections treatment guidelines, 2021. MMWR Recomm Rep. 2021;70(4):1–187. doi:10.15585/mmwr.rr7004a1.
- Tarasconi A, Perrone G, Davies J, et al. Anorectal emergencies: WSES-AAST guidelines. World J Emerg Surg. 2021;16(1):48. doi:10.1186/s13017-021-00384-x.
- Holt JD, Garrett WA, McCurry TK, Teichman JM. Common questions about chronic prostatitis. Am Fam Physician. 2016;93(4):290–296.
- Clemens JQ, Erickson DR, Varela NP, Lai HH. Diagnosis and treatment of interstitial cystitis/bladder pain syndrome. J Urol. 2022;208(1):34–42. doi:10.1097/JU.0000000000002756.
- Gupta RT, Kalisz K, Khatri G, et al. ACR Appropriateness Criteria® acute onset flank pain-suspicion of stone disease (urolithiasis). J Am Coll Radiol. 2023;20(11S):S315–S328. doi:10.1016/j.jacr.2023.08.020.
- Preminger GM, Tiselius HG, Assimos DG, et al. 2007 guideline for the management of ureteral calculi. J Urol. 2007;178(6):2418–2434. doi:10.1016/j.juro.2007.09.107.

Hematuria (Blood in Urine)

Introduction

Hematuria, defined as the presence of red blood cells in the urine, may be gross (visible) or microscopic (nonvisible, typically ≥3 RBCs per high-power field on urine microscopy). It is a common clinical finding with a prevalence ranging from 2% to 31% depending on the population and detection method. Major diagnostic considerations include distinguishing glomerular from non-glomerular sources, identifying urologic malignancy, and evaluating for other causes such as infection, stones, or trauma. The evaluation overlaps with presentations such as urinary tract infection, nephrolithiasis, and lower urinary tract symptoms, and should always include confirmation of hematuria, exclusion of contamination, and assessment for risk factors for malignancy or progressive renal disease.

Checklist DDX

Serious/life-threatening: malignancy of the urinary tract (bladder, renal cell, upper tract urothelial carcinoma), acute tubular necrosis, rapidly progressive glomerulonephritis, rhabdomyolysis, renal infarction, and trauma (renal laceration, bladder rupture, urethral rupture)

Common: urinary tract infection, nephrolithiasis, benign prostatic hyperplasia, exercise-induced hematuria, iatrogenic causes (catheterization, recent urologic procedures), renal parenchymal disease (e.g., IgA nephropathy); vaginal contamination and menstruation (non-pathologic mimics in women)

Commonly misdiagnosed: bladder cancer, glomerular hematuria (often mistaken for lower tract source), rhabdomyolysis, interstitial cystitis, exercise-induced hematuria, anticoagulant-associated hematuria (which does not exclude underlying pathology), contamination from vaginal or anal sources

Systematic DDX

- Vascular
  - Renal infarction, renal vein thrombosis, arteriovenous malformation, vasculitis (e.g., ANCA-associated)
- Infectious/inflammatory
  - Urinary tract infection, pyelonephritis, prostatitis, cystitis, schistosomiasis (in endemic regions), interstitial cystitis

- **Neoplastic**
    - Bladder cancer, renal cell carcinoma, upper tract urothelial carcinoma, prostate cancer, urethral carcinoma
- **Dysfunction**
    - Benign prostatic hyperplasia, nephrolithiasis, glomerulonephritis (IgA nephropathy, Alport syndrome, thin basement membrane disease), sickle cell nephropathy
- **Injury/trauma**
    - Blunt or penetrating trauma to the kidney/ureter/bladder/urethra, iatrogenic injury (instrumentation/surgery), exercise-induced hematuria, rhabdomyolysis
- **Compression/obstruction**
    - Ureteral or bladder calculi, obstructing tumors, urethral strictures, external compression from pelvic masses
- **Anomalies of development/aging**
    - Congenital anomalies (e.g., polycystic kidney disease, horseshoe kidney), atrophic changes in the elderly, age-related vascular fragility
- **Toxic-metabolic**
    - Drug-induced hematuria (cyclophosphamide, anticoagulants), radiation cystitis, metabolic disorders predisposing to stones
- **Everything else**
    - **Mimics:** menstrual contamination, factitious hematuria, pigmenturia (myoglobinuria, hemoglobinuria)

Notes

General considerations: The evaluation of hematuria should begin with confirmation on repeat urinalysis, exclusion of infection and contamination, and a thorough history and physical examination. Professional societies recommend risk-adapted diagnostic strategies, with cystoscopy and upper tract imaging (CT urography or ultrasound) for high-risk patients, and nephrology referral for those with glomerular features (proteinuria, dysmorphic RBCs, casts, or renal dysfunction). Anticoagulation does not preclude a full evaluation for underlying pathology.

Red flags: painless gross hematuria, diffuse edema, renal dysfunction, flank pain, hypotension, trauma

Special populations: In children, urinary tract infection and glomerulonephritis are the most common causes; family history and associated findings guide further workup. In older adults, malignancy risk is higher, especially in men and smokers. Women are at risk for delayed cancer diagnosis due to misattribution to infection.

In patients on anticoagulation, hematuria should not be attributed solely to medication without further evaluation. In endemic regions, schistosomiasis should be considered. Remember that rhabdomyolysis will be positive for blood on urine dipsticks, but negative for red blood cells on urinalysis.

Further Reading

- Wolfman DJ, Marko J, Nikolaidis P, et al. ACR Appropriateness Criteria® Hematuria. J Am Coll Radiol. 2020;17(5S):S138–S147. doi:10.1016/j.jacr.2020.01.028.
- Ingelfinger JR. Hematuria in adults. N Engl J Med. 2021;385(2):153–163. doi:10.1056/NEJMra1604481.
- Nielsen M, Qaseem A. Hematuria as a marker of occult urinary tract cancer. Ann Intern Med. 2016;164(7):488–497. doi:10.7326/M15-1496.
- Bolenz C, Schröppel B, Eisenhardt A, et al. The investigation of hematuria. Dtsch Arztebl Int. 2018;115(48):801–807. doi:10.3238/arztebl.2018.0801.
- Rai BP, Luis Dominguez Escrig J, Vale L, et al. Urothelial cancers and RCC among patients with hematuria. Eur Urol. 2022;82(2):182–192. doi:10.1016/j.eururo.2022.03.027.
- Margulis V, Sagalowsky AI. Assessment of hematuria. Med Clin North Am. 2011;95(1):153–159. doi:10.1016/j.mcna.2010.08.028.
- Horváth O, Szabó AJ, Reusz GS. Significant causes of hematuria in childhood. Pediatr Nephrol. 2023;38(8):2549–2562. doi:10.1007/s00467-022-05746-4.

Urinary Incontinence

Introduction

Urinary incontinence is defined as the involuntary loss of urine and presents as a spectrum of symptoms, including stress, urgency, overflow, and mixed incontinence. Major diagnostic considerations include distinguishing between subtypes, identifying reversible causes, and ruling out serious underlying pathology such as malignancy or neurologic disease. Overlap with other lower urinary tract symptoms (frequency, urgency, nocturia) is common, and incontinence may coexist with urinary tract infection or pelvic organ prolapse.

Checklist DDX

Serious/life-threatening: cauda equina syndrome, malignancy of the urinary tract (bladder, urethra), severe pelvic organ prolapse with urinary retention, rapidly progressive neurologic disease (e.g., spinal cord compression, multiple sclerosis)

Common: stress incontinence (involuntary loss of urine with increased abdominal pressure, often due to urethral sphincter incompetence or pelvic floor weakness), urgency incontinence (sudden compelling urge to void, often idiopathic or associated with overactive bladder), mixed incontinence, overflow incontinence (bladder outlet obstruction or impaired detrusor contractility), transient incontinence due to reversible factors (infection, medications, excessive fluid intake, constipation, or delirium)

Commonly misdiagnosed: mixed incontinence (often mistaken for pure stress or urgency incontinence), overflow incontinence (misattributed to stress or urgency), atrophic vaginitis in postmenopausal women, functional incontinence due to cognitive or mobility impairment

Systematic DDX

- **Vascular**
    - Pelvic vascular malformations, ischemic injury
- **Infectious/inflammatory**
    - Urinary tract infection, chronic cystitis, atrophic vaginitis, radiation cystitis
- **Neoplastic**
    - Bladder cancer, urethral carcinoma, pelvic malignancies with local invasion or compression

- **Dysfunction**
    - Stress incontinence (urethral sphincter incompetence, pelvic floor weakness), urgency incontinence (detrusor overactivity, overactive bladder), overflow incontinence (impaired detrusor contractility, diabetic autonomic neuropathy), neurogenic bladder (multiple sclerosis, Parkinson disease, spinal cord injury), functional incontinence (cognitive or mobility impairment)
- **Injury/trauma**
    - Pelvic or perineal trauma, obstetric injury, iatrogenic injury from pelvic surgery or radiation
- **Compression/obstruction**
    - Spinal cord compression (from malignancy or spinal epidural abscess), cauda equina syndrome, pelvic organ prolapse, urethral stricture, bladder outlet obstruction (e.g., large fibroid, pelvic mass), severe constipation
- **Anomalies of development/aging**
    - Congenital anomalies (ectopic ureter, epispadias), age-related pelvic floor atrophy, genitourinary syndrome of menopause
- **Toxic-metabolic**
    - Medication-induced incontinence (diuretics, alpha-blockers, anticholinergics, sedatives), metabolic derangements (hyperglycemia, hypercalcemia), alcohol
- **Everything else**
    - Psychogenic causes, excessive fluid intake, behavioral factors

Notes

General considerations: The initial evaluation should include a focused history, physical examination, urinalysis, and assessment of symptom severity and impact on quality of life. Management is mostly focused on identifying and treating reversible causes, such as infection, medications, and comorbid conditions (obesity, constipation, sleep apnea, cognitive impairment). Most patients do not require extensive testing before initial management, and validated questionnaires can help subtype incontinence. Urodynamics, cystoscopy, and imaging are reserved for diagnostic uncertainty, hematuria, recurrent infections, or failure of initial therapy.

Red flags: severe pain, neurologic symptoms (leg weakness, saddle anesthesia), new-onset incontinence with pain, hematuria, recurrent urinary tract infections, pelvic organ prolapse beyond the hymen, elevated postvoid residual, difficulty passing a catheter

Special populations: In older adults, functional and mixed incontinence are common, and cognitive or mobility impairment may contribute. In postmenopausal women, atrophic changes and pelvic organ prolapse are frequent contributors. In men, overflow incontinence due to bladder outlet obstruction (e.g., benign prostatic hyperplasia) is more common. In children, congenital anomalies and neurologic disorders should be considered.

Further Reading

- Lukacz ES, Santiago-Lastra Y, Albo ME, Brubaker L. Urinary incontinence in women: a review. JAMA. 2017;318(16):1592–1604. doi:10.1001/jama.2017.12137.
- Goode PS, Burgio KL, Richter HE, Markland AD. Incontinence in older women. JAMA. 2010;303(21):2172–2181. doi:10.1001/jama.2010.749.
- Cameron AP, Chung DE, Dielubanza EJ, et al. The AUA/SUFU guideline on the diagnosis and treatment of idiopathic overactive bladder. J Urol. 2024;212(1):11–20. doi:10.1097/JU.0000000000003985.
- Qaseem A, Dallas P, Forciea MA, et al. Nonsurgical management of urinary incontinence in women: a clinical practice guideline from the American College of Physicians. Ann Intern Med. 2014;161(6):429–440. doi:10.7326/M13-2410.
- Rosier P. Contemporary diagnosis of lower urinary tract dysfunction. F1000Res. 2019;8:F1000 Faculty Rev-644. doi:10.12688/f1000research.16120.1.

Urethral Discharge

Introduction

Urethral discharge presents as the spontaneous or expressed release of fluid from the urethra, most commonly in men, and is a cardinal sign of urethritis. Major diagnostic considerations include distinguishing between infectious (especially sexually transmitted) and non-infectious causes and identifying complications such as epididymitis or ascending infection. Urethral discharge may overlap with presentations of dysuria, genital ulcers, or urinary tract infection.

Checklist DDX

Serious/life-threatening: disseminated gonococcal infection, severe epididymo-orchitis with abscess, Fournier gangrene

Common: gonococcal urethritis (Neisseria gonorrhoeae), nongonococcal urethritis (Chlamydia trachomatis, Mycoplasma genitalium, Trichomonas vaginalis), chemical or irritant urethritis, trauma from instrumentation or foreign bodies

Commonly misdiagnosed: nongonococcal urethritis (often mistaken for gonococcal or missed entirely), urethral stricture (misattributed to infection), chronic prostatitis, and urinary tract infection without pyuria or bacteriuria, herpes simplex virus urethritis without ulcers

Systematic DDX

- **Vascular**
    - Ischemic injury, vasculitis (e.g., Behçet disease)
- **Infectious/inflammatory**
    - Neisseria gonorrhoeae, Chlamydia trachomatis, Mycoplasma genitalium, Trichomonas vaginalis, herpes simplex virus, bacterial urinary tract infection, fungal infection (immunocompromised), chemical or irritant urethritis
- **Neoplastic**
    - Urethral carcinoma, genitourinary malignancy with ulceration or necrosis
- **Dysfunction**
    - Urethral stricture, chronic prostatitis/chronic pelvic pain syndrome

- **Injury/trauma**
    - Urethral instrumentation, catheterization, foreign body insertion
- **Compression/obstruction**
    - Urethral stricture, external compression from pelvic mass, severe prostatic enlargement
- **Anomalies of development/aging**
    - Posterior urethral valves, urethral diverticulum
- **Toxic-metabolic**
    - Drug-induced urethritis (e.g., chemotherapeutic agents), metabolic derangements predisposing to infection
- **Everything else**
    - Factitious disorder, excessive masturbation, psychogenic causes

Notes

General considerations: Specialty societies recommend that all patients with urethral discharge undergo nucleic acid amplification testing for Neisseria gonorrhoeae and Chlamydia trachomatis, with additional testing for Mycoplasma genitalium and Trichomonas vaginalis as indicated. Gram stain of urethral secretions is highly specific for gonococcal infection in men. Urinalysis and urine culture are useful to exclude urinary tract infection, but pyuria in the absence of bacteriuria should prompt evaluation for sexually transmitted infection. Urethral stricture should be considered in patients with recurrent symptoms, poor urinary stream, or history of trauma or instrumentation.

Red flags: fever, severe pain, scrotal swelling, signs of systemic illness, inability to void, persistent or bloody discharge

Special populations: In men who have sex with men, testing should include rectal and pharyngeal sites as indicated. In women, urethral discharge is less common but may be associated with cervicitis or pelvic inflammatory disease. In children, sexual abuse must be considered in the absence of clear alternative etiology. Immunocompromised patients may have atypical or severe presentations and broader infectious differentials.

Further Reading

- Workowski KA, Bachmann LH, Chan PA, et al. Sexually transmitted infections treatment guidelines, 2021. MMWR Recomm Rep. 2021;70(4):1–187. doi:10.15585/mmwr.rr7004a1.
- Miller JM, Binnicker MJ, Campbell S, et al. Guide to utilization of the microbiology laboratory for diagnosis of infectious diseases: 2024 update

- by the IDSA and ASM. Clin Infect Dis. 2024;:ciae104. doi:10.1093/cid/ciae104.
- Wessells H, Morey A, Souter L, Rahimi L, Vanni A. Urethral stricture disease guideline amendment (2023). J Urol. 2023;210(1):64–71. doi:10.1097/JU.0000000000003482.
- Kimura K, Yamamoto T, Tsuchiya J, et al. A diagnostic approach of various urethral diseases using multimodal imaging findings. Abdom Radiol. 2024;49(12) 4416–4436. doi:10.1007/s00261-024-04435-0.
- Al Lawati H, Blair BM, Larnard J. Urinary tract infections: core curriculum 2024. Am J Kidney Dis. 2024;83(1):90–100. doi:10.1053/j.ajkd.2023.08.009.
- Nelson Z, Aslan AT, Beahm NP, et al. Guidelines for the prevention, diagnosis, and management of urinary tract infections in pediatrics and adults. JAMA Netw Open. 2024;7(11):e2444495. doi:10.1001/jamanetworkopen.2024.44495.

Extremities and Musculoskeletal

Richard J. Lozano

Long H. Tu

Samreen Vora

Joint Pain and Swelling

Introduction

The first step in evaluation of joint pain (arthralgia) or joint swelling is to distinguish between true articular symptoms and non-articular or periarticular conditions by recognizing clinical patterns through the history and physical examination. Next, it is important to determine whether symptoms are inflammatory or non-inflammatory, which can include features of synovitis such as warmth and swelling, as well as systemic symptoms. The differential diagnosis is further narrowed by classification of symptoms as monoarticular or polyarticular. The most common causes of monoarticular symptoms include overuse injuries, gout, septic arthritis, osteoarthritis, and acute rheumatoid arthritis. Polyarticular pain and swelling are commonly caused by self-limited illness, such as in viral arthritis. Common pathological conditions of polyarthritis include rheumatoid arthritis and spondyloarthropathies. If the diagnosis remains unclear or confirmation is needed, further serologic/tissue studies, imaging studies, subspecialty consultation may be obtained.

Checklist DDX

Serious/life-threatening: acute septic arthritis, acute gout, severe CPPD (Calcium pyrophosphate deposition or "peudogout"), acute hemarthrosis, osteonecrosis

Common: overuse injuries, bursitis, rheumatoid arthritis (RA), osteoarthritis (OA), gout, septic arthritis, patellofemoral pain, meniscal tear, viral arthritis

Commonly misdiagnosed: osteoarthritis, rheumatoid arthritis, CPPD, fibromyalgia, Lyme arthritis, psoriatic arthritis, lupus, hematologic malignancy, osteonecrosis, polymyalgia rheumatica

Systematic DDX

Noninflammatory
- Mechanical
    - **Overuse injury:** patellofemoral pain, patellar tendinopathy, patellar subluxation, meniscal tear
    - **Degenerative:** osteoarthritis, Charcot neuropathic osteoarthropathy (most commonly due to diabetes)
- Neoplastic
    - **Primary bone neoplasia:** osteoid osteoma, chondrosarcoma, tenosynovial giant cell tumor, osteosarcoma, Ewing sarcoma

- ○ **Hematological malignancies/disorders:** multiple myeloma, lymphoma, myelodysplastic diseases
- ○ **Other:** metastatic disease
- **Miscellaneous**
    - ○ **Metabolic:** osteomalacia (vitamin D deficiency), scurvy (vitamin C deficiency)
    - ○ **Other:** osteonecrosis, hypertrophic osteoarthropathy, transient osteoporosis, hemochromatosis, hemarthrosis (more likely in patients with hemophilia or anticoagulation therapy), acromegaly
- **Pediatric**
    - ○ **Overuse injury:** patellofemoral pain, patellar tendinopathy, iliotibial band syndrome, Osgood-Schlatter disease, osteochondritis dissecans
    - ○ **Developmental:** osteonecrosis (Legg-Calve-Perthes disease, slipped capital femoral epiphysis), benign idiopathic nocturnal pains of childhood ("growing pains")
    - ○ **Other:** joint hypermobility

Inflammatory
- **Infectious**
    - ○ **Bacterial:** acute septic arthritis (e.g., *s. aureus, streptococci*), abscess, cellulitis, osteomyelitis, infectious arthritis (e.g., gonococcal arthritis, Lyme, tuberculosis, brucellosis), Whipple disease, Q-fever, rheumatic fever
    - ○ **Viral:** HBV, HCV, EBV, HIV, parvovirus, dengue virus, rubella, mumps, influenza, alphaviruses
- **Crystal arthropathies**
    - ○ CPPD, gout
- **Rheumatological**
    - ○ **Autoimmune:** rheumatoid arthritis, lupus, Sjögren's syndrome, dermatomyositis, polymyositis
    - ○ **Spondyloarthropathies:** ankylosing spondylitis, psoriatic arthritis, reactive arthritis, enteropathic arthritis (e.g., Crohn's, ulcerative colitis, celiac)
    - ○ **Vasculitis:** polyarteritis nodosa, Behcet's disease, IgA vasculitis
    - ○ **Other:** polymyalgia rheumatica, adult-onset Still's disease, serum sickness, sarcoidosis
- **Pediatric**
    - ○ **Autoimmune:** juvenile dermatomyositis, childhood-onset lupus
    - ○ **Vasculitis:** Kawasaki disease, IgA vasculitis

- **Infection:** acute septic arthritis (e.g., Staphylococcus aureus, streptococci), reactive arthritis, acute rheumatic fever
- **Other:** juvenile idiopathic arthritis, familial mediterranean fever

Notes

General considerations: Diagnosis is primarily based on patient history and physical examination. Imaging may be indicated when presentation is atypical. Radiographic imaging of all patients with possible osteoarthritis is not recommended. In suspected cases of septic arthritis, urgent arthrocentesis should be considered.

Red flags: hot or swollen joints, unexpected rapid progression, constitutional symptoms, immunocompromised status, pre-existing chronic arthritis, age >80, prolonged joint stiffness, severe pain or greater than expected from physical findings, burning pain, numbness, paresthesias, pain at rest, prosthetic joint, recent surgery

Special populations: Evaluation of pediatric patients should involve consideration of urgent conditions such as septic arthritis, Kawasaki disease, nonaccidental trauma, and neoplasia. Osteoarthritis is common in older patients. Pregnancy can exacerbate or unmask autoimmune inflammatory arthritis or cause periarticular conditions like carpal tunnel syndrome.

Further Reading

- Keret S, Kaly L, Shouval A, Eshed I, Slobodin G. Approach to a patient with monoarticular disease. Autoimmunity Reviews 2021;20(7):102848. DOI: https://doi.org/10.1016/j.autrev.2021.102848.
- Long B, Koyfman A, Gottlieb M. Evaluation and Management of Septic Arthritis and its Mimics in the Emergency Department. Western Journal of Emergency Medicine 2019;20(2):331-341. DOI: 10.5811/westjem.2018.10.40974.
- Pujalte GG, Albano-Aluquin SA. Differential Diagnosis of Polyarticular Arthritis. Am Fam Physician 2015;92(1):35-41. (In eng).
- Singh N, Vogelgesang SA. Monoarticular Arthritis. Medical Clinics of North America 2017;101(3):607-613. DOI: https://doi.org/10.1016/j.mcna.2016.12.004.
- Pinals RS. Polyarthritis and Fever. New England Journal of Medicine 1994;330(11):769-774. DOI: doi:10.1056/NEJM199403173301108.

Muscle Pain

Introduction

Muscle pain, or myalgia, is a very common and non-specific symptom. The most common cause of myalgia is intense muscle activity or mild trauma and is often self-limited and non-pathologic. Initial evaluation of serious or pathological myalgias requires pattern recognition of clinical symptoms and signs through a careful history and physical examination. It is important to classify symptoms as inflammatory or non-inflammatory and to characterize the pattern of pain. A detailed history of medications and exposure to environmental toxins is essential. Further investigation may include laboratory testing, EMG and nerve conduction studies, imaging studies, genetic testing and muscle biopsy.

Checklist DDX

Serious/life-threatening: bacterial infection (e.g., endocarditis, sepsis, pyomyositis, necrotizing fasciitis), compartment syndrome, rhabdomyolysis

Common: muscle strain, trauma, viral infection, drug-induced myopathy, polymyalgia rheumatica (PMR), pain syndromes

Commonly misdiagnosed: fibromyalgia, hypothyroidism, vitamin D deficiency, statin-induced myopathy, viral myositis, Lyme disease, polymyalgia rheumatica

Systematic DDX

- **Vascular**
    - **Ischemic myalgia:** peripheral vascular disease, sickle cell disease
- **Infectious**
    - **Bacterial:** streptococcal infection, Lyme disease, pyomyositis, necrotizing fasciitis
    - **Viral:** influenza, coronavirus, coxsackievirus, hepatitis, dengue
    - **Parasite:** trichinella
- **Inflammatory**
    - **Autoimmune:** lupus, Sjögren's syndrome, systemic sclerosis, rheumatoid arthritis, autoimmune hepatitis
    - **Myositis:** polymyositis, dermatomyositis, idiopathic inflammatory myopathies
    - **Vasculitis:** polyarteritis nodosa, Behcet's disease, other vasculitides

- o **Other:** polymyalgia rheumatica, spondyloarthropathies, adult-onset Still's disease, sarcoidosis
- **Neoplastic**
  - o **Paraneoplastic syndromes:** lung, stomach, colon, kidney, breast
  - o **Hematological disease:** multiple myeloma, lymphoma, leukemia
  - o **Other:** primary muscle tumors (e.g. rhabdomyoscarcoma, leiomyosarcoma)
- **Neuromuscular**
  - o Myasthenia gravis, polyneuropathies, muscular dystrophies, myotonic dystrophy
- **Endocrine**
  - o Thyroid dysfunction, diabetes mellitus (neuropathy, muscle infarction), adrenal insufficiency
- **Electrolyte imbalances**
  - o Hypokalemia, hyperkalemia, hypocalcemia, hypercalcemia
- **Trauma**
  - o Muscle strain, muscle tear, contusion, hematoma, compartment syndrome, crush syndrome
- **Toxic**
  - o **Drug-induced:** alcohol, glucocorticoids, statins, antimalarials, colchicine, vincristine, amiodarone, immune checkpoint inhibitors
  - o **Toxins:** envenomation (snake venom, spider venom)
- **Metabolic**
  - o **Acquired:** osteomalacia (vitamin D deficiency), scurvy (vitamin C deficiency)
  - o **Genetic:** hemochromatosis, porphyrias, amyloidosis
- **Miscellaneous**
  - o **Pain syndromes:** fibromyalgia, chronic fatigue syndrome, myofascial pain syndrome
  - o **Psychiatric:** somatization disorder, discontinuation of serotonin reuptake inhibitors (e.g. venlafaxine, paroxetine)
- **Pediatric**
  - o **Inflammatory:** childhood-onset SLE, juvenile systemic sclerosis, juvenile dermatomyositis, familial mediterranean fever
  - o **Genetic:** muscular dystrophies, myotonic dystrophies, glycogen storage disorders, fatty acid disorders, mitochondrial myopathies
  - o **Other:** overuse syndromes, benign idiopathic nocturnal pains of childhood (growing pains), amplified musculoskeletal pain syndromes

Notes

General considerations: Diagnostic workup of myalgia should be carried out in a standardized process to avoid overlooking important information and to avoid unnecessary invasive testing. Common laboratory testing includes complete blood count, CK, renal and liver function tests, LDH, and endocrine studies.

Red flags: constitutional symptoms, objective weakness, redness, swelling, warmth, greater than expected from physical findings, presence of triggers (physical exercise, certain foods, temperature changes), atrophy, fasciculations

Special populations: In pediatric patients, consider inflammatory disorders with childhood onset and genetic conditions. In pregnant patients, muscle pain often results from mechanical strain due to weight gain, altered posture, and hormone-induced ligament laxity, particularly in the third trimester. Common causes include leg muscle cramps, carpal tunnel syndrome, and pelvic girdle pain, with inflammation or rare autoimmune myopathies also possible. In older patients, muscle pain is frequently due to sarcopenia, polymyalgia rheumatica, or inflammatory myopathies such as polymyositis, with medication-induced myopathy and toxic-metabolic causes also important considerations.

Further Reading

- Altabás-González I, Pérez-Gómez N, Pego-Reigosa JM. How to investigate: Suspected systemic rheumatic diseases in patients presenting with muscle complaints. Best Practice & Research Clinical Rheumatology 2019;33(4):101437. DOI: https://doi.org/10.1016/j.berh.2019.101437.
- Glaubitz S, Schmidt K, Zschüntzsch J, Schmidt J. Myalgia in myositis and myopathies. Best Practice & Research Clinical Rheumatology 2019;33(3):101433. DOI: https://doi.org/10.1016/j.berh.2019.101433.
- Chavez LO, Leon M, Einav S, Varon J. Beyond muscle destruction: a systematic review of rhabdomyolysis for clinical practice. Critical Care 2016;20(1). DOI: 10.1186/s13054-016-1314-5.
- Weiser P. Approach to the Patient with Noninflammatory Musculoskeletal Pain. Pediatric Clinics of North America 2012;59(2):471-492. DOI: https://doi.org/10.1016/j.pcl.2012.03.012.

Weakness

Introduction

The differential diagnosis of weakness is broad and requires distinguishing between true muscle weakness and subjective fatigue or pain-related motor impairment. The first step in evaluation is to assess for emergent or urgent conditions requiring acute intervention for impending respiratory failure. In stable patients, a comprehensive history and physical examination is necessary for narrowing the differential as the pathologic etiology may occur at any level of the neuromuscular pathway (upper motor neuron, lower motor neuron, neuromuscular junction, muscle fibers). The most common cause of unilateral weakness is acute brain infarction or ischemia and intracerebral hemorrhage. Critical illness is the most common cause of neuromuscular weakness (in settings like the intensive care unit). A systematic approach involves assessing whether the weakness is unilateral or bilateral, and determining the presence of diminished mental status, upper motor neuron (UMN) or lower motor neuron (LMN) signs, cranial nerve deficits, extremity weakness, oculomotor weakness, bulbar weakness, proximal or distal weakness, and central neurologic or peripheral nerve involvement.

Checklist DDX

Serious/life-threatening: cerebral lesion (stroke, hemorrhage, mass), spinal cord compression (stroke, hemorrhage, mass, inflammation), Guillain-Barré syndrome (GBS), tick paralysis, botulism, organophosphate poisoning, myasthenic crisis, rhabdomyolysis, endocrine crisis (diabetic ketoacidosis, myxedema coma, thyrotoxicosis, adrenal crisis), severe electrolyte abnormalities (hypokalemia, hyperkalemia)

Common: non-neuromuscular weakness (fatigue, malaise, asthenia, ataxia), cerebral lesion, Guillain-Barré syndrome, critical illness weakness, cervical spondylotic myelopathy, sarcopenia, frailty

Commonly misdiagnosed: ischemic stroke, peripheral neuropathy, radiculopathy, multiple sclerosis, thoracic myelopathy, myasthenia gravis, Guillain-Barrè syndrome

Systematic DDX

Topology*
- **Brain (UMN)**
    - **Cerebral lesion:** stroke, hemorrhage, tumor, abscess
    - **Infection:** neurocysticercosis, toxoplasmosis

- o **Inflammatory:** multiple sclerosis, acute disseminated encephalomyelitis
- o **Other:** hemiplegic migraine, postictal paralysis, cerebral palsy
- **Spinal cord (UMN)**
  - o **Spinal cord lesion:** stroke, hemorrhage, tumor, abscess
  - o **Infectious:** HSV, HIV, CMV, VZV, Lyme disease, neurosyphilis (tabes dorsalis), tuberculous spondylitis
  - o **Inflammatory:** multiple sclerosis, transverse myelitis, neuromyelitis optica, paraneoplastic syndromes, sarcoidosis
  - o **Genetic/developmental:** hereditary spastic paraplegias, Chiari malformations, tethered cord
  - o **Other:** amyotrophic lateral sclerosis, vitamin B12 deficiency (subacute combined degeneration), hepatic myelopathy (chronic liver disease), spondylotic myelopathy
- **Anterior horn cell (LMN)**
  - o Amyotrophic lateral sclerosis, poliomyelitis, west Nile virus, rabies, spinal muscular atrophy
- **Peripheral nerve and nerve root (LMN)**
  - o **Nerve/nerve root lesion:** radiculopathy, trauma (brachial, lumbar plexopathies), Erb's palsy, entrapment (e.g. carpal tunnel syndrome)
  - o **Toxins:** alcohol, heavy metals (e.g. arsenic, lead, thallium, mercury), tick paralysis
  - o **Infection:** Lyme disease, diphtheria, HIV, CMV, VZV, tuberculosis, syphilis
  - o **Inflammatory:** Guillain-Barre syndrome (recent history of c. jejuni, EBV, CMV, mycoplasma), vasculitis, arachnoiditis, sarcoidosis
  - o **Metabolic:** diabetes, porphyria, thiamine, vitamin B12, pyridoxine toxicity
  - o **Genetic:** hereditary sensorimotor disease (Charcot-Marie-Tooth disease), Friedrich ataxia
  - o **Neoplastic:** spinal cord tumors (e.g. ependymoma, astrocytoma, meningioma, nerve sheath tumor, chordoma), metastatic disease (e.g. prostate, breast, lung)
  - o **Other:** critical illness, radiation, dysautonomias (e.g. postural orthostatic tachycardia syndrome [POTS]), amyloidosis
- **Neuromuscular junction**
  - o **Autoimmune:** myasthenia gravis, Lambert-Eaton syndrome (paraneoplastic syndrome)
  - o **Toxins/drug-induced:** botulism, envenomation (snake venom, spider venom), organophosphates, neuromuscular blockade

- **Muscle fiber**
    - **Infection:** viral infection (e.g. influenza, coronavirus, coxsackievirus, EBV, HSV, VZV, hepatitis, dengue), trichinosis
    - **Inflammatory:** dermatomyositis, polymyositis, systemic sclerosis, Sjögren's syndrome, idiopathic inflammatory myositis
    - **Toxins:** alcohol myopathy, recreational drugs (e.g. cocaine, amphetamines, opioids)
    - **Endocrine** adrenal insufficiency, thyroid dysfunction, Cushing syndrome, acromegaly, primary hyperaldosteronism, endocrine crisis (e.g. DKA, myxedema coma, thyrotoxicosis, adrenal crisis)
    - **Electrolyte imbalance:** hypokalemia, hyperkalemia, hypocalcemia, hypercalcemia, hypermagnesemia, hypophosphatemia, hyponatremia
    - **Genetic:** muscular dystrophies, myotonic dystrophy, glycogen storage diseases, lipid storage diseases, mitochondrial diseases, muscle channelopathies (e.g. periodic paralysis)
    - **Drug-induced:** fluoroquinolones, glucocorticoids, statins, amiodarone, colchicine, vincristine, antiretrovirals
    - **Other:** sarcopenia, frailty, rhabdomyolysis, critical illness myopathy
- **Mimics**
    - Anemia, hypoglycemia, ACS, HF, presyncope, dehydration, COPD, carbon monoxide poisoning, infectious disorders (e.g. sepsis), neoplasms, pain syndromes (e.g. fibromyalgia), somatic symptoms, neurological functional disorder, factitious disorder

*Many entities listed present in multiple or different topographic distributions depending on disease course and individual presentation.

Notes

General considerations: Most cases of subjective weakness are not due to a neuromuscular process but rather due to fatigue or malaise attributable to medical illness. Patients with a suspected neuromuscular process should be admitted for comprehensive evaluation of pathological or life-threatening conditions.

Red flags: signs of impending respiratory failure (tachypnea, increasing generalized weakness, dysphagia, dysphonia, dyspnea, hypoxemia, accessary muscle use), altered mental status, cortical signs, unilateral or bilateral weakness or paralysis, visual symptoms, bulbar signs, UMN signs, LMN signs, fever, cranial nerve deficits, bowel/bladder dysfunction, dysautonomia, fatigability, proximal weakness

Special populations: Evaluation of acute weakness in pediatric patients should involve consideration of emergent or life-threatening conditions such as cerebral or spinal cord lesions, head trauma, and conditions causing impending respiratory failure or increased intracranial pressure. In the evaluation of older adults, sarcopenia and frailty should also be included in the differential diagnosis.

Further Reading

- Khamees D, Meurer W. Approach to Acute Weakness. Emergency Medicine Clinics of North America 2021;39(1):173-180. DOI: https://doi.org/10.1016/j.emc.2020.09.010.
- Larson ST, Wilbur J. Muscle Weakness in Adults: Evaluation and Differential Diagnosis. Am Fam Physician 2020;101(2):95-108.
- Ganti L, Rastogi V. Acute Generalized Weakness. Emergency Medicine Clinics of North America 2016;34(4):795-809. DOI: https://doi.org/10.1016/j.emc.2016.06.006.

- Latronico N, Rasulo FA, Eikermann M, Piva S. Critical Illness Weakness, Polyneuropathy and Myopathy: Diagnosis, treatment, and long-term outcomes. Critical Care 2023;27(1). DOI: 10.1186/s13054-023-04676-3.
- Oliveira R, Ramalho Rocha F, Teodoro T, Oliveira Santos M. Acute non-traumatic tetraparesis, 2013; Differential diagnosis. Journal of Clinical Neuroscience 2021;87:116-124. DOI: 10.1016/j.jocn.2021.02.024.

Neck Pain

Introduction

The differential diagnosis for neck pain is broad and can encompass musculoskeletal, neurologic, and rheumatological etiologies. Degenerative changes are common and can be found even in asymptomatic individuals, making it difficult to determine the precise cause of pain in some patients. The initial evaluation of patients with neck pain involves assessing for serious or life-threatening causes that require urgent intervention, as well as identifying red flag symptoms. Once these conditions are excluded, further investigation requires characterizing the onset, distribution, and nature of the pain. Physical examination should include observation of neck movement, range of motion, palpation of paraspinal muscles, neurologic assessment of radicular and UMN signs, and provocative maneuvers in patients with radicular symptoms.

Checklist DDX

Serious/life-threatening: cerebral lesion (stroke, mass, hemorrhage), cervical cord compression/lesion (trauma, tumor, abscess, hemorrhage, demyelinating, inflammatory), meningitis, arterial dissection, myocardial ischemia

Common: cervical strain, cervical spondylosis, cervical discogenic pain, cervical facet osteoarthritis, cervical radiculopathy

Commonly misdiagnosed: cervical strain, cervical radiculopathy, myofascial pain syndrome, referred shoulder pain, temporomandibular (TMJ) disorders, subacute thyroiditis

Systematic DDX

- Vascular
    - Angina pectoris, myocardial ischemia, arterial dissection (e.g. vertebral artery, carotid artery), vertebrobasilar insufficiency
- Infectious
    - Meningitis, abscess (epidural, extradural), discitis, osteomyelitis, peritonsillar abscess, tetanus, herpes zoster
- Inflammatory:
    - **Musculoskeletal:** rheumatoid arthritis, ankylosing spondylitis, polymyalgia rheumatica, myositis, diffuse idiopathic skeletal hyperostosis

- o **Other:** giant cell arteritis, thyroiditis
- **Neoplasm**
    - o **Spinal cord tumor:** ependymoma, astrocytoma, meningioma, nerve sheath tumor, chordoma
    - o **Metastatic disease:** prostate, breast, lung, thyroid, kidney
    - o **Hematological disease:** multiple myeloma
    - o **Other:** apical lung tumor
- **Musculoskeletal**
    - o **Trauma:** cervical strain (e.g. whiplash injury), vertebral lesion (e.g. osteoporotic crush fractures, joint dislocation), atlantoaxial subluxation (Down syndrome)
    - o **Degenerative:** cervical spondylosis (degenerative changes), cervical discogenic pain, cervical facet osteoarthritis
    - o **Other:** ossification of the posterior longitudinal ligament
- **Neurologic**
    - o **Cerebral:** tension headache, reversible cerebral vasoconstriction syndrome, Parkinson's disease, multiple system atrophy, Chiari malformations
    - o **Spinal cord:** cervical radiculopathy (cervical foraminal stenosis, herniated disc, VZV, Lyme disease, diabetes), cervical myelopathy, cervical dystonia
- **Miscellaneous**
    - o **Pain syndromes:** myofascial pain syndrome, fibromyalgia, psychogenic pain
    - o **Referred pain:** esophageal obstruction, biliary disease, referred shoulder pain, temporomandibular joint disorder, thyroiditis
    - o **Congenital:** thyroglossal duct cyst, branchial cleft cysts, dermoid cysts
    - o **Other:** thoracic outlet syndrome, stiff person syndrome

Notes

General considerations: Provocative maneuvers for evaluation of neck pain include Babinski reflex (cervical myelopathy), Hoffman sign (UMN lesion), Lhermitte sign (non-specific cervical cord compression; myelopathy, multiple sclerosis, mass, infection), Spurling test (cervical radiculopathy), and upper limb tension test (cervical radiculopathy). Most patients with atraumatic neck pain without red flag symptoms do not require imaging. CT is recommended for suspicion of cervical instability in major trauma cases. MRI is recommended for evaluation of suspected spine infection, acute neurologic compromise, or progressive neurologic symptoms. In the absence of red flag symptoms, treatment is focused on pain and function, and many patients will improve over time regardless of treatment.

Red flags: sudden-onset neck pain, recent major neck trauma (including chiropractic manipulation), diminished mental status, Lhermitte phenomenon (electrical sensation in back or limbs upon flexion of the neck), acute or progressive limb weakness, sensory abnormality, progressive gait impairment, bladder/bowel dysfunction, nuchal rigidity (Kernig's sign), abnormal neck posture, neck stiffness, tremor, anterior neck pain, fever, weight loss, malignancy, parenteral drug use, immunocompromised status, chronic glucocorticoid use

Special populations: Meningitis is especially important to consider in infants, young children, and in geriatric population. It is also important to consider acute coronary syndrome presenting as neck pain in the older adults with cardiovascular risk factors.

Further Reading

- Vijiaratnam N, Williams DR, Bertram KL. Neck pain: What if it is not musculoskeletal? Australian Journal of General Practice 2018;47(5):279-282. DOI: 10.31128/afp-10-17-4358.
- Childress MA, Stuek SJ. Neck Pain: Initial Evaluation and Management. Am Fam Physician 2020;102(3):150-156.
- Daniels AH, Alsoof D, McDonald CL, Diebo BG, Kuris EO. Clinical Examination of the Cervical Spine. New England Journal of Medicine 2023;389(17):e34. DOI: 10.1056/nejmvcm2204780.
- Theodore N. Degenerative Cervical Spondylosis. New England Journal of Medicine 2020;383(2):159-168. DOI: 10.1056/nejmra2003558.

Back Pain (Thoracic, Lumbar, Sacral)

Introduction

Back pain is a common symptom with a broad range of etiologies. Initial focus is on diagnosis of medical emergencies and identification of red flag symptoms. After exclusion of these conditions, it is helpful to narrow the diagnosis to nonspecific low back pain, pain due to radiculopathy or spinal stenosis, or pain due to specific spinal etiologies such as cancer, infection, or rheumatologic etiologies. Nonspecific low back pain accounts for 80 to 90% of all cases of low back pain in the primary care setting and many patients improve within a few weeks. A detailed medical history and physical examination is essential in the investigation of radiculopathy and specific spinal etiologies. Physical examination should include inspection of the spine, palpation of spinous processes and paraspinal muscles, range of motion, and complete neurological testing of motor function, sensation, deep tendon reflexes, and gait.

Checklist DDX

Serious/life-threatening: spinal cord compression (e.g. cauda equina syndrome), metastatic disease, spinal infection (e.g. abscess, osteomyelitis), aortic dissection, spinal epidural hematoma

Common: muscle strain, intervertebral disc disorders, facet joint arthropathy, spinal stenosis, lumbar radiculopathy, myofascial pain syndrome

Commonly misdiagnosed: lumbar radiculopathy, facet joint arthropathy, sacroiliac joint dysfunction, vertebral compression fractures, axial spondyloarthritis, pyelonephritis, vaso-occlusive disease, myofascial pain syndrome

Systematic DDX

- **Mechanical**
  - **Degenerative:** intervertebral disc disorders, facet joint arthropathy (e.g. osteoarthritis), spinal stenosis (e.g. degenerative changes, spondylolisthesis, trauma, spine surgery, metabolic disorders, endocrine disorders), sacroiliac joint dysfunction
  - **Trauma:** lumbar strain, vertebral compression fractures (e.g. osteoporosis, trauma, chronic glucocorticoid use), spondylolysis
  - **Other:** lumbar post-laminectomy syndrome, piriformis syndrome, lumbosacral transitional vertebra, apophysitis

- **Vascular**
    - Spinal epidural hematoma, spinal dural arteriovenous fistula, intraabdominal aneurysm or dissection
- **Infectious**
    - Vertebral osteomyelitis (e.g. *s. aureus*, tuberculosis), discitis, arachnoiditis, spinal abscess, herpes zoster, tuberculous spondylitis
- **Inflammatory**
    - Axial spondyloarthritis (e.g. ankylosing spondylitis, psoriatic spondylitis, reactive arthritis, inflammatory bowel disease), transverse myelitis
- **Neoplasm**
    - **Primary neoplasia:** (arising from bone or adjacent structures) meningioma, neurofibroma, schwannoma, chordoma, osteoid osteoma, Ewing sarcoma, osteochondroma
    - **Metastatic disease:** breast, prostate, lung, thyroid, kidney
    - **Hematological disorders:** multiple myeloma, leukemia, lymphoma
    - Retroperitoneal tumors
- **Metabolic**
    - Osteoporosis, osteosclerosis (Paget disease)
- **Congenital**
    - Kyphoscoliosis, spina bifida occulta, tethered spinal cord
- **Miscellaneous**
    - **Intra-abdominal visceral disease:** peptic ulcer, pancreatitis, cholecystitis, nephrolithiasis, pyelonephritis, prostatitis, endometriosis, pelvic infection, aortic aneurysm or dissection
    - **Other:** pain syndromes, vaso-occlusive pain (sickle cell disease), psychosocial distress, postural

Notes

General considerations: Physical exam maneuvers for assessing radiculopathy include ipsilateral and contralateral straight leg raise (passive lifting by the examiner of the affected or unaffected leg to an angle less than 60 degrees reproduces pain radiating distally to knee). Routine imaging in patients with nonspecific low back pain is not recommended as abnormal findings are common and may not be the cause of the pain. Diagnostic imaging is recommended in patients with severe or progressive neurologic deficits, suspected serious underlying conditions, nonresponse to standard treatments, or when surgery or steroid injection is considered.

Red flags: neurologic deficits, severe or intractable pain that interferes with function, constitutional symptoms, history of malignancy, unexplained weight loss, worse pain at night, major trauma, high infection risk (e.g. parenteral drug use, long-term glucocorticoid use), immunocompromise, fever, age >70

Special populations: In pediatric patients, back pain is commonly nonspecific and caused by benign musculoskeletal conditions and trauma. Axial spondyloarthritis should be considered in pediatric patients with chronic back pain and morning stiffness. In pregnant individuals, low back pain is common and worsens as pregnancy progresses, making diagnosis of pathological conditions more challenging. In the geriatric population, vertebral compression fractures may be missed due to gradual presentation or attribution to degenerative disease.

Further Reading

- Low Back Pain. Annals of Internal Medicine 2021;174(8):ITC113-ITC128. DOI: 10.7326/aitc202108170 %m 34370518.
- Chiarotto A, Koes BW. Nonspecific Low Back Pain. New England Journal of Medicine 2022;386(18):1732-1740. DOI: 10.1056/nejmcp2032396.
- Urits I, Burshtein A, Sharma M, et al. Low Back Pain, a Comprehensive Review: Pathophysiology, Diagnosis, and Treatment. Current Pain and Headache Reports 2019;23(3):23. DOI: 10.1007/s11916-019-0757-1.
- Achar S, Yamanaka J. Back Pain in Children and Adolescents. Am Fam Physician 2020;102(1):19-28.

Focal or Unilateral Extremity Swelling

Introduction

The differential for unilateral or focal swelling is broad, depends on the location of symptoms, and initially requires focusing on emergent conditions with identification of red flag symptoms and systemic symptoms. Once severe or life-threatening conditions are ruled out, a detailed medical history assessing associated symptoms and chronicity, and physical examination with characterization of the swelling is vital. Acute lower extremity swelling should prompt evaluation for deep venous thrombosis (DVT), initially via calculation of the Wells Score, followed by compression ultrasonography in patients with intermediate/high risk. Patients with chronic (>3 months) unilateral lower extremity swelling should undergo duplex ultrasonography with reflux for evaluation of chronic venous insufficiency and differentiation from lymphedema. Further evaluation involves narrowing the differential and more targeted evaluation for specific clinical entities.

Checklist DDX

Serious/life-threatening: compartment syndrome, necrotizing soft tissue infection, toxic shock syndrome, osteomyelitis, septic arthritis, DVT, angioedema

Common: chronic venous insufficiency (CVI), lymphedema, cellulitis, drug reaction, contact dermatitis, insect stings/bites, urticaria

Commonly misdiagnosed: cellulitis, CVI, lymphedema

Systematic DDX

- **Vascular**
    - DVT, superficial thrombophlebitis, postthrombotic syndrome, chronic venous insufficiency (i.e. venous stasis dermatitis), lymphedema, hematoma, SVC syndrome, mycotic aneurysm, erythromelalgia, calciphylaxis, vascular malformations, lymphangiomas, aortocaval fistula, May-Thurner syndrome (right iliac artery compresses the left iliac vein)
- **Infectious**
    - **Bacterial:** cellulitis, erysipelas, folliculitis, lymphadenitis, cutaneous abscess, septic arthritis, pyomyositis, erythema migrans, necrotizing, necrotizing soft tissue infection, toxic shock

syndrome, osteomyelitis, clostridial myonecrosis, medical device infection
- **Viral:** HSV, VZV, parvovirus B19, CMV
- **Fungal:** Cryptococcus neoformans, Sporothrix schenckii (e.g. nodular lymphangitis), mucormycosis
- **Parasitic:** Trypanasoma cruzii, myiasis

- **Inflammatory**
  - **Allergic:** contact dermatitis, angioedema, drug reaction, fixed drug reaction
  - **Autoimmune:** relapsing polychondritis, eosinophilic cellulitis
  - **Vasculitis:** familial mediterranean fever, polyarteritis nodosa
  - **Other:** erythema nodosum, panniculitis, cutaneous graft vs. host disease (GVHD), sarcoidosis, Sweet syndrome, pyoderma gangrenosum, hidradenitis suppurativa

- **Neoplastic**
  - Lymphoma, leukemia, Paget disease of the breast, extramammary Paget disease, inflammatory breast carcinoma, carcinoma erysipeloides

- **Trauma**
  - Compartment syndrome, pressure bullae, postcutaneous injection, IV-line infiltration

- **Miscellaneous**
  - Insect stings/bites, reaction to foreign body implant, radiation recall, epidermoid cyst, complex regional pain syndrome

Notes

General considerations: Venous stasis dermatitis often mimics cellulitis and is distinguished by its bilateral nature. Unilateral presentations can occur in patients with unilateral leg injury or anatomical variation.

Red flags: recent trauma, pain out of proportion to physical exam, pain with passive stretching of the muscle, immunocompromise, immobilization, signs of septicemia such as fever, chills, hypotension, altered mental status, other organ dysfunction, skin necrosis, neurological deficits or paresthesias, airway compromise

Special populations: Evaluation of focal swelling in the pediatric population should involve additional consideration of congenital etiologies such as epidermoid or dermoid cysts. In pregnant patients, focal or unilateral extremity swelling should raise concern for deep vein thrombosis. In older patients, unilateral extremity swelling commonly suggests venous thrombosis, cellulitis, or lymphedema.

Further Reading

- Raff AB, Kroshinsky D. Cellulitis. JAMA 2016;316(3):325. DOI: 10.1001/jama.2016.8825.
- Mortensen SJ, Vora MM, Mohamadi A, et al. Diagnostic Modalities for Acute Compartment Syndrome of the Extremities. JAMA Surgery 2019;154(7):655. DOI: 10.1001/jamasurg.2019.1050.
- McDermott J, Kao LS, Keeley JA, Grigorian A, Neville A, De Virgilio C. Necrotizing Soft Tissue Infections. JAMA Surgery 2024;159(11):1308. DOI: 10.1001/jamasurg.2024.3365.
- Patel H, Skok CJ, Demarco A. Peripheral Edema: Evaluation and Management in Primary Care. American Family Physician 2022;106(5):557-564.

Non-Pitting Edema

Introduction

Non-pitting edema is peripheral edema that does not retain an indentation after pressure is applied. It typically occurs due to increased protein-rich interstitial fluid, deposition of other substances, or tissue fibrosis. Early-stage lymphedema can exhibit pitting edema whereas chronic will exhibit non-pitting edema. Early-stage lymphedema is often misdiagnosed due to other mimics with extremity swelling. Secondary lymphedema has a prevalence of 1 in 1000 individuals. In the US, it most commonly occurs following lymphadenectomy and radiation therapy for breast cancer. Primary lymphedema is rare (prevalence of 1 in 100,000) and typically occurs in childhood. The Kaposi-Stemmer sign (a positive sign where the skin on the top of the second toe or finger cannot be pinched because it is too thick) is pathognomonic for chronic lymphedema.

Checklist DDX

Serious/life-threatening: angioedema, myxedema coma

Common: lymphedema, drug-induced edema

Commonly misdiagnosed: lymphedema, drug-induced edema

Systematic DDX

- **Inflammatory**
    - Scleroderma (scleroderma-like disorders), angioedema
- **Endocrine**
    - Hypothyroid myxedema, pretibial myxedema of Graves' disease
- **Medications**
    - **Vasodilatory:** antihypertensives (e.g. CCBs, α-adrenergic receptor blockers, vasodilators), antiepileptics (e.g. gabapentinoids), antidepressants, antipsychotics, antiparkinsonian
    - **Renal (sodium retention):** hormone therapy, glucocorticoids, NSAIDs
    - **Lymphatic:** chemotherapy
    - **Unknown:** thiazolidinediones, PPIs
- **Other**
    - **Primary lymphedema:** developmental lymphatic vascular anomalies

- **Secondary lymphedema:** disruption of lymphatic drainage from previous radiation or surgery, obesity, infection, malignancy, CVI
- Lipedema (abnormal accumulation of fat tissue in specific areas of the body, typically the legs, arms, and buttocks)

Notes

General considerations: A detailed medical history and physical should involve determining the chronicity, distribution, and symmetry of edema, obtain pertinent surgical history, and identify systemic symptoms. A careful medication history is essential as many medications can trigger or worsen edema, especially in patients with underlying lymphatic or venous disease. General laboratory evaluation of edema includes BNP, TSH, LFTs, BMP, and urine protein/creatinine ratio.

Red flags: airway compromise, previous extremity trauma, surgery, radiation, systemic symptoms, malignancy

Special populations: Evaluation of non-pitting edema in the pediatric population should involve consideration of primary lymphedema. Lipedema can occur with pubertal onset. Edema may be associated with pregnancy and should be treated with conservative measures (i.e. reducing time spent on feet, leg elevation, resting on the left side, and wearing compressive stockings).

Further Reading

- Patel H, Skok CJ, Demarco A. Peripheral Edema: Evaluation and Management in Primary Care. American Family Physician 2022;106(5):557-564.
- Grada AA, Phillips TJ. Lymphedema: Pathophysiology and clinical manifestations. Journal of the American Academy of Dermatology 2017;77(6):1009-1020. DOI: 10.1016/j.jaad.2017.03.022.
- Merli GJ, Yenser H, Orapallo D. Approach to the Patient with Non-cardiac Leg Swelling. Med Clin North Am 2023;107(5):945-961. (In eng). DOI: 10.1016/j.mcna.2023.05.009.

Skin and Subcutaneous

Carys Kenny-Howell

Long H. Tu

Leah B. Colucci

Rash (Diffuse, Focal)

Introduction

Rash refers to noticeable change in the texture or color of the skin, often presenting as an area of redness, bumps, or irritation. Rash may be accompanied by itching, swelling, or pain. There is wide range of potential etiologies, including infectious (e.g., viral exanthems, bacterial infections), inflammatory (e.g., eczema, psoriasis), allergic (e.g., contact dermatitis), and systemic (e.g., autoimmune diseases, drug reactions) processes. When evaluating a rash, it is important to consider factors such as the rash's distribution, morphology, duration, and any associated systemic symptoms. A thorough assessment includes the patient's medical history, recent exposures, and any new medications.

Checklist DDX

Serious/life-threatening: Stevens-Johnson syndrome, toxic epidermal necrolysis, meningococcemia, melanoma, disseminated intravascular coagulation, Rocky Mountain spotted fever, Kawasaki disease, necrotizing fasciitis, drug reaction with eosinophilia and systemic symptoms (DRESS)

Common: focal (contact dermatitis, cellulitis, herpes simplex virus, impetigo,), diffuse (viral exanthems, psoriasis, seborrheic dermatitis, atopic dermatitis/eczema), either (urticaria, drug eruption)

Commonly misdiagnosed: tickborne rickettsial diseases, cutaneous T-cell lymphoma

Systematic DDX

Categorized by morphology and distribution
- Macules
    - **Generalized/disseminated:** viral exanthem (measles, rubella), secondary syphilis, typhoid, pityriasis versicolor (particularly in humid climates)
    - **Localized:** leukoderma-like patches in tuberculoid leprosy, freckles (sun-exposed areas), chloasma (central face), Berloque dermatitis (photo-distributed)
    - **Mucocutaneous or specific pattern:** vitiligo (often acral and periorificial), neurofibromatosis (café-au-lait spots), Peutz-Jeghers syndrome (perioral and mucosal pigmentation)

- **Other:** allergic reaction (variable), drug eruption (variable, though often generalized), solar lentigines
- Papules and plaques
  - **Localized to skin folds and typical sites:** psoriasis (extensor surfaces), lichen planus (flexural areas), seborrheic dermatitis (scalp, nasolabial folds, eyebrows upper chest), keratosis pilaris (extensor upper arms, thighs), Darier disease/keratosis follicularis (generalized follicular), insect bites
  - **Generalized/multifocal:** scabies (interdigital webs, wrists, axilla), molluscum contagiosum (children, clustered), tinea corporis (localized or widespread), eczema (varied, often flexural in children), Kaposi's sarcoma (lower extremities, mucosa), tuberous sclerosis (facial angiofibromas)
  - **Others:** acne (face, upper back, chest), hyperlipidemia-related xanthomas (extensor surfaces, tendons), folliculitis, drug eruptions, lupus pernio
- Nodules
  - **Localized or regional:** warts (hands, feet), leprosy nodules (cooler areas), syphilis gumma, tuberculosis nodules, atypical mycobacteria, keratoacanthoma (sun-exposed areas), rheumatoid nodules (extensor surfaces), gouty tophi (around joints), epidermoid cysts (face, neck, trunk), lipoma (trunk)
  - **Generalized/systemic:** sarcoidosis (widespread nodules), pyoderma gangrenosum (any site), lymphoma and metastatic carcinoma (variable sites), erythema nodosum (shins)
- Pustules
  - **Localized:** staphylococcal impetigo (mouth, nostrils), folliculitis (hair-bearing areas), pseudomonas hot tub folliculitis (localized bathing areas), herpes simplex/zoster (dermatomal for zoster), candida (intertriginous areas), acne vulgaris (face, upper trunk)
  - **Generalized:** Behçet's disease (oral, genital mucosa, skin), pustular psoriasis (generalized or localized), dermatitis herpetiformis (extensor surfaces), hidradenitis suppurativa (axilla, groin), smallpox/monkeypox (face, extremities), disseminated gonococcal infection (extremities, palms, soles)
- Blisters
  - **Localized:** herpes simplex/zoster (dermatomal or mucocutaneous), bullous impetigo (localized erosions), burns and friction (local trauma sites), insect bites
  - **Generalized or widespread:** varicella (chickenpox), staphylococcal scalded skin syndrome, eczema (varied distribution),

- bullous pemphigoid (mainly elderly), pemphigus vulgaris (mucosal and skin), dermatitis herpetiformis (extensor surfaces), Stevens-Johnson syndrome/toxic epidermal necrolysis, coxsackievirus (hand-foot-and-mouth disease)
  - **Other:** edema-related blisters (dependent areas in congestive heart failure, renal failure, liver failure), drug-induced (variable distribution), autoimmune
- **Petechiae and purpura**
  - **Generalized:** meningococcemia, endocarditis, Rocky Mountain spotted fever, viral hemorrhagic fevers (dengue, Ebola), leukemia, disseminated intravascular coagulation, immune thrombocytopenic purpura, thrombotic thrombocytopenic purpura, IgA vasculitis (lower extremities predominant), systemic lupus erythematosus, sepsis
  - **Localized or dependent areas:** trauma, solar purpura (sun-exposed areas), liver failure, renal failure, vitamin C and K deficiencies, anticoagulant use
- **Erythema**
  - **Localized:** erythema multiforme (target lesions on hands, feet, mucosa), erythema migrans (tick bite area), erythema induratum (posterior lower legs), erythema marginatum (trunk and proximal limbs), cellulitis, contact dermatitis
  - **Generalized or symmetrical:** erythema nodosum (pretibial areas), livedo reticularis (limbs, trunk), erythematous plaques/scales (pityriasis versicolor), palmar erythema (palms, associated with systemic diseases), drug reactions, scarlet fever, rosacea (central face)

Categorized by morphology and pathophysiology
- **Macules**
  - **Infection:** viral exanthem (measles, rubella), pityriasis versicolor, secondary syphilis, tuberculoid leprosy, typhoid
  - **Developmental/congenital:** vitiligo, neurofibromatosis, Peutz-Jeghers syndrome
  - **Other:** allergic reaction, drug eruption, freckles, chloasma, Berloque dermatitis
- **Papules and plaques**
  - **Infection:** scabies, molluscum contagiosum, tinea
  - **Inflammatory:** psoriasis, lichen planus, keratosis follicularis, eczema, keratosis pilaris, seborrheic dermatitis, drug eruptions, lupus pernio
  - **Neoplastic/genetic:** Kaposi's sarcoma, tuberous sclerosis

- o **Other:** hyperlipidemia, insect bite, acne
- **Nodules**
  - o **Infectious:** warts (human papillomavirus), leprosy, syphilis, tuberculosis, atypical mycobacteria
  - o **Metabolic/inflammatory:** gouty tophi, rheumatoid nodules, sarcoidosis, pyoderma gangrenosum, erythema nodosum
  - o **Neoplastic:** keratoacanthoma, lymphoma, metastatic carcinoma
  - o **Other:** epidermoid cysts, lipoma
- **Pustules**
  - o **Infection:** staphylococcal impetigo, folliculitis, pseudomonas (hot tub), herpes simplex/zoster, candida, smallpox/monkeypox, disseminated gonococcal infection
  - o **Inflammatory:** Behçet's, pustular psoriasis, dermatitis herpetiformis, hidradenitis suppurativa, acne vulgaris
- **Blisters (vesicles/bullae)**
  - o **Infection:** herpes simplex/zoster, chickenpox, hand-foot-mouth, bullous impetigo, staphylococcal scalded skin syndrome
  - o **Inflammatory:** eczema, bullous pemphigoid, pemphigus vulgaris, dermatitis herpetiformis, porphyria, epidermolysis bullosa
  - o **Dysfunction:** edema (congestive heart failure, renal failure, liver failure)
  - o **Injury/trauma:** burns, friction, insect bites
  - o **Drug-induced:** Stevens-Johnson syndrome, toxic epidermal necrolysis, ACE inhibitors, barbiturates
- **Petechiae and purpura**
  - o **Infection:** meningococcemia, endocarditis, rocky mountain spotted fever, viral hemorrhagic fevers, sepsis
  - o **Inflammatory/hematologic:** IgA vasculitis, systemic lupus erythematosus, immune thrombocytopenic purpura, thrombotic thrombocytopenic purpura, leukemia, disseminated intravascular coagulation, hemophilia
  - o **Dysfunction/metabolic:** liver failure, renal failure, vitamin deficiency (C/scurvy, K)
  - o **Other:** trauma, aging (solar purpura), drug reaction (warfarin, steroids, non-steroidal anti-inflammatory drugs, cytotoxic agents)
- **Erythema**
  - o **Infectious:** erythema multiforme (herpes simplex, mycoplasma), erythema nodosum (tuberculosis, streptococcus), erythema migrans (Lyme disease), cellulitis
  - o **Inflammatory:** erythema multiforme (Stevens-Johnson syndrome), erythema nodosum (sarcoidosis, inflammatory bowel

disease), erythema marginatum (rheumatic fever), erythema induratum (tuberculosis), livedo reticularis (systemic lupus erythematosus, antiphospholipid syndrome), erythematous scales/plaques (pityriasis versicolor, etc.), rosacea
- **Drug/hormonal:** erythema multiforme (barbiturates, sulfonamides, penicillin's), erythema nodosum (sulfonamides, oral contraceptives)
- **Dysfunction/metabolic:** palmar erythema (liver disease, rheumatoid arthritis, pregnancy, thyrotoxicosis)

Notes

General considerations: When evaluating a rash, focus on its distribution, morphology, and timing in relation to other symptoms and exposure. A thorough history includes recent travel, new medications, and potential environmental and infectious exposures. While many rashes are benign and self-limiting, management should be guided by the most likely etiology, with careful attention to signs of a more serious pathology.

Red flags: rapid spread, systemic symptoms (fever, hypotension, etc.), respiratory distress, involvement of mucous membranes, blistering, skin detachment

Special populations: In children, rashes are frequently due to viral exanthems or allergic reactions. However, serious conditions like Kawasaki disease, meningococcemia, and immune-mediated conditions should be considered. In older adults, rashes may present atypically and can be a sign of underlying systemic disease, such as vasculitis or malignancy. Pregnant women may experience benign rashes that are hormonally mediated (urticaria), but conditions like intrahepatic cholestasis of pregnancy or pemphigoid gestationis should be considered. Immunocompromised patients are at higher risk for opportunistic infections presenting with rash. Poor hygiene, homelessness, and crowded living conditions increase risk for infestations (e.g., scabies, lice), irritant/contact dermatitis, and secondary infections.

Further Reading

- Allmon A, Deane K, Martin KL. Common Skin Rashes in Children. Am Fam Physician. 2015 Aug 1;92(3):211–6.
- McKinnon HD, Howard T. Evaluating the febrile patient with a rash. Am Fam Physician. 2000 Aug 15;62(4):804–16.
- Yan A, Madigan L, Korman A, Shearer S, Dulmage B, Patel T, et al. Morbilliform Eruptions: Differentiating Low-Risk Drug Eruptions, Severe Cutaneous Adverse Reactions, Viral Eruptions, and Acute Graft-

- Versus-Host Disease. Am J Clin Dermatol. 2025 May;26(3):379–93.
- Santistevan J, Long B, Koyfman A. Rash Decisions: An Approach to Dangerous Rashes Based on Morphology. J Emerg Med. 2017 Apr;52(4):457–71.
- Alves F, Gonçalo M. Suspected inflammatory rheumatic diseases in patients presenting with skin rashes. Best Pract Res Clin Rheumatol. 2019 Aug;33(4):101440.
- Ely JW, Seabury Stone M. The generalized rash: part I. Differential diagnosis. Am Fam Physician. 2010 Mar 15;81(6):726–34.
- Ely JW, Seabury Stone M. The generalized rash: part II. Diagnostic approach. Am Fam Physician. 2010 Mar 15;81(6):735–9.

Skin Lesion (Focal/Solitary)

Introduction

A focal or solitary skin lesion is a single, distinct area of altered skin that may vary in size, shape, color, and texture. When evaluating such a lesion, it is crucial to consider its clinical characteristics and any changes over time. Key aspects to consider include the lesion's symmetry, border, color, diameter, and evolution, often summarized by the "ABCDE" criteria for melanoma. The differential diagnosis spans benign conditions such as seborrheic keratosis and dermatofibromas to malignant lesions such as basal cell carcinoma and melanoma. It is important to obtain a comprehensive patient history, including recent trauma, cumulative sun exposure, and family history of skin cancer to guide the diagnostic process.

Checklist DDX

Serious/life-threatening: melanoma, Merkel cell carcinoma, cutaneous squamous cell carcinoma, malignant vascular tumors, cutaneous metastasis, cutaneous T-cell lymphoma

Common: dermatofibroma, seborrheic keratosis, epidermoid inclusion cyst, verruca vulgaris (warts), cherry angioma, benign melanocytic nevus, basal cell carcinoma, acrochordons (skin tags), milia

Commonly misdiagnosed: Merkel cell carcinoma, melanoma, seborrheic keratosis when inflamed, localized chronic fibrosing vasculitis

Systematic DDX

- Macule/patch
    - **Infection:** viral exanthems (measles, rubella, varicella), secondary syphilis (macular syphilide), erythrasma, tinea or pityriasis versicolor
    - **Inflammatory:** vitiligo, cutaneous lupus erythematosus, fixed drug eruption, pityriasis rosea, lichen planus
    - **Neoplastic:** benign melanocytic nevus, malignant melanoma (early), lentigo maligna, mycosis fungoides
    - **Other:** café au lait macules, solar lentigo, freckles, chloasma/melasma

- Papule
    - **Vascular/neoplastic:** cherry angioma, pyogenic granuloma, seborrheic keratosis, basal cell carcinoma (early), neurofibroma, angiofibroma, Langerhans cell histiocytosis
    - **Infection:** molluscum contagiosum, warts (human papillomavirus), scabies, folliculitis
    - **Inflammatory:** lichen planus, granuloma annulare, sarcoidosis, arthropod bite reaction, keratosis pilaris
    - **Other:** xanthomas, milia
- Plaque
    - **Vascular/neoplastic:** hemangioma (superficial), Kaposi's sarcoma, seborrheic keratosis, squamous cell carcinoma in situ, mycosis fungoides
    - **Infection:** tinea corporis, erysipelas, cutaneous leishmaniasis
    - **Inflammatory:** psoriasis, necrobiosis lipoidica, cutaneous lupus erythematosus (discoid), eczema, contact dermatitis
- Nodule
    - **Vascular/neoplastic:** hemangioma (deep), pyogenic granuloma, dermatofibroma, epidermoid cyst, basal cell carcinoma (nodular), squamous cell carcinoma (nodular), malignant melanoma (nodular), Merkel cell carcinoma
    - **Infection:** furuncle/carbuncle/abscess, leprosy
    - **Inflammatory:** rheumatoid nodule, erythema nodosum
- Vesicle/bulla
    - **Infectious:** herpes simplex virus, varicella zoster virus, bullous impetigo, herpes gestationis, coxsackievirus
    - **Inflammatory:** bullous pemphigoid, pemphigus vulgaris, dermatitis herpetiformis, erythema multiforme, epidermolysis bullosa
    - **Other:** fixed drug eruption (bullous), porphyria cutanea tarda, burns, friction blisters, insect bites
- Pustule
    - **Infection:** folliculitis, impetigo (non-bullous), staphylococcal abscess, pseudomonas (hot tub folliculitis), herpes simplex/zoster (pustular), candida, bacillary angiomatosis
    - **Inflammatory:** pustular psoriasis, Behçet's syndrome, dermatitis herpetiformis (pustular), hidradenitis suppurativa, acne vulgaris
- Ulcer/erosion
    - **Vascular/metabolic:** pyoderma gangrenosum, venous stasis ulcer, arterial ulcer, necrobiosis lipoidica (ulcerated), calciphylaxis, pressure ulcer

- o **Infection:** ecthyma, mycobacterium ulcerans (Buruli ulcer), leishmaniasis (ulcerative), cutaneous anthrax (eschar), syphilitic chancre, chancroid
- o **Neoplastic:** squamous cell carcinoma (ulcerated), basal cell carcinoma (ulcerated), cutaneous metastases (ulcerated),
- **Purpura/petechiae/ecchymosis**
  - o **Vascular/inflammatory:** vasculitis (leukocytoclastic, IgA), stasis dermatitis, systemic lupus erythematosus (vasculitic purpura)
  - o **Infection:** meningococcemia, Rocky Mountain spotted fever, infective endocarditis, dengue
  - o **Hematologic/neoplastic:** Kaposi's sarcoma (purpuric), leukemia cutis, lymphoma, thrombocytopenia (immune thrombocytopenic purpura, disseminated intravascular coagulation), coagulopathies (hemophilia)
  - o **Other:** chronic liver disease (coagulopathy), trauma (ecchymosis, hematoma), vitamin C and K deficiencies

Notes

General considerations: Initial assessment of a focal or solitary skin lesion should include a detailed history and physical examination, focusing on the lesion's duration, changes in size or color, associated symptoms (itching, pain, bleeding), and any relevant exposures or trauma. Diagnostic workup may involve skin biopsy, dermoscopy, and laboratory tests to assess for systemic involvement. Imaging studies may be warranted if deeper tissue involvement is suspected.

Red flags: rapid growth or recent change in morphology, irregular or poorly defined borders, color changes, ulceration, bleeding, associated systemic symptoms such as fever or weight loss; concerning "ABCDE" criteria for melanoma (asymmetry, border irregularity, color variation, diameter >6 mm, and evolving nature); immunocompromise, history of skin cancer

Special populations: In children, solitary skin lesions are often benign, such as hemangiomas or molluscum contagiosum. However, large congenital nevi, rapidly changing lesions or those with atypical features should be evaluated for malignancy. In older patients, new or changing lesions may suggest skin cancer, such as basal cell carcinoma or melanoma. Pregnant women may experience changes in skin lesions due to hormonal influences. Immunocompromised individuals are at increased risk for opportunistic infections, cutaneous manifestations of systemic disease, and aggressive skin cancers.

Further Reading

- Rigopoulos D, Larios G, Katsambas A. Skin signs of systemic diseases. Clin Dermatol. 2011;29(5):531–40.
- Gupta MA, Gupta AK. Self-induced dermatoses: A great imitator. Clin Dermatol. 2019;37(3):268–77.
- Mahboob A, Haroon TS. Drugs causing fixed eruptions: a study of 450 cases. Int J Dermatol. 1998 Nov;37(11):833–8.
- Higgins JC, Maher MH, Douglas MS. Diagnosing Common Benign Skin Tumors. afp. 2015 Oct 1;92(7):601–7.
- Requena L, Sangueza OP. Cutaneous vascular anomalies. Part I. Hamartomas, malformations, and dilation of preexisting vessels. J Am Acad Dermatol. 1997 Oct;37(4):523–49; quiz 549–52.
- Beacham BE. Common skin tumors in the elderly. Am Fam Physician. 1992 Jul;46(1):163–8.
- Pampena R, Lai M, Lombardi M, Mirra M, Raucci M, Lallas A, et al. Clinical and Dermoscopic Features Associated With Difficult-to-Recognize Variants of Cutaneous Melanoma: A Systematic Review. JAMA Dermatol. 2020 Apr 1;156(4):430–9.
- Pitambe HV, Schulz EJ. Life-threatening dermatoses due to metabolic and endocrine disorders. Clin Dermatol. 2005;23(3):258–66.

Hives

Introduction

Hives, also known as urticaria, presents as transient, pruritic wheals of varying size and shape. When evaluating urticaria, key factors to consider are the duration and pattern of the wheals, as well as the presence of any associated angioedema. A thorough history should include recent exposures to allergens or triggers, such as foods, medications, insect stings, and environmental exposures. It is also important to note any signs of systemic involvement, including anaphylaxis, which requires urgent intervention.

Checklist DDX

Serious/life-threatening: anaphylaxis, acute urticaria with angioedema involving the airway, hematologic cancers, drug-induced hypersensitivity, mast cell activation

Common: food allergies, insect stings, viral infections (e.g., upper respiratory infections), medications, stress, environmental triggers like cold or heat

Commonly misdiagnosed: conditions that mimic hives but have different pathophysiologic mechanisms (e.g., hereditary angioedema, erythema multiforme, urticaria pigmentosa [cutaneous mastocytosis], autoinflammatory syndromes [cryopyrin-associated periodic syndromes, Schnitzler's syndrome], Wells syndrome, Melkersson–Rosenthal syndrome, Gleich's syndrome, and bullous pemphigoid)

Systematic DDX

- Vascular
    - Urticarial vasculitis (normocomplementemic, hypocomplementemic/ McDuffie syndrome), cryoglobulinemia-associated vasculitis (HCV), immune complex vasculitis (e.g., IgA vasculitis)
- Infection
    - **Bacteria:** helicobacter pylori, streptococci, staphylococci, yersinia, mycoplasma pneumoniae
    - **Virus:** hepatitis viruses (B and C), norovirus, parvovirus B19, Epstein-Barr virus, herpes simplex virus
    - **Protozoa:** giardia lamblia, entamoeba, blastocystis, anisakis
    - **Helminths:** anisakis simplex
- Inflammatory
    - **Rheumatologic:** systemic lupus erythematosus, juvenile idiopathic arthritis

- - o **Autoinflammatory:** Schnitzler syndrome, cryopyrin-associated periodic syndromes
    - o **Mast cell disorder:** systemic mastocytosis, mast cell activation syndrome
  - **Neoplasia and hematologic**
    - o **Hematologic malignancies:** lymphoproliferative disorders (non-Hodgkin lymphoma, chronic lymphocytic leukemia, Waldenström macroglobulinemia), lymphoreticular cancers
    - o **Solid organ tumors:** ovarian, testicular, lung, colon, thyroid
  - **Dysfunction**
    - o **Hepatic:** chronic liver disease, cholestasis
    - o **Renal:** dialysis-related allergies, end-stage renal disease
    - o **Gastrointestinal disorders:** peptic ulcer disease (H. Pylori), gastritis, biliary tract inflammation, celiac disease
  - **Physical**
    - o **Injury/trauma:** Dermatographia (symptomatic dermographism), delayed pressure urticaria, vibratory urticaria
    - o **Other:** cold, cholinergic (heat/exercise), solar
  - **Anomalies of development/aging**
    - o **Genetic disorders:** hereditary angioedema due to C1-inhibitor deficiency, familial urticaria syndromes, autoinflammatory syndromes (e.g., cryopyrin-associated periodic syndromes),
    - o **Developmental:** mast cell disorders (urticaria pigmentosa/cutaneous mastocytosis, mastocytomas, telangiectasia macularis eruptiva perstans)
    - o **Age-related:** acquired C1-inhibitor deficiency, bradykinin-mediated angioedema (acquired C1-inhibitor deficiency and ACE inhibitor use)
    - o **Pregnancy related:** autoimmune progesterone dermatitis
  - **Metabolic**
    - o **Thyroid disease:** hypothyroidism and hyperthyroidism
    - o **Pheochromocytoma**
  - **Allergies**
    - o Food (nuts, shellfish, eggs, milk), insect stings (bees, wasps), latex, medications (penicillin, cephalosporins)
    - o **Non-IgE-mediated mast cell activation:** food additives, radiocontrast agents, opiates
  - **Drug-induced**
    - o **Medications:** aspirin, NSAIDs, ACE inhibitors, antibiotics, oral contraceptives
    - o Serum sickness-like reactions

Notes

General considerations: A detailed exposure history is crucial to identify potential triggers of hives. Management typically involves avoiding known triggers and using antihistamines to alleviate symptoms. In chronic or recurrent cases, further evaluation may be necessary to rule out underlying systemic conditions.

Red flags: angioedema (particularly around the eyes and lips), difficulty breathing, wheezing, dizziness, drop in blood pressure, fever, joint pain

Special populations: In children, acute urticaria is often triggered by infections or food allergies. In older adults, urticaria is more likely to have an underlying systemic cause, such as an autoimmune condition or an adverse medication reaction (related to polypharmacy). In pregnancy, it is important to consider pregnancy-specific dermatoses, such as polymorphic eruption of pregnancy.

Further Reading

- Kanazawa N. Hereditary disorders presenting with urticaria. Immunol Allergy Clin North Am. 2014 Feb;34(1):169–79.
- Davis MDP, van der Hilst JCH. Mimickers of Urticaria: Urticarial Vasculitis and Autoinflammatory Diseases. J Allergy Clin Immunol Pract. 2018;6(4):1162–70.
- Bernstein JA, Lang DM, Khan DA, Craig T, Dreyfus D, Hsieh F, et al. The diagnosis and management of acute and chronic urticaria: 2014 update. J Allergy Clin Immunol. 2014 May;133(5):1270–7.
- Zuberbier T, Aberer W, Asero R, Abdul Latiff AH, Baker D, Ballmer-Weber B, et al. The EAACI/GA²LEN/EDF/WAO guideline for the definition, classification, diagnosis and management of urticaria. Allergy. 2018 Jul;73(7):1393–414.
- Peroni A, Colato C, Zanoni G, Girolomoni G. Urticarial lesions: if not urticaria, what else? The differential diagnosis of urticaria: part II. Systemic diseases. J Am Acad Dermatol. 2010 Apr;62(4):557–70; quiz 571–2.
- Marzano AV, Maronese CA, Genovese G, Ferrucci S, Moltrasio C, Asero R, et al. Urticarial vasculitis: Clinical and laboratory findings with a particular emphasis on differential diagnosis. J Allergy Clin Immunol. 2022 Apr;149(4):1137–49.

Breast Pain

Introduction

Breast pain, or mastalgia, is the second most common breast-related complaint leading to medical evaluation in primary care. It is typically categorized into cyclic and noncyclic in nature. Cyclic pain is generally diffuse, bilateral, and may radiate to the axilla. It often correlates with the luteal phase of the menstrual cycle due to increased breast sensitivity from hormonal changes. Noncyclic pain is often localized and unilateral. It can be associated with factors such as oral contraceptive use, hormone therapy, tumors, trauma, infection, or ligamentous strain. Additionally, it is crucial to consider that breast pain can be referred from nearby structures, including the heart, lungs, and gastrointestinal tract.

Checklist DDX

Serious/life-threatening: inflammatory breast cancer, locally advanced or metastatic breast carcinoma, mastitis, breast abscess, acute coronary syndrome (myocardial ischemia referred to the breast), pulmonary embolism, aortic dissection, tension pneumothorax

Common: hormonal variations, fibrocystic changes, medications (oral contraceptive pills [OCPs], spironolactone), breast cysts, pregnancy or lactational breast engorgement, fat necrosis, improperly fitting bra

Commonly misdiagnosed: costochondritis or other musculoskeletal chest wall pain, cervical radiculopathy or other neuropathic referred pain, gastroesophageal reflux disease or esophageal spasm, macromastia

Systematic DDX

Cyclic mastalgia
- Hormonal fluctuations during the menstrual cycle (estrogen, progesterone), fibrocystic changes, altered pituitary regulation (latent hyperprolactinemia), dietary factors (high dietary fat intake and increased high-density lipoprotein cholesterol during the luteal phase)

Noncyclic mastalgia
- Vascular
  - Superficial thrombophlebitis of the breast (Mondor disease)
  - **Systemic vasculitis involving the breast:** polyarteritis nodosa, granulomatosis with polyangiitis, and giant cell arteritis

- o **Venous congestion:** superior vena cava syndrome, congestive heart failure
- o **Vascular tumors:** angiosarcoma, hemangioma (may also be considered under neoplastic processes)
- Infection
  - o **Mastitis:** acute lactational mastitis, breast abscess, non-lactational (periductal) mastitis, subacute mastitis
  - o **Infectious agents:** bacterial (staphylococcus aureus, coagulase-negative staphylococci, streptococci, anaerobes), viral (herpes zoster virus, shingles), fungal (candida, commonly implicated in "mammary candidiasis,")
  - o **Rare granulomatous or chronic infections:** tuberculosis, other fungal or parasitic infections
- Inflammatory
  - o **Autoimmune mastitis:** systemic lupus erythematosus, Sjögren's disease, IgG4-related disease
  - o **Structural inflammatory changes:** duct ectasia, fat necrosis
  - o **Granulomatous conditions:** idiopathic granulomatous mastitis, vasculitis involving the breast
- Neoplasia and hematologic
  - o **Benign:** breast tumors (fibroadenoma, intraductal papilloma, benign phyllodes tumor, sclerosing adenosis), breast cysts
  - o **Inflammatory breast cancer:** invasive ductal carcinoma, invasive lobular carcinoma, inflammatory breast cancer
  - o **Hematologic:** sickle cell anemia
- Dysfunction/extramammary referred pain
  - o **Cardiac:** myocardial ischemia, angina, pericarditis
  - o **Gastrointestinal:** gastroesophageal reflux disease, esophageal spasm, peptic ulcer disease, cholecystitis
  - o **Pulmonary:** pleurisy, pulmonary embolism
  - o **Musculoskeletal:** costochondritis, Tietze syndrome, pectoral strain, shoulder pain
  - o **Nerve:** cervical radiculopathy, shingles
- Injury/trauma
  - o Blunt trauma to the breast causing hematoma, fat necrosis, local inflammation; chest wall trauma, rib fracture
  - o **Iatrogenic:** post operative pain after lumpectomy, biopsy, or cosmetic surgery; post-radiation pain
- Compression/obstruction
  - o **Mechanical compression:** ill-fitting or unsupportive bras
  - o **Obstruction:** venous congestion (superior vena cava syndrome), duct ectasia, space occupying lesions

- Anomalies of development/aging
    - Macromastia (large-breast traction pain), pregnancy or lactational breast engorgement, breast involution associated with menopause
- Toxic-metabolic
    - **Endocrine:** thyroid (hypothyroidism, hyperthyroidism), hyperprolactinemia
    - **Medications:** hormone therapies (oral contraceptives, hormone replacement therapy, fertility treatments), psychotropic medications (serotonin reuptake inhibitors, antipsychotic agents), cardiovascular agents (diuretics, digitalis, methyldopa), antimicrobial (ketoconazole, metronidazole)
- Everything else
    - **Psychiatric disorders:** anxiety, depression, post-traumatic stress disorder, panic disorder, eating disorders, somatization
    - Breast implant-associated pain (capsular contracture, implant rupture)

Notes

General considerations: Evaluation of breast pain (mastalgia) should focus on distinguishing benign from malignant causes, with attention to the patient's age, menstrual cycle, and any associated symptoms such as lumps, skin changes, or discharge. Although most women with mastalgia do not have radiological findings, diagnostic imaging may be appropriate for those with non-cyclical, focal breast pain, aligning with the American College of Radiology Appropriateness Criteria. Treatment is often conservative, involving reassurance, lifestyle modifications, proper supportive garments, and pain management, unless an underlying pathology is identified.

Red flags: focal, persistent, progressive pain; palpable mass or inflammatory changes; unilateral pain, skin changes, nipple discharge, systemic symptoms such as weight loss or fever

Special populations: In premenopausal women, cyclic breast pain is commonly linked to hormonal fluctuations. Postmenopausal women have greater risk for malignancy. Pregnant and lactating women may experience breast pain due to hormonal changes, engorgement, or mastitis. In men, breast pain should prompt evaluation for gynecomastia, medication side effects or underlying malignancy, especially if accompanied by a mass.

Further Reading

- Holbrook AI, Moy L, Akin EA, Baron P, Didwania AD, Heller SL, et al. ACR Appropriateness Criteria® Breast Pain. Journal of the American College of Radiology. 2018 Nov 1;15(11):S276–82.
- Stachs A, Stubert J, Reimer T, Hartmann S. Benign Breast Disease in Women. Dtsch Arztebl Int. 2019 Aug 9;116(33–34):565–74.
- Preece PE, Mansel RE, Bolton PM, Hughes LM, Baum M, Gravelle IH. Clinical syndromes of mastalgia. Lancet. 1976 Sep 25;2(7987):670–3.
- Smith RL, Pruthi S, Fitzpatrick LA. Evaluation and Management of Breast Pain. Mayo Clinic Proceedings. 2004 Mar 1;79(3):353–72.
- Scott DM. Inflammatory diseases of the breast. Best Pract Res Clin Obstet Gynaecol. 2022 Sep;83:72–87.
- Jiménez E, Arroyo R, Cárdenas N, Marín M, Serrano P, Fernández L, et al. Mammary candidiasis: A medical condition without scientific evidence? PLoS One. 2017;12(7):e0181071.
- Goulabchand R, Hafidi A, Van de Perre P, Millet I, Maria ATJ, Morel J, et al. Mastitis in Autoimmune Diseases: Review of the Literature, Diagnostic Pathway, and Pathophysiological Key Players. J Clin Med. 2020 Mar 30;9(4):958.
- Chetlen AL, Kapoor MM, Watts MR. Mastalgia: Imaging Work-up Appropriateness. Acad Radiol. 2017 Mar;24(3):345–9.

Breast Lump

Introduction

The evaluation of a breast lump begins with a thorough history, including associated symptoms such as pain, skin changes, or nipple discharge It is important to assess hormonal factors, family history of breast cancer, and prior breast conditions. The differential diagnosis ranges from benign processes like cysts and fibroadenomas to malignant conditions such as breast carcinoma. Key factors that guide the likelihood of each diagnosis include the patient's age, the duration, the evolution of the lump, and any history of trauma or breast surgery.

Checklist DDX

Serious/life-threatening: primary breast malignancy (invasive ductal carcinoma, invasive lobular carcinoma, malignant phyllodes tumors, primary breast lymphoma, primary breast sarcoma), metastatic disease to the breast (melanoma, lung, ovarian cancers)

Common: simple cysts, fibrocystic changes, fibroadenoma, fat necrosis (following trauma or surgery), lipomas

Commonly misdiagnosed: fat necrosis, fibroadenoma in older women, complex cysts, papillary lesions, inflammatory breast carcinoma

Systematic DDX

- Vascular
    - **Benign vascular tumors:** hemangiomas (capillary, cavernous, perilobular), angiolipomas, papillary endothelial hyperplasia
    - **Malignant vascular tumors:** primary angiosarcoma of the breast, hemangiopericytoma, epithelioid hemangioendothelioma
    - **Non-neoplastic:** vasculitis involving the breast, thrombophlebitis (Mondor's disease), vascular malformations (arteriovenous malformations, venous varices)
- Infection
    - **Bacterial:** mastitis, abscess, non-puerperal mastitis, subareolar abscesses, actinomycosis of the breast, commonly staphylococcus aureus and streptococci
    - **Mycobacterial:** breast tuberculosis, mycobacterium gordonae
    - **Fungal:** cryptococcal mastitis
    - **Parasitic:** filariasis, hydatid disease

- **Inflammatory**
  - Idiopathic granulomatous mastitis, periductal mastitis, duct ectasia, lymphocytic mastopathy, sarcoidosis, granulomatosis with polyangiitis, vasculitis, foreign body granuloma, amyloidosis, necrobiotic xanthogranulomatosis, IgG4-related mastitis
- **Neoplasia and hematologic**
  - **Benign neoplasms:** fibroadenoma, benign phyllodes tumor, intraductal papilloma, lipoma, hamartoma, benign vascular tumors (as above)
  - **Malignant neoplasms:** primary (invasive ductal carcinoma, invasive lobular carcinoma, other invasive breast carcinomas, ductal carcinoma in situ, malignant phyllodes tumors, primary breast lymphoma, primary breast sarcoma, Paget disease of the breast), metastatic disease to the breast (melanoma, lung, ovarian cancer)
  - **Hematologic:** primary and secondary breast lymphomas (diffuse large B-cell lymphoma, follicular lymphoma, marginal zone lymphoma, T-cell lymphomas), plasmacytoma, myeloid sarcoma
  - **Iatrogenic breast malignancies:** radiation-associated angiosarcoma, breast implant-associated anaplastic large cell lymphoma
- **Dysfunction**
  - Chronic renal failure (vascular calcifications in the breast, amyloidosis)
- **Injury/trauma**
  - Breast hematoma, fat necrosis, post-traumatic pseudolipoma, traumatic exacerbation of pre-existing benign lesions (e.g., fibroadenoma)
- **Compression/obstruction**
  - Duct ectasia, blocked ducts, inspissated secretions, galactocele, periductal mastitis
- **Anomalies of development/aging**
  - **Development:** developmental breast cysts, hamartomas, pseudoangiomatous stromal hyperplasia, gynecomastia, ectopic (accessory breast tissue), supernumerary nipples
  - **Aging:** fibrocystic changes, simple cysts, epithelial hyperplasia (with or without atypia), papilloma, adenosis
- **Toxic-metabolic**
  - **Medications associated with gynecomastia/glandular hypertrophy:** antipsychotics, antidepressants, prokinetic agents (metoclopramide, domperidone), hormonal therapies (hGH, estrogens, hCG, anti-androgens, GnRH analogs and 5-α reductase inhibitors), spironolactone, cimetidine, ketoconazole

- o **Endocrine:** hyperprolactinemia, thyroid dysfunction, diabetes mellitus (diabetic mastopathy)
- **Everything else**
  - o Post-surgical or post-radiation changes, foreign body granuloma, chest wall lesions (costochondral joint swelling, rib exostoses, chondrosarcoma)

Notes

General considerations: The evaluation of a breast lump begins with clinical assessment, often followed by imaging (mammography and/or ultrasound) to further characterize the lump. If features are suspicious or indeterminate, tissue sampling via biopsy may be necessary to determine the nature of the lump. While the majority of breast lumps are benign, it is important to have a high index of concern for malignancy in patients over 40 or with a family history of breast cancer.

Red flags: hard mass, immobile mass, irregular or poorly defined borders, overlying skin changes such as dimpling, nipple retraction or inversion, bloody nipple discharge, rapid growth, axillary lymphadenopathy, systemic symptoms such as weight loss

Special populations: In children and adolescents, breast lumps are often benign and related to hormonal changes, such as fibroadenomas. Older patients have a greater risk of malignancy and warrant more urgent evaluation. During pregnancy and lactation, breast lumps are often due to benign conditions like galactoceles or mastitis; breast cancer is still possible in this population however. In immunocompromised patients, infections such as abscesses may present as breast lumps and require appropriate management.

Further Reading

- Sterns EE. Age-related breast diagnosis. Can J Surg. 1992 Feb;35(1):41–5.
- Sargent RE, Sener SF. Benign Breast Disease: Periareolar Mastitis, Granulomatous Lobular Mastitis, and Lymphocytic or Diabetic Mastopathy. Surg Clin North Am. 2022 Dec;102(6):1007–16.
- Gatta G, Pinto A, Romano S, Ancona A, Scaglione M, Volterrani L. Clinical, mammographic and ultrasonographic features of blunt breast trauma. Eur J Radiol. 2006 Sep;59(3):327–30.
- Reisenbichler E, Hanley KZ. Developmental disorders and malformations of the breast. Semin Diagn Pathol. 2019 Jan;36(1):11–5.
- Deepinder F, Braunstein GD. Drug-induced gynecomastia: an evidence-based review. Expert Opin Drug Saf. 2012 Sep;11(5):779–95.

- Bennett DL, Buckley A, Lee MV. Fibrocystic Change. Radiol Clin North Am. 2024 Jul;62(4):581–92.
- Morcomb EF, Dargel CM, Anderson SA. Mastitis: Rapid Evidence Review. Am Fam Physician. 2024 Aug;110(2):174–82.
- Ferris-James DM, Iuanow E, Mehta TS, Shaheen RM, Slanetz PJ. Imaging approaches to diagnosis and management of common ductal abnormalities. Radiographics. 2012;32(4):1009–30.

Palpable Soft Tissue Abnormality (Other)

Introduction

Palpable soft tissue abnormalities encompass a broad range of etiologies from benign conditions such as lipomas and cysts to more concerning pathologies like sarcomas and lymphomas. These soft tissue masses are classified as mesenchymal tumors, skin appendageal lesions, metastatic tumors, other tumors and tumorlike lesions, inflammatory lesions or infectious processes. It is often useful to consider the patient age group (adults vs children and adolescents), the depth of the lesion (cutaneous, subcutaneous, or fascial layers), and the anatomic location (extremity, head and neck, or trunk).

Checklist DDX

Serious/life-threatening: soft tissue sarcoma, lymphoma, metastatic cancer, necrotizing fasciitis, pseudoaneurysm

Common: lipoma, fibroma, epidermoid/sebaceous cyst, ganglion cyst, pilonidal cyst, post-traumatic hematoma or seroma, abscess, lymphadenopathy

Commonly misdiagnosed: benign peripheral nerve sheath tumors, dermatofibromas, soft tissue sarcoma, pseudoaneurysm

Systematic DDX

- Vascular
    - **Arterial:** pseudoaneurysm, true arterial aneurysm
    - **Venous:** superficial venous varicosities, venous malformations, superficial thrombophlebitis
    - **Vascular tumors or malformations:** hemangiomas, angioleiomyoma, high-flow arteriovenous malformation or fistula
- Infection
    - **Skin and soft tissue infections:** cellulitis, erysipelas, furuncles, carbuncles, abscess, infected cyst (common pathogens: staphylococcus aureus including MRSA, streptococcus pyogenes)
    - **Necrotizing soft tissue infections:** necrotizing fasciitis and clostridial myonecrosis (gas gangrene)
    - **Pathogens in the immunocompromised:** gram-negative bacteria, fungi (e.g., aspergillus), viruses (e.g., herpes simplex, varicella zoster)

- - Less common: mycobacterial (e.g., mycobacterium marinum), deep fungal infections, parasitic infestations (e.g., cutaneous myiasis)
- Inflammatory
  - Inflammatory myopathies: polymyositis, dermatomyositis, focal myositis
  - Granulomatous diseases: sarcoidosis, rheumatoid nodules, ANCA-associated vasculitides (e.g., granulomatosis with polyangiitis, eosinophilic granulomatosis with polyangiitis)
  - Fibrosclerotic and pseudotumor disorders: retroperitoneal fibrosis, sclerosing mediastinitis, orbital pseudotumor, inflammatory pseudotumor
  - Soft-tissue and rheumatic conditions: tendinitis, bursitis, myositis ossificans
  - Lymphadenopathy
- Neoplasia and hematologic
  - Benign neoplastic: lipoma, schwannoma, neurofibroma, hemangioma, leiomyoma, angiomyoma, fibroma of tendon sheath, benign fibrous histiocytoma, pilomatricoma
  - Intermediate (locally aggressive/rarely metastasizing): desmoid fibromatosis, giant cell tumor of tendon sheath, inflammatory myofibroblastic tumor, dermatofibrosarcoma protuberans
  - Malignant neoplastic: soft tissue sarcomas (undifferentiated pleomorphic sarcoma, synovial sarcoma, leiomyosarcoma, myxofibrosarcoma, fibrosarcoma, liposarcoma, rhabdomyosarcoma), angiosarcoma, malignant peripheral nerve sheath tumor, myxoid variants of several sarcomas
  - Hematologic: extramedullary hematopoiesis (thalassemia, sickle cell disease, myelofibrosis, leukemia), hematologic malignancies (lymphoma, leukemia, multiple myeloma), histiocytic disorders (hemophagocytic lymphohistiocytosis), soft tissue swelling due to bleeding (hemophilia) or immune complex deposition (cryoglobulinemia)
- Dysfunction
  - Abdominal wall dysfunction: hernia (inguinal, femoral, umbilical)
- Injury/trauma
  - Hematoma, seroma, fat necrosis, post-traumatic lipoma, muscle tear or contusion, myositis ossificans, Morel-Lavallée lesion, fibrocartilaginous pseudotumor

- **Compression/obstruction**
    - Lymphedema, venous congestion (deep vein thrombosis, chronic venous insufficiency), acute compartment syndrome, deep-tissue pressure injury
- **Anomalies of development/aging**
    - **Developmental:** congenital cysts (branchial cleft cysts, thyroglossal duct cysts), vascular malformations, accessory or anomalous muscles, benign hamartomatous lesions
    - **Aging:** mucoid degeneration (tendons, ligaments, articular discs), elastofibroma dorsi, Dupuytren's contracture, trigger finger
- **Toxic-metabolic**
    - **Toxic myopathies:** statins, alcohol, corticosteroids, antiretroviral agents, colchicine, some chemotherapeutics
    - **Toxic tendinopathies:** fluoroquinolone antibiotics, glucocorticoids, statins, aromatase inhibitors
    - **Metabolic:** diabetes mellitus, familial hypercholesterolemia, cerebrotendinous xanthomatosis, gout, alkaptonuria, hypophosphatasia, tumoral calcinosis
- **Everything else**
    - **Other dermatologic lesions:** dermatofibroma, seborrheic keratosis, acrochordon (skin tag), sebaceous hyperplasia, cherry angioma, epidermal inclusion cysts, pilar cysts, keratoacanthoma, pyogenic granuloma, basal cell carcinoma, squamous cell carcinoma, melanoma

Notes

General considerations: Initial evaluation should focus on the characteristics of the mass, such as size, consistency, mobility, location and tenderness, history of trauma, and any associated systemic symptoms. Imaging and biopsy may be warranted for definitive diagnosis, particularly if the mass is rapidly growing, firm, painful, fixed to underlying structures or associated with systemic symptoms.

Red flags: rapid growth, fixation to underlying structures, ulceration, associated systemic symptoms (fever, weight loss, or night sweats), recurrence after excision

Special populations: In children, soft tissue masses are often benign but can include serious tumors such as sarcomas or lymphomas. In older patients, the likelihood of malignancy increases, and masses may be related to metastatic disease. Pregnant patients may experience changes in soft tissue due to hormonal influences. Immunocompromised individuals are at higher risk for infectious causes, including atypical mycobacterial infections, deep fungal infections, and abscesses. Post-surgical or radiation patients can develop benign masses like fat necrosis or scar tissue, but also malignancies like radiation-induced angiosarcoma.

Further Reading

- Ahmed Malik F, Roy Chaudhary S, Edwards N, Rajasekaran RB, Chari B. Non-neoplastic pathologies mimicking sarcoma - Experience from a tertiary referral centre multidisciplinary team. Eur J Radiol. 2022 Nov;156:110510.
- Achar S, Yamanaka J, Oberstar J. Soft Tissue Masses: Evaluation and Treatment. Am Fam Physician. 2022 Jun 1;105(6):602–12.
- Beaman FD, Kransdorf MJ, Andrews TR, Murphey MD, Arcara LK, Keeling JH. Superficial soft-tissue masses: analysis, diagnosis, and differential considerations. Radiographics. 2007;27(2):509–23.
- Beaman FD, Kransdorf MJ, Andrews TR, Murphey MD, Arcara LK, Keeling JH. Superficial Soft-Tissue Masses: Analysis, Diagnosis, and Differential Considerations. RadioGraphics. 2007 Mar;27(2):509–23.
- Gaddey HL, Riegel AM. Unexplained Lymphadenopathy: Evaluation and Differential Diagnosis. Am Fam Physician. 2016 Dec 1;94(11):896–903.
- Schaefer IM, Fletcher CDM. Recent advances in the diagnosis of soft tissue tumours. Pathology. 2018 Jan;50(1):37–48.

Neurologic

Carys Kenny-Howell

Susan L. Giampalmo

Long H. Tu

Headache

Introduction

Headache is a common symptom that can present with a variety of accompanying features such as nausea, photophobia, or aura. The differential diagnosis for headache encompasses a wide range of conditions, from benign primary headaches like tension-type or migraines to more serious secondary causes. When the cause is unclear ("headache of unknown origin"), consider vascular events, intracranial pathologies, infections, and medication side effects. Special scenarios, including immunocompromised states, recent trauma, and pregnancy, require careful evaluation due to their associations with specific etiologies.

Checklist DDX

Serious/life-threatening: intracranial hemorrhage, thromboembolic (stroke may rarely present as headache, cavernous sinus thrombosis, venous sinus thrombosis), other vascular (vasospasm, hypertensive emergency, internal carotid or vascular artery dissection), intracranial mass lesion (brain tumor), increased intracranial pressure (obstructive hydrocephalus, herniation, idiopathic intracranial hypertension – also vision related, as below), neuro-ophthalmic/vision related (acute angle closure glaucoma, temporal arteritis), infectious (meningitis, encephalitis, brain abscess), toxic (carbon monoxide, heavy metals)

Common: primary headache (e.g., tension, migraine, cluster), musculoskeletal/referred (e.g., TMJ, muscle strain), viral/benign infectious (e.g., sinusitis), post-traumatic, iatrogenic (e.g., post-lumbar puncture)

Commonly misdiagnosed: idiopathic intracranial hypertension, spontaneous intracranial hypertension, medication-overuse headache

Systematic DDX

Primary headache (no underlying cause)
- Migraine, tension headache, cluster headache; headache from cough, exercise, primary stabbing headache, occipital neuralgia

Secondary headache
- Vascular
  - **Hemorrhagic:** intracranial hemorrhage (epidural, subdural, subarachnoid, parenchymal), aneurysm (including sentinel), arteriovenous malformation, pituitary apoplexy

- o **Ischemic or vaso-occlusive:** ischemic stroke, internal carotid artery or vertebral artery dissection, cerebral venous thrombosis
- o **Vasculopathies:** reversible cerebral vasoconstriction syndrome (RCVS), posterior reversible encephalopathy syndrome (PRES)
- o **Blood pressure-related:** hypertensive emergency, pre-eclampsia, eclampsia

- Infection
  - o **Central nervous system:** meningitis, encephalitis, brain abscess
  - o **Paranasal and contiguous:** sinusitis, otitis media, mastoiditis, dental abscesses, orbital cellulitis
  - o **Systemic:** Influenza, COVID-19
- Inflammatory
  - o **Vasculitis:** giant cell arteritis, systemic lupus erythematosus, polyarteritis nodosa, Takayasu arteritis, eosinophilic granulomatosis with polyangiitis (Churg-Strauss)
  - o Optic neuritis
- Dysfunction
  - o Cervicogenic headaches, temporomandibular joint disease, spontaneous intracranial hypotension
- Neoplasia and hematologic
  - o **Brain tumor:** glioblastoma, meningioma, hemangioblastoma, schwannoma, pituitary adenoma
- Injury/trauma
  - o Traumatic brain injury, concussion, post-concussive syndrome, dural tear producing intracranial hypotension (e.g., post-procedural)
- Compression/obstruction
  - o Hydrocephalus, idiopathic intracranial hypertension, glaucoma, trigeminal neuralgia, third ventricle colloid cysts
- Anomalies of development/aging
  - o Paget disease of bone, temporomandibular joint disease
- Toxic-metabolic
  - o Alcohol use or withdrawal, caffeine withdrawal, opioid withdrawal, sympathomimetics
  - o Carbon monoxide poisoning
  - o **Medication overuse:** analgesics, triptans, opioids, ergotamines, nifedipine, glyceryl trinitrate
  - o **Metabolic:** hypoglycemia, hypoxemia, hypothyroidism, dehydration
  - o Menstrual-related headache

- **Everything else**
    - Psychosis, depression, stress

Special scenarios (which overlap with above)
- **Infection in HIV/immunocompromised patients**
    - Toxoplasmosis, HSV encephalitis, bacterial abscess, cryptococcus, tuberculosis, malignancy (lymphoma)
- **Postpartum headache**
    - Post-dural puncture headache, other vascular causes

Notes

General considerations: Many common causes of headache involve lifestyle factors such as hydration, sleep, alcohol/tobacco consumption, and stress, so modification is often recommended alongside supportive treatment for these cases of primary headache. Expectations about headaches and their possible reoccurrence should also be managed to help patients recognize the patterns of their symptoms and the meanings behind them. Often times, in the absence of red flag symptoms, emergency imaging is not required for headache.

Red flags: (SNOOP mnemonic) systemic symptoms, neurological symptoms, onset >50 years old, onset is sudden, and pattern changes of headache; subacute or progressive headache in an older patient, onset associated with sneezing or coughing, rash, fever, meningismus, pregnancy; history of trauma, eye pain, painkiller overuse, malignancy

Special populations: Patients with a malignancy can have a higher risk of cerebral venous sinus thrombosis and ischemic stroke. Immunocompromised patients are more susceptible to infectious etiologies of headache. In pregnancy or postpartum, new or worsening headaches may indicate conditions like preeclampsia, cerebral venous sinus thrombosis, or subarachnoid hemorrhage. Patients over 50 are at increased risk for vascular and oncologic etiologies.

Further Reading

- Viera AJ, Antono B Acute Headache in Adults: A Diagnostic Approach. Am Fam Physician. 2022 Sep;106(3):260–8.
- Robbins MS. Diagnosis and Management of Headache: A Review. JAMA. 2021 May 11;325(18):1874–85.
- Walling A. Frequent Headaches: Evaluation and Management. Am Fam Physician. 2020 Apr 1;101(7):419–28.
- Kopel D, Peeler C, Zhu S. Headache Emergencies. Neurologic Clinics.

2021 May 1;39(2):355–72.
- Dodick D. Pearls: Headache. Semin Neurol. 2010 Feb;30(01):074–81.
- Tintinalli, J. E., & Ma, O. J. (2020). Headaches. Tintinalli's emergency medicine: A comprehensive study guide (9th edition). McGraw-Hill.

Focal Weakness

Introduction

When diagnosing focal weakness, it is important to consider the onset and site of weakness, as well as any possible precipitating factors, such as trauma. Nerve injuries may be the result of external insult, internal insult, intrinsic lesion, or increased susceptibility to injury through another disease process. While some nerve injuries may recover over time, others may not recover and even progress to further weakness and paralysis.

Checklist DDX

Serious/life-threatening: vascular (ischemic or hemorrhagic stroke, spinal cord infarction), infectious (spinal epidural abscess, encephalitis, myelitis), and neoplastic/oncologic emergencies (spinal cord compression due to metastatic disease, primary brain tumors)

Common: peripheral nerve compression syndromes (e.g., carpal tunnel syndrome, ulnar neuropathy), musculoskeletal injuries (e.g., rotator cuff tear, lumbar radiculopathy), and minor cerebrovascular events (e.g., transient ischemic attacks)

Commonly misdiagnosed: functional neurological disorders, early-stage neurodegenerative diseases (e.g., amyotrophic lateral sclerosis), and atypical presentations of migraine or seizure disorders

Systematic DDX

Pathophysiologic approach
- Vascular
    - Stroke (ischemic, hemorrhagic), aneurysmal subarachnoid hemorrhage, spinal cord infarction, nerve infarction, reversible cerebral vasoconstriction syndrome (RCVS)
- Infection
    - Poliomyelitis, diphtheria, viral myositis, infectious radiculopathy, spinal abscess, post-infectious (e.g., acute flaccid myelitis)
- Inflammatory
    - Transverse myelitis, inflammation of nerve root or plexus, inflammatory myopathy

- **Neoplasia and hematologic**
    - Central nervous system tumor (brain, spinal cord), tumor infiltration of plexus, paraneoplastic syndromes (e.g., Lambert Eaton myasthenic syndrome)
- **Dysfunction**
    - **Acquired neuromuscular diseases:** amyotrophic lateral sclerosis, Guillain-Barré syndrome, myasthenia gravis
    - **Musculoskeletal:** disuse atrophy, tendon rupture
    - Seizures (post-ictal state/Todd's paralysis)
- **Injury/trauma**
    - Spinal cord transection, trauma, laceration, surgery, injections
- **Compression/obstruction**
    - Compressive myelopathy: epidural abscess, hematoma, tumor; entrapment neuropathy
- **Anomalies of development/aging**
    - **Hereditary neuromuscular diseases:** spinal muscular atrophy, Charcot-Marie-Tooth disease, congenital myasthenia, Duchenne muscular dystrophy
- **Toxic-metabolic**
    - **Neuromuscular toxins:** botulinum, tetrodotoxin, ciguatoxin, bungarotoxins, thallium, arsenic
    - **Medication-induced myopathies:** statins, corticosteroid
    - **Endocrine:** diabetic amyotrophy, porphyria
    - **Metabolic:** thiamine deficiency, electrolyte disturbances
- **Everything else**
    - Functional weakness, period of unconsciousness (anesthetic or other), tick toxicosis/paralysis

Localization approach
- **Brain**
    - Ischemic stroke, intracranial hemorrhage, mass lesions
- **Spinal cord (myelopathy)**
    - Transverse myelitis, spinal infection, compressive myelopathies
- **Anterior horn cell (motor neuron disorders)**
    - Amyotrophic lateral sclerosis, poliomyelitis
- **Nerve root (radiculopathy)**
    - Disc herniation, fractures, abscess
- **Plexus (plexopathy)**
    - Idiopathic plexitis, compressive plexopathies

- **Peripheral nerve (neuropathy)**
  - Demyelinating (Guillain-Barré syndrome), infectious (diphtheria), nutritional (thiamine deficiency), toxic (thallium, arsenic), metabolic (porphyria)
- **Neuromuscular junction**
  - Myasthenia gravis, Lambert Eaton syndrome, botulism, envenomation
- **Muscle (myopathy)**
  - Inflammatory myopathy, viral myositis

Notes

General considerations: Imaging studies, such as MRI or CT scans, are often necessary to identify structural lesions or vascular events. Laboratory tests may be needed to rule out metabolic or infectious causes of focal weakness. Treatment should be guided by the specific diagnosis, with urgent intervention required for conditions like stroke or spinal cord compression.

Red flags: sudden onset weakness, progression/deterioration, altered mental status, severe headache, loss of bowel or bladder control

Special populations: In children, focal weakness may be due to congenital conditions, infections, or inflammatory processes such as Guillain-Barré syndrome. In older adults, it is often associated with cerebrovascular accidents or degenerative diseases like Parkinson's. Pregnant women may experience focal weakness due to hormonal changes or vascular events such as stroke. Immunocompromised individuals are at increased risk for opportunistic infections affecting the nervous system, while those with severe social/economic risks may have delayed presentations due to limited access to healthcare.

Further Reading

- Virmani T, Agarwal A, Klawiter EC. Clinical Reasoning: A young adult presents with focal weakness and hemorrhagic brain lesions. Neurology. 2011 May 31;76(22):e106–9.
- El-Sherif Y, Sarva H, Valsamis H. Clinical Reasoning: An unusual lung mass causing focal weakness. Neurology. 2012 Jan 10;78(2):e4–7.
- Tarulli A. Focal Limb Weakness. In: Tarulli A, editor. Neurology: A Clinician's Approach [Internet]. Cham: Springer International Publishing; 2021 [cited 2024 Jul 8]. p. 159–69. Available from: https://doi.org/10.1007/978-3-030-55598-6_11
- Fuller G. Focal Peripheral Neuropathies. Journal of Neurology,

Neurosurgery & Psychiatry. 2003 Jun 1;74(90002):20ii–24.
- Larson ST, Wilbur J. Muscle Weakness in Adults: Evaluation and Differential Diagnosis. Am Fam Physician. 2020 Jan 15;101(2):95–108.
- Sivadasan A, Cortel-LeBlanc MA, Cortel-LeBlanc A, Katzberg H. Peripheral nervous system and neuromuscular disorders in the emergency department: A review. Academic Emergency Medicine. 2024;31(4):386–97.
- Werhahn KJ. Weakness and focal sensory deficits in the postictal state. Epilepsy & Behavior. 2010 Oct 1;19(2):138–9.

Focal Paresthesia

Introduction

Focal paresthesia, characterized by abnormal sensations such as burning, tingling, prickling, cutting, or "pins and needles," requires careful evaluation of its onset, duration, and distribution. Paresthesia can arise from a variety of causes, ranging from benign to serious, and may indicate underlying neurological or systemic conditions. Vascular and nerve compression etiologies are common. Some causes require emergent attention, such as stroke and acute spinal cord compression.

Checklist DDX

Serious/life-threatening: vascular events (stroke), acute spinal cord compression (e.g., tumor), inflammatory disorder (e.g., multiple sclerosis)

Common: peripheral nerve compression (e.g., carpal tunnel syndrome), musculoskeletal issues (e.g., cervical or lumbar radiculopathy), metabolic disorders (diabetes mellitus)

Commonly misdiagnosed: atypical presentations of migraines or seizure disorders, early degenerative disorders (e.g., multiple sclerosis), functional neurologic disorders

Systematic DDX

- Vascular
    - **Ischemic:** ischemic stroke, transient ischemic attack, cerebral venous sinus thrombosis, anterior spinal artery infarct
    - **Hemorrhagic:** subarachnoid, intracerebral hemorrhage
    - **Vasculitis:** polyarteritis nodosa, granulomatosis with polyangiitis
    - **Vascular malformations:** arteriovenous malformations, cavernous angiomas
- Infection
    - Herpes zoster (reactivation of varicella-zoster), Lyme disease (Borrelia burgdorferi), neurosyphilis, Tuberculosis with central nervous system or nerve involvement
    - **HIV-associated:** HIV sensory neuropathy, progressive multifocal leukoencephalopathy with focal demyelination

- **Inflammatory**
    - Multiple sclerosis, Guillain-Barré syndrome, transverse myelitis, neurosarcoidosis, vasculitic neuropathies, systemic lupus erythematosus, chronic inflammatory demyelinating polyneuropathy
- **Neoplasia and hematologic**
    - **Central nervous system tumor:** meningioma, astrocytic tumor
    - **Nerve sheath tumors:** schwannoma
    - Paraneoplastic syndromes
- **Organ dysfunction**
    - Seizure
- **Injury/trauma**
    - Peripheral nerve injury (laceration, stretch injury), spinal cord trauma, post-surgical
- **Compression/obstruction**
    - **Compression of spinal cord, peripheral nerves, nerve roots:** by tumor, abscess, hematoma, degenerative change, or anatomic variation
    - **Vascular compression:** thoracic outlet syndrome
- **Anomalies of development/aging**
    - **Developmental:** Chiari malformations, tethered cord, anomalous innervation patterns
    - **Aging:** cervical spondylosis with radiculopathy
- **Toxic-metabolic**
    - **Medication-induced neuropathy:** chemotherapy (platinum compounds, taxanes), isoniazid, metronidazole
    - **Toxins:** lead, arsenic
    - **Endocrine:** diabetes mellitus, hypothyroidism
    - **Deficiencies:** Vitamin B12, B6, E
- **Everything else**
    - Functional neurologic disorder, referred pain

Notes

General considerations: It is important to note the onset and duration of the paresthesia, as well as location and distribution, associated symptoms, and precipitating factors. A thorough physical and neurological examination as well as any relevant imaging studies should be conducted if a nervous system pathology is suspected.

Red flags: weakness or speech difficulties, progressive symptoms, systemic symptoms such as fever, unexplained weight loss, night sweats

Special populations: Older adults have a higher risk of vascular events and degenerative changes. Diabetic patients are particularly prone to peripheral neuropathy, necessitating regular monitoring for sensory changes to prevent complications. Immunocompromised individuals, including those with HIV or undergoing chemotherapy, have an increased susceptibility to infections such as herpes zoster, which can present with focal paresthesia.

Further Reading

- De Kock L, Van der Cruyssen F, Gruijthuijsen L, Politis C. Facial Paresthesia, a Rare Manifestation of Hereditary Neuropathy With Liability to Pressure Palsies: A Case Report. Front Neurol. 2021;12:726437.
- Brigo F, Tomelleri G, Bovi P, Bovi T. Hemiparesthesias in lacunar pontine ischemic stroke. Neurol Sci. 2012 Jun;33(3):619–21.
- Gwathmey KG, Smith AG. Immune-Mediated Neuropathies. Neurol Clin. 2020 Aug;38(3):711–35.
- Gwathmey KG, Tracy JA, Dyck PJB. Peripheral Nerve Vasculitis: Classification and Disease Associations. Neurol Clin. 2019 May;37(2):303–33.
- Beachy N, Satkowiak K, Gwathmey KG. Vasculitic Neuropathies. Semin Neurol. 2019 Oct;39(5):608–19.

Speech Abnormalities

Introduction

Speech abnormalities encompass a range of disorders affecting the ability to produce or comprehend spoken language. These can manifest as difficulties in articulation, fluency, voice, or language processing. Speech abnormalities can result from a variety of causes, including neurological, structural, or psychological factors, and may significantly impact communication and quality of life. A comprehensive evaluation is essential to determine the underlying cause and guide appropriate management.

Checklist DDX

Serious/life-threatening: stroke, neurodegenerative diseases (ALS, multiple sclerosis), brain tumors

Common: developmental speech and language disorders (articulation disorders, language delays), dysarthria and aphasia (stroke, traumatic brain injury), vocal cord pathologies (nodules, polyps), neurodegenerative diseases (Parkinson's disease), intoxication

Commonly misdiagnosed: functional speech disorders, muscle tension dysphonia, spasmodic dysphonia.

Systematic DDX

- **Vascular**
    - Stroke, transient ischemic attack; thoracic aortic aneurysm or dissection (Ortner's syndrome)
- **Infection**
    - Oral thrush, laryngitis, encephalitis (varicella zoster virus, herpes simplex virus), meningitis
- **Inflammatory**
    - **Demyelinating disease:** multiple sclerosis
    - Autoimmune encephalitis
- **Neoplasia and hematologic**
    - Brain tumor, oral/pharyngeal tumor
- **Dysfunction**
    - Orofacial myofunctional disorders, amyotrophic lateral sclerosis, seizure/post-ictal

- **Injury/trauma**
  - Traumatic brain injury, concussion
- **Compression/obstruction**
  - **Recurrent laryngeal nerve compression:** thyroid enlargement (multinodular goiter, thyroid carcinoma), esophageal carcinoma, mediastinal or paratracheal lymphadenopathy, large anterior mediastinal masses (thymoma), cervical or retropharyngeal hematoma
  - **Vocal cord compression:** laryngeal tumors (laryngeal squamous cell carcinoma)
  - **Glottic obstruction:** vocal fold nodules or polyps
- **Anomalies of development/aging**
  - **Development:** childhood apraxia of speech, autism spectrum disorder, attention deficit hyperactivity disorder, Down syndrome
  - **Congenital structural abnormalities:** cleft palate, cerebral palsy
  - **Dementia:** Parkinson's disease, Alzheimer's disease
- **Toxic-Metabolic**
  - **Metabolic encephalopathies:** hypoglycemia, hepatic encephalopathy
  - **Endocrine:** hypothyroidism, Wilson's disease,
  - **Medication-induced:** antipsychotics, sedatives, anticholinergics, neurotoxic agents
  - **Toxins:** alcohol or drug intoxication, heavy metal poisoning
- **Everything else**
  - Hearing impairment
  - **Psychiatric disorders:** mood disorders, psychosis, schizophrenia, catatonia

Notes

General considerations: Speech-language pathologists often play a crucial role in the assessment and management of speech disorders. Diagnostic imaging, such as MRI or CT scans, and other tests may be necessary to identify underlying neurological or structural causes. Treatment should be tailored to the specific etiology, with a focus on improving communication abilities and addressing any underlying conditions.

Red flags: sudden onset, hemiparesis, facial droop, altered consciousness, progressive speech difficulties with cognitive decline

Special populations: In children, early identification and intervention for speech and language disorders are crucial. Older adults have a higher risk of stroke and neurodegenerative diseases. Individuals with a history of head trauma or neurological disorders require ongoing monitoring for speech changes, as these may indicate progression or complications of their underlying condition.

Further Reading

- Allison KM, Cordella C, Iuzzini-Seigel J, Green JR. Differential Diagnosis of Apraxia of Speech in Children and Adults: A Scoping Review. J Speech Lang Hear Res. 2020 Sep 15;63(9):2952–94.
- Lott PR, Guggenbühl S, Schneeberger A, Pulver AE, Stassen HH. Linguistic analysis of the speech output of schizophrenic, bipolar, and depressive patients. Psychopathology. 2002;35(4):220–7.
- Gumus M, Koo M, Studzinski CM, Bhan A, Robin J, Black SE. Linguistic changes in neurodegenerative diseases relate to clinical symptoms. Front Neurol. 2024;15:1373341.
- Rusz J, Bonnet C, Klempíř J, Tykalová T, Baborová E, Novotný M, et al. Speech disorders reflect differing pathophysiology in Parkinson's disease, progressive supranuclear palsy and multiple system atrophy. J Neurol. 2015;262(4):992–1001.
- Haley KL, Jacks A. Three-Dimensional Speech Profiles in Stroke Aphasia and Apraxia of Speech. Am J Speech Lang Pathol. 2023 Aug 17;32(4S):1825–34.
- Noffs G, Perera T, Kolbe SC, Shanahan CJ, Boonstra FMC, Evans A, et al. What speech can tell us: A systematic review of dysarthria characteristics in Multiple Sclerosis. Autoimmun Rev. 2018 Dec;17(12):1202–9.

Facial Asymmetry

Introduction

Facial asymmetry, referring to an imbalance in the appearance of the two sides of the face, exists very commonly at a subclinical level. It can become clinical when it interferes with function or causes esthetic concerns. It can be congenital or acquired, and may involve differences in the size, shape, or position of facial features. Stroke and tumors are most serious acquired etiologies. More benign etiologies such as nerve palsies (e.g., Bell's palsy) can produce facial asymmetric, as can soft tissue or bone deformation from trauma, infection, and other disease processes.

Checklist DDX

Serious/life-threatening: stroke, cavernous sinus thrombosis, brain tumor, other malignant tumors, necrotizing fasciitis of the face or neck

Common: idiopathic facial nerve palsy, temporomandibular joint disorders, dental malocclusion, post-traumatic facial bone fracture or soft tissue injury

Commonly misdiagnosed: Parry-Romberg syndrome, temporomandibular joint disorders, Bell's palsy, congenital muscular torticollis

Systematic DDX

- Vascular
    - **Ischemic:** stroke, transient ischemic attack, cavernous sinus thrombosis
    - **Port-wine stains (capillary malformations):** Sturge-Weber syndrome, Klippel-Trenaunay syndrome
    - **Vasculitis:** granulomatosis with polyangiitis, giant cell arteritis (e.g., producing nerve palsies, neuropathy, or tissue damage)
    - **Other:** hemangiomas, vascular malformations
- Infection
    - **Direct nerve inflammation:** Bell's palsy (commonly caused by herpes simplex virus), Ramsay Hunt syndrome (herpes zoster oticus, varicella zoster virus re-activation), Lyme neuroborreliosis cranial neuritis (Borrelia burgdorferi)
    - **Involvement from adjacent structures:** acute otitis media with mastoiditis, parotiditis (mumps, influenza, Epstein-Barr virus, herpes simplex virus), osteomyelitis

- **Inflammatory**
    - Sarcoidosis, juvenile idiopathic arthritis, polychondritis, Melkersson-Rosenthal syndrome
- **Neoplasia and hematologic**
    - Benign tumors (e.g., osteomas), malignant tumors (e.g., osteosarcoma), brain tumor (e.g., cerebellopontine angle, brainstem)
- **Dysfunction**
    - Hemifacial spasm, temporomandibular joint dysfunction (e.g., condylar resorption or growth disturbance)
- **Injury/trauma**
    - Post-traumatic facial bone fracture, soft tissue injury
- **Compression/obstruction**
    - Compression by space occupying lesions (e.g., cysts, tumors, lymphadenopathy), severe nasal septal deviation
- **Anomalies of development/aging**
    - **Congenital structural abnormalities:** oculoauriculovertebral spectrum, craniosynostosis, Parry-Romberg Syndrome, congenital muscular torticollis
    - **Developmental:** neurofibromatosis, hemi-mandibular hyperplasia/elongation, unilateral cleft lip and palate, hemifacial microsomia, unilateral condylar hyperplasia, fibrous dysplasia
- **Toxic-Metabolic**
    - **Medication-induced:** corticosteroids, antipsychotics (tardive dyskinesia)
    - **Endocrine:** acromegaly, Cushing's syndrome
- **Everything else**
    - Psychogenic facial movement disorders, radiotherapy in children, dental malocclusion

Notes

General considerations: The evaluation of facial asymmetry should focus on distinguishing between acute and chronic presentations, with attention to associated symptoms such as pain, weakness, or sensory changes. Diagnostic tools often used include a neurological examination and imaging studies, such as MRI or CT, to identify potential lesions or structural abnormalities.

Red flags: sudden onset or symptom progression, other neurological deficits such as limb weakness or speech difficulties, developmental delays, visual issues, long-term use of antipsychotic medications

Special populations: In children, facial asymmetry may be congenital or the result of birth trauma, with acute presentations often linked to infections or inflammatory conditions. In older adults, asymmetry is frequently due to cerebrovascular accidents or degenerative diseases. Pregnant women may experience facial asymmetry due to hormonal changes or vascular events. Immunocompromised individuals are at increased risk for infections affecting the facial nerve, such as herpes zoster.

Further Reading

- Kim JY, Jung HD, Jung YS, Hwang CJ, Park HS. A simple classification of facial asymmetry by TML system. J Craniomaxillofac Surg. 2014 Jun;42(4):313–20.
- Thiesen G, Gribel BF, Freitas MPM. Facial asymmetry: a current review. Dental Press J Orthod. 2015 Dec;20:110–25.
- Cheong YW, Lo LJ. Facial asymmetry: etiology, evaluation, and management. Chang Gung Med J. 2011;34(4):341–51.
- Fasano A, Valadas A, Bhatia KP, Prashanth LK, Lang AE, Munhoz RP, et al. Psychogenic facial movement disorders: clinical features and associated conditions. Mov Disord. 2012 Oct;27(12):1544–51.
- Ogul H, Kiziloglu A. Unusual Cause of Facial Asymmetry: Sturge-Weber Syndrome. J Craniofac Surg. 2019 Oct;30(7):e585–6.

Ataxia

Introduction

Ataxia is a neurological sign characterized by a lack of voluntary coordination of muscle movements, which can affect gait, speech, and eye movements. Clinical evaluation of ataxia includes motor coordination, balance, and gait, and is often supplemented by neurological examination and imaging studies to identify the underlying cause. Ataxia can be sporadic, hereditary, or acquired, and is often a result of cerebellar, sensory, or vestibular dysfunction.

Checklist DDX

Serious/life-threatening: cerebellar ischemic or hemorrhagic stroke, posterior fossa mass lesions, benzodiazepine or sedative-hypnotic overdose, acute alcohol intoxication, underlying malignancy/paraneoplastic syndrome, infection (cerebellitis, encephalitis)

Common: alcohol or drug intoxication (benzodiazepines, anticonvulsants, other sedatives), peripheral vestibular dysfunction/vertigo (vestibular neuritis, Meniere's disease, ototoxic medications), hereditary or degenerative cerebellar ataxias, vitamin deficiencies (Wernicke's encephalopathy)

Commonly misdiagnosed: immune-mediated ataxias (e.g., gluten ataxia), multiple system atrophy cerebellar type, late-onset genetic ataxias; mimickers include clumsiness, developmental delay, psychogenic movement disorders

Systematic DDX

- Vascular
    - **Ischemic or hemorrhagic stroke:** cerebellar (posterior inferior cerebellar artery, superior cerebellar artery, anterior inferior cerebellar artery), brainstem (cerebellar peduncles, dorsolateral medulla), lacunar infarcts (pons, internal capsule),
    - **Vasculitis:** primary central nervous system vasculitis, systemic vasculitis with central nervous system involvement
- Infection
    - **Acute viral cerebellitis:** acute, post-infectious (varicella zoster virus, Epstein-Barr virus, influenza A, cytomegalovirus, rotavirus, herpes simplex virus, hepatitis A)

- o **Acute bacterial central nervous system infection:** meningitis, encephalitis (Streptococcus pneumoniae, Neisseria meningitidis, Listeria monocytogenes)
- o **Chronic central nervous system infection:** HIV, progressive multifocal leukoencephalopathy, or neurosyphilis
- o Brownell-Oppenheimer sporadic Creutzfeldt-Jakob disease
- Inflammatory
  - o Primary autoimmune cerebellar ataxia
  - o **Specific antibody-mediated autoimmune:** Gluten ataxia, anti-GAD65 ataxia, Miller Fisher syndrome (anti-GQ1b)
  - o **Systemic autoimmune disease with cerebellar involvement:** systemic lupus erythematosus, Sjögren's syndrome, Hashimoto's encephalopathy
  - o Autoimmune encephalitis with cerebellar involvement, opsoclonus-myoclonus-ataxia syndrome, opsoclonus-myoclonus syndrome
- Neoplasia and hematologic
  - o Primary brain tumors, especially in the posterior fossa (medulloblastoma, astrocytoma, hemangioblastoma)
  - o Metastatic lesions to the cerebellum
  - o Paraneoplastic cerebellar degeneration (most commonly associated with gynecologic, breast, small-cell lung, and Hodgkin lymphoma, mediated by anti-Yo, anti-Hu, and anti-Tr onconeural antibodies)
- Dysfunction
  - o **Neurologic:** demyelinating disease (multiple sclerosis), Parkinson's disease, peripheral neuropathy/loss of proprioception
  - o **Peripheral vestibular dysfunction/vertigo:** vestibular neuritis, Meniere's disease
  - o Liver failure (hepatic encephalopathy), hypothyroidism (Hashimoto encephalopathy), renal failure (uremic encephalopathy), musculoskeletal or joint problem
- Injury/trauma
  - o Traumatic brain injury or concussion (direct or indirect cerebellar involvement), injury to the cortico-ponto-cerebellar tract, cerebellar contusion or laceration, and traumatic hemorrhage affecting the cerebellum or its connections
- Compression/obstruction
  - o Posterior fossa mass (tumor, abscess, hematoma, cystic lesion), large cerebellar infarct with edema, normal pressure

hydrocephalus (NPH), cervical spondylosis or other causes of spinal cord compression
- **Anomalies of development/aging**
  - **Structural abnormalities:** cerebellar hypoplasia, Dandy-Walker malformation
  - **Hereditary ataxias:** autosomal dominant (spinocerebellar ataxias), autosomal recessive (Friedrich's ataxia, ataxia-telangiectasia, X-linked, mitochondrial
  - **Degenerative ataxias:** multiple system atrophy of cerebellar type, idiopathic late-onset cerebellar ataxia
  - **Late-onset hereditary ataxias:** fragile X-associated tremor/ataxia syndrome, spinocerebellar ataxia type 6 (SCA6), late-onset Friedrich's ataxia
- **Toxic-Metabolic**
  - **Drugs/toxins:** alcohol intoxication, chronic alcohol use, heavy metals (lead, mercury), recreational drugs (cocaine, heroin, phencyclidine, amphetamines)
  - **Medications:** antiepileptics (phenytoin, valproic acid, carbamazepine), sedative-hypnotic agents, benzodiazepines, lithium, antineoplastic agents (cytarabine, 5-fluorouracil, ifosfamide), amiodarone, metronidazole, some immunosuppressants
  - **Vitamin deficiencies:** vitamin B12 (subacute combined degeneration), vitamin E, thiamine (Wernicke's encephalopathy)
  - **Endocrine:** hypothyroidism, Hashimoto encephalopathy

Notes

General considerations: The time course and onset of ataxia (acute, subacute, or chronic) should be established. Acute ataxia often suggests toxic ingestion, stroke, infection, or post-infectious cerebellitis, while chronic progressive ataxia is more likely to be degenerative or genetic. Imaging, particularly brain MRI, is often used to identify structural, inflammatory, or degenerative changes, and to rule out causes such as tumors or stroke.

Red flags: focal neurological deficits (such as hemiparesis or cranial nerve palsies), meningeal signs, hyporeflexia or areflexia, ophthalmoplegia, visual impairment, altered consciousness (including decreased Glasgow Coma Scale), new-onset headache, persistent vomiting, seizures, the presence of "cerebellar plus" symptoms (e.g., limb or facial weakness, hypotonia, opsoclonus, myoclonus, torticollis, or vertigo), prolonged or progressive symptom duration

Special populations: In the elderly, ataxia is often multifactorial, with contributions from polypharmacy, sensory deficits, and cerebrovascular disease. In children, ataxia is often from genetic disorders, infections, or post-infectious syndromes such as acute cerebellar ataxia. Patients with a family history of ataxia may have hereditary ataxias, necessitating genetic counseling and testing.

Further Reading

- Teive HAG, Ashizawa T. Primary and secondary ataxias. Current Opinion in Neurology. 2015 Aug;28(4):413.
- van Gaalen J, Kerstens FG, Maas RPPWM, Härmark L, van de Warrenburg BPC. Drug-induced cerebellar ataxia: a systematic review. CNS Drugs. 2014 Dec;28(12):1139–53.
- Lieto M, Roca A, Santorelli FM, Fico T, De Michele G, Bellofatto M, et al. Degenerative and acquired sporadic adult onset ataxia. Neurol Sci. 2019 Jul;40(7):1335–42.
- Ercoli T, Defazio G, Muroni A. Cerebellar Syndrome Associated with Thyroid Disorders. Cerebellum. 2019 Oct;18(5):932–40.
- Hadjivassiliou M, Martindale J, Shanmugarajah P, Grünewald RA, Sarrigiannis PG, Beauchamp N, et al. Causes of progressive cerebellar ataxia: prospective evaluation of 1500 patients. J Neurol Neurosurg Psychiatry. 2017 Apr;88(4):301–9.
- Lin CYR, Kuo SH. Ataxias: Hereditary, Acquired, and Reversible Etiologies. Semin Neurol. 2023 Feb;43(1):48–64.
- Caffarelli M, Kimia AA, Torres AR. Acute Ataxia in Children: A Review of the Differential Diagnosis and Evaluation in the Emergency Department. Pediatric Neurology. 2016 Dec 1;65:14–30.
- Mariotti C, Fancellu R, Di Donato S. An overview of the patient with ataxia. J Neurol. 2005 May 1;252(5):511–8.

Delirium

Introduction

Delirium is an acute, fluctuating disturbance in attention and cognition, often accompanied by altered levels of consciousness. It is a common and serious condition, particularly in hospitalized and elderly patients; 20-25% of all hospitalized adults will develop delirium, increasing to over 70% in intensive care units. Not all altered mental status is delirium; the disturbance in attention and awareness in delirium is 1) acute, 2) fluctuating, and 3) not better explained by another preexisting, established, or evolving neurocognitive disorder. The presentation of delirium can be hyperactive, hypoactive, and mixed. Delirium usually has a complex, multifactorial etiology and can include anything that disturbs the homeostatic processes in a patient with sufficient risk factors. Those with lower cognitive reserve will require a smaller disturbance to develop delirium.

Checklist DDX

Serious/life-threatening: sepsis, acute organ failure (e.g., hepatic, renal), withdrawal (alcohol, benzodiazepines), acute neurological events (stroke, intracranial hemorrhage), serotonin syndrome, neuroleptic malignant syndrome

Common: infections (urinary tract infections, pneumonia), metabolic imbalances (electrolyte disturbances, hypoglycemia), medication effects (anticholinergics, benzodiazepines, opioids), dehydration, sleep deprivation, sensory impairments (vision/hearing loss)

Commonly misdiagnosed: hypoactive delirium; in general, delirium is commonly mistaken for dementia, depression, or psychosis

Systematic DDX

- Vascular
    - **Acute and chronic cerebrovascular disease:** acute stroke (ischemic or hemorrhagic), transient ischemic attack, cerebral small vessel disease
    - Central nervous system vasculitis
- Infection
    - **Central nervous system infections:** meningitis, encephalitis
    - **Other:** urinary tract infections, pneumonia, skin and soft tissue infections ascending cholangitis and intra-abdominal infections; sepsis, HIV, COVID-19

- **Inflammatory**
    - **Autoimmune encephalitis: associated** with neural autoantibodies anti-NMDA receptor, anti-LGI1, anti-GAD65, anti-CASPR2); systemic lupus erythematosus (neuropsychiatric lupus)
    - **Systemic inflammation:** from infection/sepsis, trauma, surgery
- **Neoplasia and hematologic**
    - Brain tumor, paraneoplastic syndromes, severe anemia
- **Dysfunction**
    - **Cardiorespiratory dysfunction:** hypoxemia (chronic obstructive pulmonary disease), hypoxia (heart failure, myocardial infarction, anemia), hypercapnia (respiratory failure), hypotension (shock, dehydration), arrythmia
    - **Neurologic dysfunction:** seizures (post-ictal state, non-convulsive status epilepticus), neurodegeneration (dementia), coma
    - Hepatic or renal failure
- **Injury/trauma**
    - Traumatic brain injury, concussion, major non-cranial injuries (e.g., hip fracture), fall, long lie
- **Compression/obstruction**
    - **Genitourinary:** urinary retention, constipation, fecal impaction
    - **Neurologic:** acute hydrocephalus, space-occupying brain lesions (tumor, abscess, hematoma), cerebral edema
- **Anomalies of development/aging**
    - **Reduced brain functional reserve:** advanced age, frailty, dementia, pre-existing cognitive impairment, multiple comorbidities
- **Toxic-Metabolic**
    - **Medication-induced:** serotonin syndrome, neuroleptic malignant syndrome, anticholinergics, opioids, sedatives, psychoactive mediations
    - **Substance intoxication or withdrawal:** alcohol illicit drugs, benzodiazepines, particularly withdrawal from long-term sedative use
    - **Endocrine:** thyroid dysfunction
    - **Nutrition/electrolyte disturbances:** poor dietary intake, dehydration, sodium imbalance, vitamin B12 deficiency, thiamine deficiency

- **Everything else**
  - **Sensory impairments:** vision, hearing loss
  - **Environmental factors:** immobility (confined to bed, restraints), sleep disturbance (sleep deprivation, day-night disorientation)
  - **Psychiatric:** severe depression, acute psychosis, paranoia, catatonia
  - **Iatrogenic:** surgery, anesthesia, poorly controlled pain

Notes

General considerations: Identifying and addressing underlying factors is crucial for effective management of delirium. This may involve reviewing medications, treating infections, correcting metabolic imbalances, and providing supportive care. Non-pharmacological interventions, such as reorientation, ensuring adequate hydration and nutrition, and optimizing the environment are key components of management. Some strategies to optimize the environment may include mobilizing the patient out of bed to a chair, reducing clutter and noise, adequate lighting, and encouraging family to bring familiar objects from home.

Red flags: rapid onset of symptoms, severe agitation, hallucinations, focal neurological signs, signs of systemic infection such as fever and hypotension

Special populations: Older age, polypharmacy, sensory impairments, and pre-existing cognitive decline increase the risk of delirium. In children, delirium is less common but can occur in the context of severe illness or medication effects. Patients in intensive care units are at high risk due to the complexity of their medical conditions and the ICU environment.

Further Reading

- Wilson JE, Mart MF, Cunningham C, Shehabi Y, Girard TD, MacLullich AMJ, et al. Delirium. Nat Rev Dis Primers. 2020 Nov 12;6(1):1–26.
- Marcantonio ER. Delirium in Hospitalized Older Adults. New England Journal of Medicine. 2017 Oct 12;377(15):1456–66.
- Saxena S, Lawley D. Delirium in the elderly: a clinical review. Postgraduate Medical Journal. 2009 Aug 1;85(1006):405–13.
- Hansen N, Krasiuk I, Titsch T. Neural autoantibodies in delirium. J Autoimmun. 2021 Dec;125:102740.
- Ormseth CH, LaHue SC, Oldham MA, Josephson SA, Whitaker E, Douglas VC. Predisposing and Precipitating Factors Associated With Delirium: A Systematic Review. JAMA Netw Open. 2023 Jan

3;6(1):e2249950.
- Cerejeira J, Nogueira V, Luís P, Vaz-Serra A, Mukaetova-Ladinska EB. The cholinergic system and inflammation: common pathways in delirium pathophysiology. J Am Geriatr Soc. 2012 Apr;60(4):669–75.
- Cerejeira J, Lagarto L, Mukaetova-Ladinska EB. The immunology of delirium. Neuroimmunomodulation. 2014;21(2–3):72–8.

Coma

Introduction

Coma is a state of prolonged unconsciousness in which a person cannot be awakened and fails to respond to external stimuli. It can be caused by traumatic, metabolic, infectious, and neurological etiologies. It is a medical emergency that requires immediate evaluation and intervention including stabilization of the airway, breathing, and circulation (the "ABCs"), followed by physical exam and additional investigations such as labs and imaging. Toxic causes of coma are more common in younger patients, and older patients are at higher risk for severe outcomes.

Checklist DDX

Serious/life-threatening: stroke, traumatic brain injury, intracranial hemorrhage, metabolic disturbances (hypoglycemia, diabetic ketoacidosis, severe electrolyte imbalances), meningitis, drug overdose/toxic causes

Common: drug intoxications/overdose (sedatives, opioids), metabolic disturbances (hypoglycemia), traumatic brain injury, stroke, systemic infections with multi-organ failure

Commonly misdiagnosed: mimics (mistaken for coma) include locked-in syndrome/eyelid opening apraxia, psychogenic unresponsiveness/catatonia, and severe toxic states with altered consciousness

Systematic DDX

- Vascular
  - **Vaso-occlusion:** ischemic stroke (including brainstem/basilar artery territory, large territory strokes with cerebral edema causing herniation, thalamic infarct, e.g., related to artery of Percheron), venous thrombosis
  - **Bleeding:** intracerebral hemorrhage, subarachnoid hemorrhage, epidural hematoma, pituitary apoplexy
  - **Other:** global cerebral hypoperfusion/hypoxic ischemic brain injury (e.g., following cardiorespiratory arrest), hypertensive encephalopathy, posterior reversible encephalopathy syndrome, primary or secondary central nervous system vasculitis

- Infection
  - **Direct brain involvement:** bacterial meningitis, bacterial meningoencephalitis, viral encephalitis, cerebral malaria, Creutzfeldt-Jakob disease
  - **Abscesses:** brain parenchymal abscess, subdural empyema, epidural abscess,
  - Sepsis-associated encephalopathy
- Inflammatory
  - Acute disseminated encephalomyelitis, autoimmune encephalitis, Hashimoto encephalopathy, neuropsychiatric systemic lupus erythematosus, neurosarcoidosis, fulminant multiple sclerosis, Behcet's disease
- Neoplasia and hematologic
  - Primary or metastatic brain tumor, leptomeningeal infiltration/metastases, paraneoplastic limbic encephalitis
- Dysfunction
  - **Organ failure:** cardiac/circulatory, respiratory, hepatic encephalopathy, renal/uremia
  - **Endocrine dysfunction:** thyroid, adrenal dysfunction, diabetes
  - **Neurologic dysfunction:** seizures, non-convulsive status epilepticus, stroke (basilar, bi-hemispheric)
- Injury/trauma
  - **Traumatic brain injury:** diffuse axonal injury, extradural/epidural/subdural hemorrhage, intracerebral hemorrhage, cerebral contusion, secondary brainstem injury
- Compression/obstruction
  - **Mass effect:** herniation syndromes from intracranial mass lesions (tumor, abscess, large stroke with edema), acute subdural or epidural hematoma
  - **Fluid outflow obstruction:** obstructive hydrocephalus
  - Spontaneous or iatrogenic intracranial hypertension
- Anomalies of development/aging
  - **Severe congenital malformations:** holoprosencephaly spectrum abnormalities, large midline defects
  - **Advanced neurodegenerative diseases:** late-stage Alzheimer's disease, advanced Parkinson's disease with parkinsonism-hyperpyrexia syndrome, end-stage multisystem atrophy
  - **Inherited metabolic, degenerative disorders:** leukodystrophies, mitochondrial disorders, fatal familial insomnia
- Toxic-metabolic
  - **Medication-induced:** sedative-hypnotics agents (benzodiazepines, barbiturates, baclofen, gamma-hydroxybutyrate), opioids

(heroin, morphine, oxycodone, hydrocodone), dissociative agents (phencyclidine, ketamine), psychiatric medications (tricyclic antidepressants, selective serotonin reuptake inhibitors), serotonin syndrome, neuroleptic malignant syndrome, immune check-point related neurotoxicity (ICANS)
    - **Toxic:** alcohol, toxic alcohols, carbon monoxide poisoning, simple asphyxiants (nitrogen), agents of histotoxic hypoxia (cyanide, clonidine)
    - **Endocrine:** hypoglycemia, diabetic ketoacidosis, hyperosmolar hyperglycemic state, thyroid disorders (myxedema coma), adrenal dysfunction
    - **Electrolyte and metabolic disturbances:** sodium, calcium, glucose, acid-base disorders, hyperammonemia, thiamine deficiency
- **Everything else**
    - High altitude cerebral edema (HACE), hypothermia

Notes

General considerations: Management of coma should focus on stabilizing the patient, addressing the underlying cause, and preventing complications. Multidisciplinary care, including input from neurologists, intensivists, and other specialists, is often required. Diagnostic imaging, such as CT or MRI scans, is often used to identify, or rule out, structural causes of coma. Laboratory tests can also be helpful to detect metabolic or toxic etiologies.

Red flags: rapid deterioration in consciousness (particularly when associated with signs of increased intracranial pressure such as bradycardia, hypertension, and irregular respiration), following head trauma (especially with preceding focal neurological deficits), fever and neck stiffness

Special populations: In children, metabolic disorders, infections, and non-accidental trauma are important considerations. In the elderly, the risk of stroke, medication-related coma, and metabolic disturbances is higher, necessitating careful assessment. Pregnant women may experience coma due to eclampsia or other pregnancy-related complications. Individuals with a history of substance abuse or psychiatric disorders require thorough evaluation to differentiate between toxic, metabolic, and psychogenic causes.

Further Reading

- Cooksley T, Rose S, Holland M. A systematic approach to the unconscious patient. Clin Med (Lond). 2018 Feb;18(1):88–92.
- Churchill's Pocketbook of Differential Diagnosis.
- Huff JS, Tadi P. Coma. In: StatPearls [Internet]. Treasure Island (FL): StatPearls Publishing; 2024 [cited 2024 Jul 8]. Available from: http://www.ncbi.nlm.nih.gov/books/NBK430722/
- Kondziella D, Bender A, Diserens K, van Erp W, Estraneo A, Formisano R, et al. European Academy of Neurology guideline on the diagnosis of coma and other disorders of consciousness. European Journal of Neurology. 2020;27(5):741–56.
- Andour H, Rostoum S, Regragui Y, Fikri M, Jiddane M, Touarsa F. Fulminant Susac syndrome—a rare cause of coma: The history of the fatal course in a young man. SAGE Open Medical Case Reports. 2023 Jan 1;11:2050313X221149826.
- Traub SJ, Wijdicks EF. Initial Diagnosis and Management of Coma. Emergency Medicine Clinics. 2016 Nov 1;34(4):777–93.
- Posner, J. B., Saper, C. B., Schiff, N. D., & Claassen, J. (2019). Plum and Posner's diagnosis and treatment of stupor and coma (5th ed.). Oxford University Press

Psychiatric

Ramtin Hajibeygi

Long H. Tu

Leah B. Colucci

Depression

Introduction

Depression, clinically referred to as major depressive disorder (MDD), is a common and serious mood disorder characterized by persistent sadness, loss of interest or pleasure in activities, and a range of cognitive and physical symptoms that interfere with daily functioning. It is estimated that up to one in four individuals in the US may experience depression during their lifetime. Prevalence is higher among women, younger individuals, and those facing socioeconomic challenges. Depression is described as a depressed mood or loss of interest/pleasure in combination with additional symptoms such as unexpected weight changes, sleep disturbances, fatigue, feelings of worthlessness, and thoughts of death, suicidal ideation, or suicide attempts. These symptoms must cause significant social or occupational impairment and must not be attributable to the effects of a substance or other medical condition.

The differential diagnosis for depression includes medical conditions that can present with similar mood or cognitive changes such as hypothyroidism, vitamin B12 deficiency, or neurodegenerative disease. Depression must also be distinguished from other psychiatric conditions including psychotic disorders, bipolar disorder, generalized anxiety disorder, and adjustment disorder.

Checklist DDX

Serious/life-threatening: stroke, subdural hematoma, hypercalcemia, hyponatremia, HIV infection, primary brain tumors (e.g., glioblastoma), metastatic brain tumors, pancreatic cancer, Addison's disease, Cushing's syndrome, myxedema coma

Common: diabetes, thyroid disorders (hypothyroidism, hyperthyroidism), alcohol use, stimulant withdrawal (e.g., cocaine, amphetamines), steroid use, antihypertensives (e.g., beta-blockers), sedatives/hypnotics (e.g., benzodiazepines), vitamin D deficiency, vitamin B12 deficiency, folate deficiency, Parkinson disease, Alzheimer disease, dysthymia, bereavement, adjustment disorder with depressed mood, anxiety disorder

Commonly misdiagnosed: thyroid disorders, vitamin deficiencies, neurological diseases

Systematic DDX

- **Psychiatric**
    - **Primary mood disorders:** major depressive disorder (unipolar depression), persistent depressive disorder (dysthymia), bipolar disorder (depressive phase), depressive disorder with mixed features
    - **Trauma and stress-related disorders:** adjustment disorder with depressed mood, post-traumatic stress disorder (PTSD)
    - **Psychotic spectrum:** psychotic depression, depression due to schizophrenia
    - **Atypical and seasonal subtypes:** atypical depression, seasonal affective disorder
    - **Substance-related and comorbid psychiatric conditions:** substance-induced mood disorder, depression secondary to anxiety disorders
- **Neurological**
    - **Vascular disorders:** cerebrovascular accident (stroke), subdural hematoma
    - **Degenerative diseases:** Parkinson's disease, Alzheimer's disease, Huntington's disease, Lewy Body dementia, other dementias
    - **Space-occupying lesions:** brain tumors (primary or metastatic)
    - **Other:** multiple sclerosis, epilepsy, traumatic brain injury
- **Infection**
    - **Chronic viral infections:** HIV/AIDS, hepatitis C
    - **Bacterial infections with neuropsychiatric impact:** neurosyphilis, Lyme disease, tuberculosis
- **Autoimmune and inflammatory disorders**
    - **Systemic autoimmune conditions:** systemic lupus erythematosus (SLE), rheumatoid arthritis
    - **Vasculitis disorders:** systemic and CNS vasculitis syndromes
- **Endocrine and metabolic**
    - **Thyroid disorders:** hypothyroidism, hyperthyroidism
    - **Adrenal disorders:** Cushing's disease/syndrome, Addison's disease
    - **Glucose metabolism:** diabetes mellitus
    - **Parathyroid and calcium-related disorders:** parathyroid disorders, hypercalcemia
    - **Electrolyte imbalances:** hyponatremia, other electrolyte disturbances

- - o **Vitamin deficiencies:** vitamin B12 deficiency, vitamin B6 deficiency, vitamin D deficiency, folate deficiency, iron deficiency anemia
- **Substance-related causes**
  - o **Substance misuse:** alcohol use disorder, illicit drug use (cocaine, amphetamines, opioids)
  - o **Medication-induced:** corticosteroids, beta-blockers, antihypertensives, isotretinoin, interferons, anticonvulsants
  - o **Withdrawal states:** alcohol withdrawal, benzodiazepine withdrawal
  - o **Sedative/hypnotic effects:** benzodiazepines, sleep medications
- **Other**
  - o **Sleep disorders:** obstructive sleep apnea
  - o **Oncologic conditions:** pancreatic cancer, other malignancies, paraneoplastic syndromes
  - o **Chronic systemic conditions:** chronic pain syndromes
  - o **Psychosocial stressors and trauma:** bereavement, social isolation, unemployment, relationship breakdown

Notes

General considerations: Accurate diagnosis of depression relies on thorough clinical assessment according to DSM criteria supported by detailed history-taking, mental status examination, and the exclusion of organic causes through appropriate laboratory and imaging investigations. Misdiagnosis may be avoided by carefully evaluating symptom duration, severity of functional impairment, and considering other psychiatric conditions that may mimic depression.

Red flags: suicidal ideation, psychotic symptoms (e.g., hallucinations, delusions), rapid mood swings suggestive of bipolar disorder, significant functional decline, refusal to eat or drink, new-onset confusion in older adults

Special populations: In children, consider ADHD, anxiety, conduct disorders, and chronic medical conditions, which are common and can complicate diagnosis. In older adults, consider dementia, delirium, medication side effects, chronic medical illnesses (e.g., hypothyroidism), and bereavement-related grief. In pregnant/post-partum women, consider pregnancy-related emotional changes, thyroid disorders, anemia, and medical conditions such as preeclampsia. Postpartum depression and bipolar disorder may emerge due to hormonal and psychosocial changes. In patients with chronic illness, depression may be masked or mimicked by somatic symptoms of the illness itself or by side effects of the medical therapies.

Further Reading

- Malhi GS, Mann JJ. Depression. Lancet. 2018 Nov 24;392(10161):2299-2312. doi: 10.1016/S0140-6736(18)31948-2. Epub 2018 Nov 2. PMID: 30396512.
- Bradley RG, Binder EB, Epstein MP, Tang Y, Nair HP, Liu W, Gillespie CF, Berg T, Evces M, Newport DJ, Stowe ZN, Heim CM, Nemeroff CB, Schwartz A, Cubells JF, Ressler KJ. Influence of child abuse on adult depression: moderation by the corticotropin-releasing hormone receptor gene. Arch Gen Psychiatry. 2008 Feb;65(2):190-200. doi: 10.1001/archgenpsychiatry.2007.26. PMID: 18250257; PMCID: PMC2443704.
- Green JG, McLaughlin KA, Berglund PA, Gruber MJ, Sampson NA, Zaslavsky AM, Kessler RC. Childhood adversities and adult psychiatric disorders in the national comorbidity survey replication I: associations with first onset of DSM-IV disorders. Archives of general psychiatry. 2010 Feb 1;67(2):113-23.

Anxiety

Introduction

Anxiety is defined as a state of apprehension, tension, or uneasiness arising from the anticipation of potential danger. It is important to recognize that although anxiety and fear share similar physiological manifestations, their definitions are distinct: fear represents an emotional response to an identifiable threat, whereas anxiety denotes a fear response in the absence of a real or imminent danger. Careful assessment evaluating for anxiety is essential, as approximately 2% to 4% of the general population experience symptoms severe enough to meet criteria for an anxiety disorder. The diagnosis requires exclusion of underlying medical conditions such as hyperthyroidism, cardiac arrhythmias, and substance use or withdrawal, which may produce similar somatic presentations. Additionally, psychiatric disorders including depression, post-traumatic stress disorder (PTSD), and obsessive-compulsive disorder (OCD) may either mimic or co-occur with anxiety disorders, warranting a thorough evaluation.

Checklist DDX

Serious/life-threatening: acute myocardial infarction, arrythmias, pulmonary embolism, seizures, brain tumors, hypoglycemia, and substance overdose or withdrawal

Common: genetic predisposition, personality traits (e.g., neuroticism), psychosocial stressors, and coexisting psychiatric conditions such as depression, PTSD, and OCD, as well as substance use (e.g., caffeine, nicotine, alcohol)

Commonly misdiagnosed: hyperthyroidism or cardiac arrhythmias, depression, PTSD

Systematic DDX

- **Psychiatric**
    - **Primary anxiety disorders:** generalized anxiety disorder (GAD), panic disorder, social anxiety disorder (social phobia), specific phobias, agoraphobia, OCD, PTSD
    - **Adjustment and trauma-related disorders:** adjustment disorder with anxiety, PTSD (if not classified under primary), panic attacks triggered by natural fears or situational stressors

- o **Substance-induced and comorbid psychiatric causes:** substance-induced anxiety disorder, anxiety due to other psychiatric conditions (e.g., major depressive disorder, bipolar disorder)
- **Neurological**
    - o **Seizure-related conditions:** epilepsy (especially temporal lobe epilepsy)
    - o **Headache and pain syndromes:** migraine
    - o **Demyelinating and inflammatory:** multiple sclerosis
    - o **Traumatic or vascular causes:** traumatic brain injury, cerebrovascular accident (stroke)
    - o **Structural CNS lesions:** brain tumors
- **Infection**
    - o HIV/AIDS, neurosyphilis, Lyme disease, chronic infections (e.g., tuberculosis), hepatitis C
- **Autoimmune and inflammatory**
    - o **Systemic autoimmune disorders:** systemic lupus erythematosus (SLE), rheumatoid arthritis
    - o **Vasculitis:** systemic or CNS vasculitis syndromes
- **Cardiopulmonary**
    - o **Cardiac conditions:** mitral valve prolapse, cardiac arrhythmias, congestive heart failure
    - o **Pulmonary conditions:** chronic obstructive pulmonary disease (COPD), asthma, pulmonary embolism
- **Endocrine and metabolic**
    - o **Thyroid disorders:** hyperthyroidism, hypothyroidism
    - o **Adrenal disorders and catecholamine excess:** pheochromocytoma, Cushing's syndrome, Addison's disease
    - o **Glucose metabolism:** diabetes mellitus (hypoglycemia)
    - o **Electrolyte and metabolic disturbances:** hyponatremia, hypernatremia, hypocalcemia, others as relevant
    - o **Nutritional deficiencies:** vitamin B12 deficiency, folate deficiency, iron deficiency anemia
- **Substance-related**
    - o **Stimulant and substance intoxication:** caffeine intoxication, illicit drug use (e.g., cocaine, amphetamines), stimulant medications
    - o **Withdrawal states:** alcohol, benzodiazepine and opioid withdrawal
    - o **Medication side effects:** corticosteroids, beta agonists, bronchodilators stimulants, thyroid hormone

- **Other**
    - **Psychosocial causes**: psychological trauma, severe psychosocial stressors (e.g., bereavement, unemployment, relational stress)
    - Chronic pain syndromes, obstructive sleep apnea, insomnia

Notes

General considerations: When diagnosing anxiety, it is essential to distinguish it from medical and psychiatric conditions that may mimic its presentation while considering contextual, age-related, and physiological factors. Clinicians should avoid attributing physical symptoms physical symptoms solely to anxiety without thorough evaluation. Comprehensive assessment includes identifying symptom triggers, characteristic patterns (e.g., excessive worry, panic attacks, phobias), and the degree of impairment to daily functioning, to ensure that the diagnosis aligns with established criteria such as those outlined in the DSM.

Red flags: persistent restlessness or agitation, sleep disturbances, sudden or unexplained onset of anxiety symptoms, rapid worsening of anxiety over a short period, coexisting depression or mood changes, current or past substance use or withdrawal

Special populations: In children anxiety often presents with somatic complaints such as stomach aches and may be challenging to distinguish from normative childhood fears or other conditions such as ADHD, depression, autism spectrum disorder, or medical illnesses. In elderly adults, anxiety should be differentiated from dementia, depression, medication side effects and age-related cognitive changes. In pregnant patients, anxiety must be distinguished from physiological changes of pregnancy (palpitations, dyspnea), underlying medical conditions like hyperthyroidism or anemia, and coexisting mood disorders such as depression.

Further Reading

- Hawken T, Turner-Cobb J, Barnett J. Coping and adjustment in caregivers: A systematic review. Health psychology open. 2018 Nov;5(2):2055102918810659.
- Domhardt M, Geßlein H, von Rezori RE, Baumeister H. Internet-and mobile-based interventions for anxiety disorders: A meta-analytic review of intervention components. Depression and anxiety. 2019 Mar;36(3):213-24.
- Uhde TW, Singareddy R. Biological research in anxiety disorders. Psychiatry as a Neuroscience. 2002 Apr 15:237-86.

Psychosis

Introduction

Psychosis is a common and functionally impairing symptom observed across a broad spectrum of psychiatric, neurodevelopmental, neurologic, and medical conditions. Psychosis is characterized by the presence of delusions, hallucinations without insight, or both. They are clearly defined ordinary symptoms of psychosis in both psychiatric disease and neurologic disorders. Psychosis is the hallmark symptom of schizophrenia spectrum disorders, a common but variable symptom of mood and substance use disorders, and fairly common symptom of a broad range of developmental, acquired, and degenerative neurologic and medical disorders. In all of these conditions, psychosis is both a cause of impairment and a barrier to productivity and social participation.

Checklist DDX

Serious/life-threatening: ischemic stroke, brain neoplasm, limbic encephalitis (paraneoplastic or autoimmune), Wilson disease (hepatolenticular degeneration), alcohol withdrawal

Common: schizophrenia spectrum disorders, mood disorders with psychotic features, substance-induced psychosis, obsessive-compulsive disorder, Alzheimer's disease, Parkinson disease, Lewy body dementia, dopaminergic agents, anticholinergics

Commonly misdiagnosed: Alzheimer's disease, Parkinson disease, epilepsy, substance-induced psychosis

Systematic DDX

- **Psychiatric causes**
    - **Primary psychotic disorders:** schizophrenia, schizoaffective disorder, brief psychotic disorder, delusional disorder
    - **Mood disorders with psychotic features:** bipolar disorder (with psychotic features), major depressive disorder with psychotic features
    - **Substance/medication-induced psychotic disorders:** substance-induced psychotic disorder medication-induced psychosis
    - **Psychosis secondary to other psychiatric conditions:** severe PTSD, severe anxiety disorders

- **Neurological causes**
  - **Structural brain abnormalities:** brain tumors, traumatic brain injury
  - **Neurodegenerative disorders:** Parkinson's disease, Huntington's disease, Dementia (e.g., Alzheimer's disease, Lewy body dementia, frontotemporal)
  - **Other:** cerebrovascular accident (stroke), epileptic disorders (e.g., temporal lobe epilepsy), demyelinating disorders (e.g., multiple sclerosis)
- **Infectious**
  - **Viral infections:** HIV/AIDS, herpes simplex virus encephalitis
  - **Bacterial infections:** neurosyphilis, tuberculosis, Lyme disease
  - **Fungal infections:** cryptococcal meningitis
- **Autoimmune and inflammatory**
  - **Autoimmune encephalitis:** anti-NMDA receptor encephalitis, other autoimmune/paraneoplastic encephalitis
  - **Systemic autoimmune diseases:** systemic lupus erythematosus (SLE), vasculitis syndromes (e.g., CNS vasculitis)
- **Endocrine and metabolic**
  - **Thyroid disorders:** hypothyroidism, hyperthyroidism
  - **Adrenal disorders:** Cushing's syndrome, Addison's disease
  - **Liver or kidney disorders:** hepatic or uremic encephalopathy
  - **Metabolic disturbances:** hypoglycemia, electrolyte imbalances
  - **Vitamin deficiencies:** vitamin B12 deficiency, thiamine deficiency (e.g., Wernicke's encephalopathy), niacin deficiency (pellagra)
- **Substance-related**
  - **Substance intoxication:** alcohol, cocaine, amphetamines, hallucinogens (e.g., LSD, PCP), cannabis, synthetic cannabinoids
  - **Substance withdrawal:** alcohol, benzodiazepines, other sedatives
  - **Medication-induced:** corticosteroids, anticholinergics, dopaminergic agents (e.g., L-DOPA)
- **Other**
  - **Psychosocial causes:** severe psychosocial stressors or trauma
  - Severe sleep deprivation

Notes

General considerations: The workup of psychosis requires a comprehensive clinical assessment, incorporating a detailed psychiatric and medical history focusing on symptom onset and progression, nature (such as hallucinations, delusions, and disorganized thought), the impact on daily functioning, and safety concerns (risk to self or others). Medical and laboratory testing are conducted to rule out the underlying conditions that may cause or mimic psychosis. These tests include complete blood count, metabolic panels, toxicology screens, thyroid function tests, and pregnancy tests when relevant. Early recognition and intervention are critical to improve patient outcomes. Equally important is the involvement of patient families and support systems, both in gathering collateral history and incorporating into ongoing care.

Red Flags: sudden onset of psychotic symptoms, history of polypharmacy or recent changes in medication, presence of neurologic symptoms (confusion, seizures, focal deficits)

Special populations: In children, consider mood disorders with psychotic features, medical causes, and developmental phenomena such as vivid imagination or trauma-related symptoms. In older adults, it is crucial to differentiate psychosis from delirium, dementia-related psychosis, medication side effects, and neurodegenerative disorders. In pregnant women, the differential should include delirium due to medical conditions or substance use, mood disorders with psychotic features, and rare but severe conditions like postpartum psychosis.

Further Reading

- Courvoisie H, Labellarte MJ, Riddle MA. Psychosis in children: diagnosis and treatment. Dialogues in clinical neuroscience. 2001 Jun 30;3(2):79-92.
- Friedman SH, Reed E, Ross NE. Postpartum psychosis. Current psychiatry reports. 2023 Feb;25(2):65-72.
- Arciniegas DB. Psychosis. CONTINUUM: lifelong learning in neurology. 2015 Jun 1;21(3):715-36.

Endocrine

Maad Galal

Long H. Tu

Nickolas Srica

Heat Intolerance

Introduction

Heat intolerance is the inability to tolerate warm temperatures, often due to an abnormal physiological response to heat. This condition can result from either congenital or acquired factors and can lead to a permanent or temporary susceptibility to heat. Distinguishing between permanent and transient heat intolerance indicates varying underlying causes, allowing tailored interventions for each type of heat intolerance. Some individuals may develop severe or even life-threatening symptoms in response to heat exposure. Heat intolerance is linked to heat-related illnesses such as heat stroke. It is important to distinguish elevated body temperature due to heat intolerance, which can commonly occur in the setting of environmental or thermoregulatory issues, from true fever, which often occurs due to infectious (and other) etiologies.

Checklist DDX

Serious/life-threatening: heat stroke, heat exhaustion, encephalitis, thyroid storm, carcinoid syndrome, pheochromocytoma

Common: hyperthyroidism, autonomic dysfunction, multiple sclerosis, dehydration, obesity, menopause, caffeine, medication-induced, psychogenic

Commonly misdiagnosed: ectodermal dysplasia, chronic idiopathic anhidrosis

Systematic DDX

- **Vascular**
  - **Cardiovascular:** heart failure, coronary artery disease, arrhythmia
  - **Others:** chronic kidney disease, stroke
- **Infection**
  - Encephalitis (meningoencephalitis), sepsis, tetanus
- **Inflammatory**
  - Psoriasis, irritable bowel syndrome
- **Neoplasia and hematologic**
  - Sickle cell disease, pheochromocytoma, carcinoid syndrome
- **Dysfunction**
  - **Central nervous system:** multiple sclerosis, seizure disorder, Parkinson's disease

- o **Peripheral/autonomic nervous system**: postural orthostatic tachycardia syndrome, Guillain-Barré syndrome, diabetic neuropathy
- **Injury/trauma**
  - o Burns, previous heat injuries (heat stroke, heat cramps, heat exhaustion, heat rash), spinal cord injuries, x-ray irradiation, rhabdomyolysis
- **Toxic-metabolic**
  - o **Drugs**: diuretics, antihistamines, antipsychotics, anticholinergics, beta-blockers, stimulants (amphetamine), angiotensin-converting enzyme inhibitors, alcohol, atropine, anabolic steroids, hormonal replacement therapy
  - o **Endocrine**: hyperthyroidism, thyroid storm, diabetic ketoacidosis, menopause, adrenal insufficiency
- **Anomalies of development/aging**
  - o **Congenital/genetic**: ectodermal dysplasia, idiopathic anhidrosis, TRPV1 mutation
- **Everything else**
  - o Pregnancy, caffeine, obesity, dehydration, anxiety disorders, fibromyalgia

Notes

General considerations: When approaching the diagnosis of heat intolerance in the geriatric population, it is important to consider their diminished thermoregulatory responses, which increase vulnerability to heat-related complications, particularly in the presence of comorbid cardiovascular or respiratory conditions. In contrast, athletes involved in high-intensity sports are at higher risk of heat intolerance because of prior exertional heat injuries, with training and competing in high temperatures and humidity further exacerbating their heat stress risk.

Red flags: hyperthermia (>40.5 °C), tachycardia, sweating, flushing, fatigue, lightheadedness, headache, and paresthesia, progressing to weakness, muscle cramps, oliguria, anhidrosis, nausea, agitation, hypotension, syncope, confusion, delirium, seizures, coma

Special populations: Children may uncommonly have heat intolerance from congenital thermoregulatory disorders (e.g., ectodermal dysplasia). Older adults often have reduced circulation and multiple comorbidities that exacerbate heat intolerance. Pregnant women have increased metabolic heat production and may be especially susceptible to heat stress, though mild subjective heat intolerance in pregnancy is not necessarily concerning. Patients with neurological disease (e.g., multiple sclerosis) or endocrine disorders may manifest more severe heat sensitivity.

Further Reading

- Achebak H, Rey G, Chen Z, Lloyd SJ, Quijal-Zamorano M, Méndez-Turrubiates RF, et al. Heat exposure and cause-specific hospital admissions in Spain: a nationwide cross-sectional study. Environ Health Perspect. 2024;132(5).
- Gauer R, Meyers BK. Heat-related illnesses. Am Fam Physician. 2019;99(8):482–9.
- Lee SY, Pearce EN. Hyperthyroidism: a review. Jama. 2023 Oct 17;330(15):1472-83.
- Ikäheimo TM, Jokelainen J, Hassi J, Hiltunen L, Keinänen-Kiukaanniemi S, Laatikainen T, et al. Diabetes and impaired glucose metabolism is associated with more cold-related cardiorespiratory symptoms. Diabetes Res Clin Pract. 2017;129:116–25.
- Epstein Y. Heat intolerance: predisposing factor or residual injury? Med Sci Sports Exerc. 2024;22(1).
- Moran DS, Eli-Berchoer L, Heled Y, Mendel L, Schocina M, Horowitz M. Heat intolerance: does gene transcription contribute? J Appl Physiol. 2006;100(4):1370–6.
- Richards N, Dilley A. Contribution of hyperpolarization-activated channels to heat hypersensitivity and ongoing activity in the neuritis model. Neuroscience. 2014;284:87–98.
- Leiva DF, Church B. Heat Illness. PubMed. Treasure Island (FL): StatPearls Publishing; 2024 [cited 2025 Jul 14]

Cold Intolerance

Introduction

Cold intolerance represents a nonspecific clinical symptom characterized by abnormal or exaggerated responses to cool environmental temperatures. Patients typically experience a constellation of symptoms including pain, paresthesia, numbness, rigors, joint stiffness, weakness, edema, or cutaneous color changes upon cold exposure. The Cold Intolerance Symptom Severity (CISS) scale provides standardized assessment and risk stratification for symptom severity. The underlying pathophysiology encompasses several mechanisms: impaired thermogenesis (commonly seen in hypothyroidism), abnormal vascular reactivity (as in Raynaud's phenomenon), or altered sensory processing (associated with neuropathy or fibromyalgia). Contributing factors include reduced body mass, decreased metabolic rate, and autonomic nervous system dysfunction. Clinical evaluation requires systematic history-taking and physical examination, with particular attention to symptom chronicity, environmental triggers, and associated manifestations to guide appropriate diagnostic workup.

Checklist DDX

Serious/life-threatening: myxedema coma (severe hypothyroidism), adrenal insufficiency/crisis, hypopituitarism, environment-induced hypothermia, frostbite

Common: hypothyroidism, fibromyalgia, anemia, peripheral vascular disease, atherosclerosis, Raynaud's disease, diabetes mellitus, low body weight, malnutrition, vitamin B12 deficiency, medication-induced, diseases of the hypothalamus, paroxysmal cold hemoglobinuria, autonomic dysfunction, chronic kidney disease, trench foot, upper extremity trauma or surgery

Commonly misdiagnosed: hypothyroidism, hypopituitarism, Raynaud's phenomenon, acrocyanosis, pernio (chilblains), early connective tissue diseases (e.g., scleroderma, lupus), peripheral neuropathy, psychiatric illness, substance-use disorders, eating disorders (e.g., anorexia nervosa), cold agglutinin disease

Systematic DDX

- Vascular
    - Peripheral artery disease, atherosclerosis, arterial injury, hypothalamic stroke, congestive heart failure, Raynaud's disease, acrocyanosis

- **Infectious/inflammatory**
    - **Infection:** poliomyelitis, leprosy
    - **Inflammatory:** rheumatoid arthritis, multiple sclerosis, cryoglobulinemia, rheumatoid arthritis
- **Neoplasia and hematologic**
    - Anemia, paroxysmal cold hemoglobinuria, Waldenstrom's macroglobulinemia, cold agglutinin disease, polycythemia vera
    - Hypothalamic lesions (e.g., brain tumors)
- **Dysfunction**
    - **Seizure-related:** epilepsy
    - **Peripheral nerve dysfunction:** peripheral neuropathy (e.g., carpal tunnel syndrome), autonomic dysfunction
- **Injury/trauma**
    - Nonfreezing cold injuries (immersion/trench foot, chilblains, panniculitis, cold urticaria), frostbite, upper limb surgery (flexor tendon repair, amputations), traumatic hand injury (fracture), hand-arm vibration syndrome, complex regional pain syndrome (CRPS)
- **Anomalies of development/aging**
    - **Inherited:** Fabry disease, TRPA1 mutation, TRPM8 channel polymorphism
    - **Neurodegenerative:** Wernicke's encephalopathy, Parkinson's disease
- **Toxic-metabolic**
    - **Endocrine:** hypothyroidism, diabetes mellitus, hypopituitarism, adrenal insufficiency
    - **Drugs:** oxaliplatin (chemotherapy), opioid withdrawal, beta-blockers, nicotine
    - **Metabolic:** vitamin B12 deficiency
    - **Toxic:** alcohol-use disorder, substance-use disorders
- **Everything else**
    - Fibromyalgia, chronic kidney disease, anorexia nervosa, bulimia nervosa, hyperemesis gravidarum, environmental (e.g., housing instability)

Notes

General considerations: Initial evaluation may include baseline studies such as CBC, TSH, and iron panels, with additional testing guided by clinical presentation. Cold intolerance should not be dismissed as benign, particularly in elderly patients or those with systemic symptoms, as it may represent a treatable underlying pathology. Management centers on addressing the root cause while implementing environmental modifications. Individual factors including age, gender, and injury type significantly influence cold tolerance, with emerging research highlighting genetic determinants of cold-induced pain sensitivity. This condition substantially impacts quality of life and represents a leading cause of disability following hand trauma or surgery.

Red flags: sudden or unexplained onset, unexplained weight loss or severe fatigue, new paresthesia, chest pain, or dyspnea

Special populations: Women, older adults, and individuals of African-American or Afro-Caribbean descent demonstrate higher prevalence and symptom severity, likely reflecting physiological and genetic variations in cold response. Pregnancy and postpartum periods warrant evaluation for thyroid dysfunction or iron deficiency when cold intolerance develops. Occupational exposures such as vibrating tools and social factors including inadequate housing can worsen or reveal latent cold sensitivity. These populations may require targeted screening and tailored interventions.

Further Reading

- Magistroni E, Parodi G, Fop F, Battiston B, Dahlin LB. Cold intolerance and neuropathic pain after peripheral nerve injury in upper extremity. J Peripher Nerv Syst. 2020;25(2):184–90.
- Saenz Ibarra B, Meeker J, Jalali O, Lynch MC. Cold-induced dermatoses. Am J Dermatopathol. 2018;40(4):291–4.
- Stjernbrandt A, Carlsson D, Pettersson H, Liljelind I, Nilsson T, Wahlström J. Cold sensitivity and associated factors: a nested case–control study performed in Northern Sweden. Int Arch Occup Environ Health. 2018;91(7):785–97.
- Stjernbrandt A, Björ B, Pettersson H, Lundström R, Liljelind I, Nilsson T, et al. Manifestations of cold sensitivity: a case series. Int J Circumpolar Health. 2020;79(1):1749001.
- Christogianni A, Bibb R, Filingeri D. Body temperatures, thermal comfort, and neuropsychological responses to air temperatures ranging between 12°C and 39°C in people with multiple sclerosis. Physiol Behav. 2023;266:114179.
- Zafren K, Hollis S, Weiss EA, Danzl D, Wilburn J, Kimmel N, et al. Prevention and treatment of nonfreezing cold injuries and warm water immersion tissue injuries: supplement to Wilderness Medical Society clinical practice guidelines for the prevention and treatment of frostbite. Wilderness Environ Med. 2023;34(2):172–81.

Excessive Thirst (Polydipsia)

Introduction

Polydipsia is defined as excessive thirst with abnormally high fluid intake, typically exceeding 3 liters daily, and often serves as an important clinical indicator of underlying pathology. This condition affects 6-17% of patients with chronic psychiatric illness and can lead to serious complications, including life-threatening hyponatremia. Polydipsia is fundamentally classified into primary (behavioral/psychiatric) and secondary (medical) etiologies. Primary polydipsia originates from psychological factors, while secondary forms result from identifiable conditions such as diabetes mellitus or diabetes insipidus that disrupt normal physiological regulation of thirst and fluid balance. Accurate diagnosis requires systematic evaluation incorporating clinical history, physical examination, and targeted laboratory studies. Standardized assessment tools, including the Polydipsia Diagnostic Criteria and Polydipsia Severity Scale, aid clinicians by incorporating key indicators such as fluid intake patterns, serum sodium levels, and urine specific gravity to distinguish between etiologies and guide appropriate management. It is also important to note that polydipsia is often accompanied by polyuria, which is an increased volume of urine output exceeding 3 liters per day in adults, and either of these symptoms warrants further investigation.

Checklist DDX

Serious/life-threatening: hyperosmolar hyperglycemic state and diabetic ketoacidosis (severe diabetes mellitus complications), primary polydipsia (psychogenic water intoxication), untreated diabetes insipidus, severe electrolyte derangements (e.g., hypercalcemia, hypernatremia), intracranial lesions (brain tumors causing central diabetes insipidus), adrenal insufficiency

Common: diabetes mellitus, syndrome of inappropriate antidiuretic hormone (SIADH), primary (psychogenic) polydipsia in psychiatric illness (e.g., schizophrenia), chronic kidney disease

Commonly misdiagnosed: poorly controlled diabetes mellitus, central vs. nephrogenic diabetes insipidus, adrenal insufficiency, psychogenic polydipsia

Systematic DDX

Pathophysiologic approach
- Vascular
    - Chronic heart failure, organ ischemia
- Infection
    - **Bacterial:** meningitis, tuberculosis, syphilis
    - **Viral:** encephalitis (herpes, cytomegalovirus)
    - **Parasitic:** toxoplasmosis
- Neoplasia and hematologic
    - Pituitary adenoma, craniopharyngioma, meningioma, metastatic disease
- Dysfunction
    - **Renal:** chronic kidney disease
    - **Neurogenic/psychiatric:** primary (psychogenic) polydipsia (schizophrenia, anxiety)
- Injury
    - Head trauma
- Toxic-metabolic
    - **Endocrine:** hyperthyroidism, hyperparathyroidism, hyperaldosteronism (Conn's disease), Cushing's disease
    - **Metabolic:** diabetes mellitus, hyperosmolar hyperglycemic state, nephrogenic diabetes insipidus, electrolyte imbalance (hypercalcemia, hypernatremia, hypokalemia), adrenal insufficiency, gestational diabetes
    - **Drugs:** diuretic, lithium, anticholinergic, demeclocycline
- Everything else
    - Sarcoidosis, Langerhans cell histiocytosis

Primary vs secondary
- Primary polydipsia
    - **Psychogenic polydipsia:** schizophrenia, bipolar disorder, depression, anxiety, obsessive compulsive disorder (OCD), anorexia nervosa, alcoholism
    - **Neurodevelopmental disorders:** autism, intellectual disability
    - **Habitual or compulsive water drinking:** health-conscious individuals, athletes
    - **Dipsogenic polydipsia:** hypothalamic lesions or dysfunction, cerebral lesions, granulomatous diseases (sarcoidosis), infectious causes (e.g., tuberculous meningitis), vascular conditions (vasculitis), psychological stress, and trauma affecting the thirst center

- **Secondary polydipsia**
    - **Lack of antidiuretic hormone:** central diabetes insipidus
    - **Renal insensitivity to antidiuretic hormone:** primary nephrogenic diabetes insipidus (congenital or familial), secondary nephrogenic diabetes insipidus, renal failure, hyperadrenocorticism, hypoadrenocorticism, hypoadrenocorticism, hypoadrenocorticism, hypokalemia, hypercalcemia, pyelonephritis, liver failure, pyometra
    - **Increased renal tubular solute load:** diabetes mellitus, renal glycosuria, renal failure, hypoadrenocorticism, post-obstructive diuresis, diuretics
    - **Decreased medullary tonicity:** hepatic failure, low-protein diets, hypokalemia, hyponatremia

Notes

General considerations: The assessment of polydipsia requires a structured approach to distinguish between primary behavioral causes and secondary medical conditions, as management strategies and clinical outcomes differ significantly. A detailed clinical history should evaluate psychiatric comorbidities, medication use, and any underlying systemic disease. Initial laboratory workup should include serum and urine osmolality, electrolyte levels, and glucose testing. Current diagnostic standards prioritize copeptin-based testing over traditional water deprivation, offering superior accuracy and patient safety—particularly in differentiating central diabetes insipidus from primary polydipsia.

Red flags: dehydration, headache, recurrent vomiting, visual field loss, confusion, lethargy, seizures, dry mucous membranes, hypotension, tachycardia

Special populations: Patients with chronic psychiatric disorders frequently experience excessive thirst and fluid intake, which can lead to dangerously low sodium levels. Careful distinction from diabetes insipidus is essential to prevent inappropriate desmopressin treatment. Geriatric patients present unique challenges due to multiple medications, cognitive changes, social factors, and various health conditions that increase their susceptibility to excessive fluid intake. These factors require thoughtful assessment before proceeding with dynamic testing protocols. In children, genetic causes are more prevalent, and copeptin-based testing offers a safer alternative to traditional water deprivation tests, which carry greater risks in pediatric patients. Pregnant patients also go through various physiologic changes that can lead to excessive thirst, but depending on severity this can be a sign of something more significant, such as gestational diabetes, which warrants evaluation.

Further Reading

- Mahon M, Amaechi G, Slattery F, Sheridan AL, Roche EF. Fifteen-minute consultation: polydipsia, polyuria, or both. Arch Dis Child Educ Pract Ed. 2019;104(3):141–5.
- Sakuma M, Misawa F, Maeda M, Fujii Y, Uchida H, Mimura M, et al. Development of diagnostic criteria and severity scale for polydipsia: a systematic literature review and well-experienced clinicians' consensus. Psychiatry Res. 2021;297:113708.
- Atila C, Beck J, Refardt J, Erlic Z, Drummond JB, Sailer CO, et al. Psychopathological characteristics in patients with arginine vasopressin deficiency (central diabetes insipidus) and primary polydipsia compared to healthy controls. Eur J Endocrinol. 2024;190(5):354–62.
- Chamberlain L. Hyponatremia caused by polydipsia. Crit Care Nurse. 2012;32(3):e11–20.
- Rowe M, Patel N, Jeffery J, Flanagan D. Use of copeptin in interpretation of the water deprivation test. Endocrinol Diabetes Metab. 2023;6(3).
- Carr AC. Diabetes insipidus and other polyuric syndromes. In: Encyclopedia of Endocrine Diseases. 2nd ed. Elsevier; 2014. p.637–51.e3
- Hillier TA, Pedula KL, Ogasawara KK, Vesco KK, Oshiro CE, Lubarsky SL, Van Marter J. A pragmatic, randomized clinical trial of gestational diabetes screening. New England Journal of Medicine. 2021 Mar 11;384(10):895-904.

Excessive Hunger (Polyphagia)

Introduction

Polyphagia (or hyperphagia) refers to excessive appetite and food intake, which is generally indicative of an underlying health issue. It differs from normal variations in appetite by its persistence, the rapid return of hunger after meals, and obsessive focus on food. The differential diagnosis of polyphagia encompasses several major categories, including endocrine disorders, neurological conditions, and metabolic derangements. Appetite changes should be interpreted within the context of weight change – whether the patient is gaining, losing, or maintaining weight – as this provides essential diagnostic clues.

Checklist DDX

Serious/life-threatening: diabetic ketoacidosis, thyroid storm, insulinoma

Common: diabetes mellitus (type 1 and 2), hyperthyroidism, bulimia nervosa, binge-eating disorder, medication and drug-induced (corticosteroids, cannabis), premenstrual syndrome

Commonly misdiagnosed: Prader-Willi syndrome, Kleine-Levin syndrome, polycystic ovary syndrome (PCOS), atypical depression, Cushing's syndrome, hypothalamic mass lesions

Systematic DDX

Pathophysiologic approach
- **Vascular**
    - Stroke (thalamic or hypothalamic)
- **Infection**
    - Post-acute COVID-19 syndrome, tapeworm, Helicobacter pylori
- **Neoplasia and hematologic**
    - Hypothalamic lesions, pheochromocytoma, pancreatic cancer (insulinoma, glucagonoma), craniopharyngioma, insulinoma, or other intracranial tumors
- **Dysfunction**
    - Frontotemporal dementia, eating disorders (bulimia nervosa, binge-eating disorder)

- Toxic-metabolic
    - **Endocrine:** hyperthyroidism (Graves' disease), Cushing's syndrome
    - **Metabolic:** diabetes mellitus, hypoglycemia
    - **Drugs:** corticosteroids, antipsychotics, antidepressants, cannabinoids
    - **Toxic:** alcohol, cannabis
- Anomalies of development/aging
    - Alstrom syndrome, WAGR syndrome, Fragile X syndrome, Bardet–Biedl syndrome, obesity syndromes (Prader-Willi syndrome, MC4R deficiency)
- Everything else
    - Premenstrual syndrome, polycystic ovary syndrome, atypical depressive disorder, stress, and anxiety

Primary vs. secondary

- Primary polyphagia
    - **Destruction of satiety center:** mass lesion, trauma, infection, inflammation
    - **Other:** psychogenic, stress
- Secondary polyphagia
    - **Physiologically increased metabolic rate:** cold temperatures, pregnancy, lactation, growth, exercise, burns
    - **Pathologically increased metabolic rate:** hyperthyroidism, infection, neoplasia
    - **Decreased energy supply:** diabetes mellitus, exocrine pancreatic insufficiency, infiltrative bowel disease
    - **Decreased intake:** low-calorie diet, hypoglycemia
- Drug-induced polyphagia
    - Glucocorticoids, phenobarbital, antihistamines, progestins, benzodiazepines, cyproheptadine, mirtazapine, clozapine

Notes

General considerations: Assessment of polyphagia requires a multidisciplinary approach, integrating behavioral, metabolic, and hormonal evaluations. Patient history and symptom diaries can be instrumental in identifying triggers, patterns, and severity of hunger episodes. Commonly used tools include the Eating Disorder Examination Questionnaire and the Dykens' Hyperphagia Questionnaire, particularly in cases with suspected genetic or psychiatric etiology. Laboratory tests—such as glucose, thyroid function, cortisol, and insulin levels—are crucial for identifying endocrine and metabolic contributors. Standardized scales like the Three-Factor

Eating Inventory and the Dutch Eating Behavior Questionnaire provide structured insights into hyperphagic behaviors. Screening for mood disorders, substance use, and metabolic syndromes is essential, particularly when appetite changes are abrupt or extreme.

Red flags: extreme thirst, weight loss, frequent urination, severe psychiatric symptoms, suspicion for underlying genetic syndrome

Special populations: In children and adolescents, evaluation should consider normal appetite increases during growth and puberty, while also assessing for underlying causes such as genetic syndromes (e.g., Prader-Willi, Bardet-Biedl), hypothalamic dysfunction, or medication effects. Management may involve family-centered behavioral strategies and, when appropriate, pharmacologic intervention. In pregnant or lactating women, heightened appetite is often physiologic; however, assessment should rule out gestational diabetes and thyroid disorders, with a focus on supporting both maternal and fetal nutritional needs. For individuals on appetite-stimulating medications (e.g., atypical antipsychotics, corticosteroids), routine monitoring of weight and metabolic health is advised.

Further Reading

- Kaggwa MM, Favina A, Najjuka SM, Zeba Z, Mamun MA, Bongomin F. Excessive eating, and weight gain:A rare post-acute COVID-19 syndrome. Diabetes & Metabolic Syndrome: Clinical Research & Reviews. 2021 Sep;15(5):102252.
- Khabbazi A, Farzaneh R, Mahmoudi M, Shahi M, Jabbaripour Sarmadian A, Babapour E, et al. Cold intolerance, and associated factors: a population study. Scientific Reports. 2022 Oct 27;12(1).
- Heymsfield SB, Avena NM, Baier L, Brantley P, Bray GA, Burnett LC, et al. Hyperphagia: Current Concepts and Future Directions Proceedings of the 2nd International Conference on Hyperphagia. Obesity (Silver Spring, Md). 2014 Feb 1;22(0 1): S1–17.
- Stefanaki K, Karagiannakis DS, Peppa M, Vryonidou A, Kalantaridou S, Goulis DG, et al. Food Cravings and Obesity in Women with Polycystic Ovary Syndrome: Pathophysiological and Therapeutic Considerations. Nutrients. 2024 Jan 1;16(7):1049.
- Arnouk L, Hélène Chantereau, Courbage S, Tounian P, Clément K, Poitou C, et al. Hyperphagia and impulsivity: use of self-administered Dykens' and in-house impulsivity questionnaires to characterize eating behaviors in children with severe and early-onset obesity. Orphanet Journal of Rare Diseases. 2024 Feb 23;19(1)

- Attia E, Walsh BT. Eating Disorders: A Review. JAMA. 2025 Apr 8;333(14):1242–52.
- US Preventive Services Task Force. Screening for Eating Disorders in Adolescents and Adults: US Preventive Services Task Force Recommendation Statement. JAMA. 2022 Mar 15;327(11):1061–7.
- Hampl SE, Hassink SG, Skinner AC, Armstrong SC, Barlow SE, Bolling CF, et al. Clinical Practice Guideline for the Evaluation and Treatment of Children and Adolescents With Obesity. Pediatrics. 2023 Jan 9;151(2):e2022060640.

Hematologic and Lymphatic

Ahmed Kertam

Long H. Tu

Nurudeen L. Osumah

Easy Bruising or Bleeding

Introduction

Easy bruising and abnormal bleeding represent frequent clinical presentations encountered across various healthcare settings. While often attributable to benign causes such as minor trauma or vascular fragility, these symptoms can also serve as the initial manifestation of serious, potentially life-threatening underlying hematologic disorders or systemic illnesses. A systematic evaluation is essential to differentiate normal variations from pathological conditions and to identify the specific etiology, which can range from inherited coagulation defects to acquired disorders to medication side effects. It is noteworthy that a significant proportion of healthy individuals, between 26% and 45%, report a history of symptoms such as epistaxis, easy bruising, or gum bleeding. These symptoms do not automatically signify pathology. Clinicians must assess the frequency, severity, location, and context of presentation. This distinction is crucial for avoiding over-investigation of benign cases while ensuring that true bleeding disorders are not overlooked.

Checklist DDX

Serious/life-threatening: inherited coagulopathies: hemophilia A (factor VIII deficiency) or hemophilia B (factor IX deficiency), acquired coagulopathies (e.g., disseminated intravascular coagulation [DIC], liver failure with associated coagulopathy), thrombocytopenia (e.g., thrombotic thrombocytopenic purpura [TTP] or acute leukemia with bone marrow failure), non-accidental trauma

Common: minor accidental trauma, medication effects (e.g., non-steroidal anti-inflammatory drugs [NSAIDs], antiplatelet agents [e.g., aspirin], and anticoagulants [e.g., warfarin, direct oral anticoagulants]), purpura simplex, mild forms of von Willebrand disease, primary immune thrombocytopenia

Commonly misdiagnosed: mild inherited bleeding disorders (e.g., mild von Willebrand disease or mild factor deficiencies), non-accidental trauma (NAT), early stages of liver disease, subclinical vitamin K deficiency, heparin induced thrombocytopenia

Systematic DDX

- **Vascular**
  - **Vasculitis:** Henoch-Schönlein purpura, microscopic polyangiitis, polyarteritis nodosa, etc.

- o **Inherited connective tissue disorders:** Ehlers-Danlos syndrome, pseudoxanthoma elasticum, etc.
  - o **Others:** amyloidosis, hereditary hemorrhagic telangiectasia, purpura simplex (easy bruising)
- **Infection**
  - o Sepsis and disseminated intravascular coagulation (DIC), meningococcemia, Rocky Mountain spotted fever, endocarditis)
- **Inflammatory/autoimmune**
  - o Immune thrombocytopenia (ITP), thrombotic thrombocytopenic purpura (TTP), hemolytic uremic syndrome (HUS), systemic lupus erythematosus
- **Neoplasia and hematologic**
  - o **Hematologic malignancies:** leukemias (especially acute promyelocytic leukemia [APL] causing DIC), myelodysplastic syndromes, multiple myeloma, lymphomas, myeloproliferative neoplasms
  - o **Solid tumors:** metastatic carcinoma with bone marrow infiltration, paraneoplastic syndromes (e.g., Trousseau's syndrome with associated bleeding)
- **Dysfunction**
  - o **Organ failure:** liver failure (impaired synthesis of coagulation factors, thrombocytopenia), renal failure (uremic platelet dysfunction), HELLP syndrome (hemolysis, elevated liver enzyme levels, low platelet count syndrome)
- **Injury/trauma**
  - o Accidental trauma, non-accidental trauma (NAT), iatrogenic injury (e.g., post-surgical bleeding, complications of invasive procedures)
- **Toxic-metabolic**
  - o **Medication-induced:** anticoagulants (warfarin, direct oral anticoagulants), antiplatelets (aspirin, clopidogrel), non-steroidal anti-inflammatory drugs (NSAIDs), certain antibiotics, valproic acid, selective serotonin reuptake inhibitors (SSRIs)
  - o **Nutritional deficiencies:** vitamin K deficiency, vitamin C deficiency (scurvy)
  - o **Systemic conditions:** uremia (platelet dysfunction), Alcoholism chronic lead exposure
- **Anomalies of development/aging**
  - o **Inherited bleeding disorders:** hemophilia A (Factor VIII deficiency), hemophilia B (Factor IX deficiency), von Willebrand disease (vWD), rare factor deficiencies (e.g., Factor VII deficiency, Factor XIII deficiency)

- o **Inherited platelet disorders:** inherited giant platelet disorders (e.g., Sebastian syndrome, May-Hegglin anomaly, Bernard-Soulier syndrome), Glanzmann thrombasthenia
- o **Inherited connective tissue disorders:** Ehlers-Danlos syndrome (vascular type)
- o **Aging-related:** senile purpura
- Everything else
    - o Factitious bleeding (self-inflicted injury), psychiatric conditions (e.g., Munchausen syndrome, self-harm), environmental exposures

Notes

General considerations: Evaluation requires detailed personal and family history, medication review, and physical examination. History should cover bleeding type, frequency, site, and triggers. Physical examination should assess lesion type (e.g., petechiae, purpura, ecchymoses, hematomas) and distribution. Initial laboratory evaluation includes complete blood count (CBC) with peripheral blood smear, prothrombin time (PT), and activated partial thromboplastin time (aPTT). The International Society on Thrombosis and Hemostasis (ISTH) bleeding assessment tool can be useful. For vitamin K deficiency and early liver cell failure, PT is prolonged and PTT might be normal, as Factor VII is depleted first. Renal failure often shows normal platelet count but increased bleeding time (BT).

Red flags: spontaneous deep tissue bleeding (e.g., hemarthroses, large hematomas), intracranial hemorrhage, severe mucocutaneous bleeding (e.g., persistent epistaxis requiring packing or transfusion, menorrhagia with hemodynamic instability), bleeding disproportionate to trauma, new onset bleeding in elderly patients, bleeding with systemic illness (e.g., fever, unexplained weight loss, generalized lymphadenopathy, jaundice)

Special populations: In children, consider severe inherited bleeding disorders and non-accidental trauma; vitamin K deficiency is common. Elderly patients are at increased risk due to polypharmacy (anticoagulants, antiplatelet agents), liver/renal dysfunction, myelodysplastic syndromes, and senile purpura. Pregnant women may have increased bleeding due to hormonal changes and vascularity; evaluate severe bleeding for coagulopathies (e.g., von Willebrand disease), placental abnormalities, or preeclampsia/HELLP syndrome. Purpura simplex is a normal finding in women, typically on the upper arms and thighs. Immunocompromised patients have a higher bleeding risk due to infections (e.g., sepsis-induced DIC), chemotherapy-induced myelosuppression, or specific opportunistic infections.

Further Reading

- Doherty TM, Kelley A. Bleeding disorders. In: StatPearls [Internet]. Treasure Island (FL): StatPearls Publishing; 2025 Jan–. Available from: https://www.ncbi.nlm.nih.gov/books/NBK541050/. Accessed 2025 Jul 30.
- Muncie HL Jr, Sirmans SM, James E. Easy bruising and bleeding: primary care evaluation. Am Fam Physician. 2016 Feb 15;93(4):279-86. Available from: https://www.aafp.org/pubs/afp/issues/2016/0215/p279.html. Accessed 2025 Jul 30.
- Duggan A, et al. Bleeding and bruising: primary care evaluation. PubMed. 2023 Nov 15. Available from: https://pubmed.ncbi.nlm.nih.gov/39556633/. Accessed 2025 Jul 30.
- Al-Samkari H. Bruising and bleeding in infants and children: a practical approach. ResearchGate. 2016 Jan. Available from: https://www.researchgate.net/publication/7138643_Bruising_and_bleeding_in_infants_and_children_-_A_practical_approach. Accessed 2025 Jul 30.
- Sebastian syndrome. Indian J Dermatol Venereol Leprol. 2016 Mar-Apr;82(2):224-6. Available from: https://ijdvl.com/easy-bruising-due-to-giant-platelet-possibly-myh9-related-sebastian-syndrome/. Accessed 2025 Jul 30.
- Verywell Health. Could you have a vitamin C deficiency? 10 symptoms to watch for. 2025 Jul 24. Available from: https://www.verywellhealth.com/vitamin-c-deficiency-symptoms-11760476. Accessed 2025 Jul 30.

Pallor

Introduction

Pallor, or paleness of the skin and mucous membranes, is a common clinical sign that frequently indicates anemia, a condition characterized by a reduction in red blood cell mass or hemoglobin concentration. However, pallor can also result from other non-anemic causes, such as vasoconstriction due to shock, syncope, or even anxiety. Anemia itself is a symptom, not a diagnosis, and its evaluation requires a systematic and thorough approach to identify the underlying etiology, which can range from nutritional deficiencies and chronic diseases to acute blood loss or primary hematologic disorders. While pallor itself is a clinical finding, it is not synonymous with anemia. Pallor is a physical sign observed during clinical examination, while anemia is a specific laboratory diagnosis defined by reduced hemoglobin or red blood cell count. Clinicians must confirm anemia with objective laboratory tests and, if is absent, investigate other potential causes of pallor; this ensures a comprehensive diagnostic approach to avoid premature closure.

Checklist DDX

Serious/life-threatening: acute severe hemorrhage (e.g., gastrointestinal bleeding or ruptured ectopic pregnancy), aplastic anemia, acute hemolytic crises (e.g., severe glucose-6-phosphate dehydrogenase (G6PD) deficiency or autoimmune hemolytic anemia), acute leukemia, severe disseminated malignancy with bone marrow infiltration

Common: iron deficiency anemia, anemia of chronic disease or inflammation (e.g., chronic infections, autoimmune disorders, malignancies), vitamin B12 deficiency, folate deficiency, mild blood loss (e.g., from heavy menstrual bleeding or minor gastrointestinal blood loss), thalassemia trait, chronic kidney disease, drug induced anemia (e.g. hydroxyurea, zidovudine, chemotherapy), sickle cell anemia

Commonly misdiagnosed: early stages of chronic blood loss (e.g., occult gastrointestinal bleeding), mild thalassemias, anemia of chronic kidney disease, myelodysplastic syndromes, sideroblastic anemia, drug-induced anemias, subtle hemolytic anemias

Systematic DDX

- **Reduced red blood cell mass**
  - **Blood loss**
    - **Acute haemorrhage:** trauma, gastrointestinal bleed, ruptured ectopic pregnancy, postpartum haemorrhage
    - **Chronic blood loss:** peptic ulcer disease, colorectal cancer, angiodysplasia, inflammatory bowel disease, hemorrhoids, hookworm infestation, heavy menstrual bleeding
  - **Reduced production of RBCs**
    - **Nutrient deficiencies:** iron deficiency anemia, vitamin B12 deficiency (pernicious anemia, malabsorption, vegan diet), folate deficiency (malnutrition, alcoholism, methotrexate use)
    - **Bone marrow disorders:** aplastic anemia, myelodysplastic syndrome, pure red cell aplasia, marrow infiltration by leukemia or lymphoma or metastases, myelofibrosis
    - **Chronic disease and inflammation:** anemia of chronic disease (rheumatoid arthritis, tuberculosis, chronic infections), chronic kidney disease, chronic liver disease, hypothyroidism, adrenal insufficiency, hypopituitarism
    - **Infections suppressing erythropoiesis:** parvovirus B19, HIV, babesiosis
    - **Other:** Early iron deficiency (normocytic before becoming microcytic), alcoholism, uremia, dilutional anemia (pregnancy, fluid overload), severe protein–energy malnutrition
  - **Increased destruction of RBCs (hemolysis)**
    - **Intrinsic RBC defects:** hemoglobinopathies (sickle cell disease, thalassemia), enzyme deficiencies (G6PD deficiency, pyruvate kinase deficiency), membrane defects (hereditary spherocytosis, hereditary elliptocytosis), paroxysmal nocturnal hemoglobinuria
    - **Extrinsic RBC defects:** autoimmune hemolytic anemia, transfusion reactions, microangiopathic hemolytic anemia (thrombotic thrombocytopenic purpura, hemolytic uremic syndrome, disseminated intravascular coagulation), infections (malaria, babesiosis, clostridium perfringens sepsis), toxins and venoms (snake bites,

certain mushrooms, chemical agents), mechanical trauma (prosthetic heart valves, exercise-induced hemolysis)
- **Reduced peripheral blood flow**
  - **Generalized hypoperfusion**
    - Shock (hypovolemic, cardiogenic, septic, anaphylactic, obstructive), severe heart failure
  - **Localized hypoperfusion**
    - Peripheral arterial disease, acute limb ischemia (embolus, thrombosis), acute compartment syndrome, vasospasm (Raynaud's phenomenon, cold exposure, emotional stress), drug-induced vasoconstriction (alpha-agonists, cocaine, amphetamines)
- **Reduced oxygen saturation**
  - Severe hypoxemia (acute respiratory distress syndrome massive pulmonary embolism, pneumonia, pulmonary edema),
  - Carbon monoxide poisoning
  - Methemoglobinemia (nitrates, dapsone, local anesthetics)
- **Pigment & skin disorders mimicking pallor**
  - Albinism, severe cachexia (advanced malignancy, chronic illness), chronic liver disease

Notes

General considerations: Initial evaluation involves CBC with red blood cell indices, peripheral blood smear, and reticulocyte count. Further investigations include iron studies, vitamin B12 and folate levels, and hemolysis tests. A bone marrow biopsy may be needed. Anemia classification by MCV is fundamental for narrowing the differential diagnosis.

Red flags: acute severe pallor/anemia, hemodynamic instability (tachycardia, hypotension, dizziness), chest pain/dyspnea with anemia, neurological symptoms (e.g., severe vitamin B12 deficiency with subacute combined degeneration), petechiae/purpura; unexplained weight loss, fever, or lymphadenopathy accompanying anemia

Special populations: In children, common causes include iron deficiency (especially in toddlers and adolescents), thalassemia's, and other inherited anemias; acute severe anemia may suggest hemolytic uremic syndrome, parvovirus B19 aplastic crisis, or acute leukemia. In older adults, anemia is often multifactorial (anemia of chronic disease, iron deficiency from occult GI bleeding, myelodysplastic syndromes); it is not a normal part of aging. Physiologic anemia of pregnancy is common due to plasma volume expansion; however, true iron deficiency and folate deficiency are also highly prevalent. Anemia of chronic disease is highly prevalent in individuals with chronic inflammatory conditions, infections, autoimmune disorders, and malignancies. Chronic kidney disease is a particularly common cause due to decreased erythropoietin production.

Further Reading

- Duggan A, et al. Anemia. In: StatPearls [Internet]. Treasure Island (FL): StatPearls Publishing; 2025 Jan–. Available from: https://www.ncbi.nlm.nih.gov/books/NBK499994/ [cited 2025 Jul 30].
- Means RT. Anemia of chronic disease. N Engl J Med. 2012 Oct 11;367(15):1461-2.
- DeFrances CJ, Podgornik MN. 2004 National Hospital Discharge Survey. Adv Data. 2006 Jun 27;(371):1-19.
- Kaushansky K. The anemia of chronic disease. N Engl J Med. 2005 Feb 24;352(10):1032-4.

Swollen Glands or Lymph Nodes

Introduction

Swollen glands, or lymphadenopathy, refer to enlarged lymph nodes and are a common clinical finding that can arise from a wide array of underlying conditions. Lymph nodes are integral components of the immune system, acting as filters and sites for immune cell activation. Their enlargement typically signifies an active immune response to infection, inflammation, or malignancy. The clinical significance of lymphadenopathy varies greatly, ranging from benign, self-limiting reactive processes to serious, life-threatening systemic diseases. Lymphadenopathy should never be dismissed without careful clinical evaluation.

Checklist DDX

Serious/life-threatening: malignancies (e.g., lymphomas, leukemias, metastatic carcinomas), disseminated infections (e.g., AIDS, tuberculosis, cryptococcosis, sepsis) autoimmune diseases (e.g., systemic lupus erythematosus, sarcoidosis, Kawasaki disease)

Common: viral infections (e.g., common cold, infectious mononucleosis caused by Epstein-Barr virus, cytomegalovirus, rubella), bacterial infections (e.g., streptococcal pharyngitis, localized skin infections, cat scratch disease), generalized reactive lymphadenopathy from local inflammation or recent vaccination

Commonly misdiagnosed: atypical infections (e.g., tuberculosis, toxoplasmosis, atypical mycobacteria), early-stage lymphomas (especially indolent types), sarcoidosis, drug-induced lymphadenopathy, less common inflammatory conditions (e.g., Kikuchi-Fujimoto disease [histiocytic necrotizing lymphadenitis])

Systematic DDX

Generalized lymphadenopathy
- Infectious/inflammatory
    - **Infections:** Lyme disease, leprosy, leishmaniasis, trypanosomiasis, histoplasmosis, coccidioidomycosis.
    - **Inflammatory:** rheumatoid arthritis, multiple sclerosis, and cryoglobulinemia, poliomyelitis, SLE.
- Neoplasia and hematologic
    - Anemia, paroxysmal cold hemoglobinuria, Waldenstrom's macroglobulinemia, hypothalamic lesions (e.g., brain tumors)

- **Dysfunction**
  - **Seizure-related:** epilepsy
  - **Peripheral nerve dysfunction:** peripheral neuropathy (e.g., carpal tunnel syndrome)
- **Injury/trauma**
  - Nonfreezing cold injuries (immersion/trench foot, chilblains, panniculitis, cold urticaria), frostbite, upper limb surgery (flexor tendon repair, amputations), traumatic hand injury (fracture), hand-arm vibration syndrome, complex regional pain syndrome (CRPS)
- **Anomalies of development/aging**
  - **Inherited:** Fabry disease, TRPA1 mutation, TRPM8 channel polymorphism
  - **Neurodegenerative:** Wernicke's encephalopathy, Parkinson's disease
- **Toxic-metabolic**
  - **Endocrine:** hypothyroidism, diabetes mellitus
  - **Drugs:** oxaliplatin, opioid withdrawal, beta-blockers, nicotine
  - **Metabolic:** vitamin B12 deficiency
- **Everything else**
  - Fibromyalgia, anorexia nervosa

Localized lymphadenopathy

- **Head and cervical**
  - **Infection:** acute and self-limiting viral illnesses (children), staphylococcal and streptococcal infections, atypical mycobacteria, cat-scratch disease
  - **Inflammatory:** Kikuchi lymphadenitis, sarcoidosis, Kawasaki disease
  - **Malignancy:** supraclavicular adenopathy (high risk of intra-abdominal malignancy, especially in adults >40 years)
- **Axillary**
  - **Infections/ injuries:** upper extremities infections/injuries, cat-scratch disease, tularemia, sporotrichosis
  - **Malignancy:** Hodgkin lymphoma, non-Hodgkin lymphoma, metastasis (e.g., breast, lung, thyroid, stomach, colorectal, pancreatic, ovarian, kidney, skin cancers including malignant melanoma)
  - **Other:** silicone breast implants (inflammatory reaction)
- **Epitrochlear**
  - Lymphoma, melanoma, infections of the upper extremity, sarcoidosis, secondary syphilis

- **Inguinal**
    - **Infections:** sexually transmitted infections (e.g., herpes simplex, lymphogranuloma venereum, chancroid, syphilis), lower extremity skin infections
    - **Malignancy:** penile and vulvar squamous cell carcinomas, melanoma

> Notes

General considerations Evaluation relies on detailed history and physical examination. History should cover localizing symptoms, constitutional symptoms (fever, weight loss, fatigue, night sweats), epidemiologic clues (occupational exposures, recent travel, high-risk behaviors), and medication use. Physical examination should focus on location (regional vs. generalized), size (e.g., >1 cm generally enlarged; epitrochlear >0.5 cm, inguinal >1.5 cm abnormal), consistency (stony-hard for metastatic cancer, firm/rubbery for lymphoma, softer for infections/inflammation, fluctuant for suppurant, "shotty" for small viral nodes), tenderness, and mobility (fixed vs. mobile). Matting can be benign or malignant. Anatomic location helps narrow diagnosis – e.g., supraclavicular nodes, especially left-sided Virchow's node, have a high malignancy risk; paraumbilical (Sister Joseph's) node suggests abdominal/pelvic neoplasm. Persistent or progressively enlarging lymphadenopathy warrants further investigation. A 3-4 week observation period is prudent for localized nodes with a benign clinical picture. Excisional biopsy of the most abnormal node is preferred for definitive diagnosis when indicated.

Red flags: supraclavicular lymphadenopathy (especially left-sided); hard, fixed, non-tender, or rapidly growing nodes; generalized lymphadenopathy with systemic "B symptoms" (unexplained fever, drenching night sweats, unexplained weight loss); lymphadenopathy in immunocompromised patients or in children with signs of serious systemic illness (e.g., persistent fever, rash, conjunctivitis suggestive of Kawasaki disease)

Special populations: In children, lymphadenopathy is common due to viral infections; consider also Kawasaki disease, cat scratch disease, lymphomas, or leukemias. In older patients, there is higher likelihood of malignancy (e.g., lymphoma, chronic lymphocytic leukemia, metastatic disease) or chronic inflammatory conditions. In pregnancy, lymphadenopathy is commonly reactive to infections; severe or persistent lymphadenopathy requires evaluation for toxoplasmosis or lymphoma. In immunocompromised individuals, consider opportunistic infections (e.g., atypical mycobacteria, fungal infections) and lymphoproliferative disorders (e.g., post-transplant lymphoproliferative disorder [PTLD]).

Further Reading

- Goldsmith SM, Forouhar F. Approach to lymphadenopathy. Clin Lab Med. 2018 Jun;38(2):183-201.
- Bazemore AW, Smucker DR. Lymphadenopathy and malignancy. Am Fam Physician. 2002 Dec 1;66(12):2103-10. Available from: https://www.aafp.org/pubs/afp/issues/2002/1201/p2103.html. Accessed 2025 Jul 30.
- Ioannidis I. Lymphadenopathy in children. Curr Opin Pediatr. 2013 Feb;25(1):112-7.
- Naik R, Varma S. Approach to lymphadenopathy. Indian J Med Res. 2017 Aug;146(2):172.
- Ferrer R. Lymphadenopathy: differential diagnosis and evaluation. Am Fam Physician. 1998 Oct 15;58(6):1313-20. Available from: https://www.aafp.org/pubs/afp/issues/1998/1015/p1313.html. Accessed 2025 Jul 30.

Allergy

Roshan Singh

Long H. Tu

Jon Heavey

Frequent Sneezing

Introduction

Frequent sneezing is defined as repeated, excessive, or uncontrollable expulsion of air from the nose and mouth, often due to irritation of the nasal mucosa. While sneezing is a normal protective reflex to clear nasal passages of irritants, allergens, or infections; persistent or recurrent sneezing may signal underlying pathology such as allergic, infectious, or structural causes. Identifying the etiology is essential, as some causes are benign while others may be serious or life-threatening.

Checklist DDX

Serious/life-threatening: anaphylaxis (severe allergic reaction), asthma exacerbation (especially in the context of allergy), angioedema (especially if involving airway compromise)

Common: allergic rhinitis (seasonal or perennial), nonallergic rhinitis (including vasomotor, gustatory, hormonal, atrophic, medication-induced, senile, occupational, nonallergic rhinitis with eosinophilia syndrome [NARES], emotional, and exercise-induced variants), viral upper respiratory infections (common cold), bacterial sinusitis

Commonly misdiagnosed: allergic rhinitis mistaken for viral infection or nonallergic rhinitis, nonallergic rhinitis subtypes (such as vasomotor or medication-induced) misdiagnosed as allergy, structural abnormalities (nasal polyps, deviated septum), chronic sinusitis, occupational exposures, neurological conditions (e.g., trigeminal neuralgia), other systemic diseases (e.g., gastroesophageal reflux disease [GERD])

Systematic DDX

- **Vascular**
    - Vasculitis involving nasal vessels (e.g., granulomatosis with polyangiitis) may cause chronic nasal symptoms including sneezing
- **Infectious/inflammatory**
    - **Viral:** rhinovirus, influenza, respiratory syncytial virus (RSV), SARS-CoV-2 (COVID-19), others
    - **Bacterial:** acute or chronic sinusitis, secondary bacterial infection of allergic/inflamed mucosa

- o **Fungal:** rare, but possible in immunocompromised hosts
- o **Allergic rhinitis:** IgE-mediated response to environmental allergens (pollen, dust mites, pet dander, mold spores, cockroach antigen)
- o **Nonallergic rhinitis:** includes vasomotor, gustatory, hormonal, atrophic, medication-induced, senile, occupational, NARES, emotional, exercise-induced subtypes
- **Neoplastic**
  - o **Nasal tumors:** benign or malignant, e.g., inverted papilloma, squamous cell carcinoma
- **Dysfunction**
  - o **Systemic diseases:** hypothyroidism (may cause mucosal edema), GERD/laryngopharyngeal reflux (reflex sneezing due to irritation), oral allergy syndrome (cross-reactivity with foods and pollens)
- **Injury/trauma**
  - o **Nasal trauma:** fracture, foreign body, iatrogenic injury (may trigger acute or recurrent sneezing)
- **Compression/obstruction**
  - o **Nasal polyps:** non-cancerous growths causing obstruction, congestion, sneezing
  - o **Deviated nasal septum:** anatomical displacement (causing turbulent airflow and irritation)
  - o Foreign body (especially in children, may cause persistent or unilateral sneezing)
- **Anomalies of development/aging**
  - o **Congenital:** rare anatomical variants
  - o **Aging:** senile rhinitis (watery rhinorrhea and sneezing in elderly; often triggered by environmental stimuli)
- **Toxic-metabolic**
  - o **Medication-induced:** oral contraceptives, aspirin, ACE inhibitors, beta-blockers, overuse of topical decongestants (rhinitis medicamentosa), and other drugs
  - o **Environmental exposures/toxins:** smoke, perfumes, air pollution, occupational irritants (latex, flour, chemicals)
- **Everything else**
  - o **Emotional/psychosocial:** emotional stress, anxiety, excitement (emotional rhinitis)
  - o Cerebrospinal fluid leak (rare, but may cause rhinorrhea and sneezing), exercise-induced (especially in cold or polluted air)

Notes

General considerations: Careful history—including onset, duration, frequency, triggers, associated symptoms (e.g., congestion, rhinorrhea, ocular symptoms), and environmental or occupational exposures—is crucial. Physical examination should assess for structural abnormalities, signs of allergy, or infection. Diagnostic workup may include allergy testing, nasal cytology, and imaging (sinus radiograph or CT scan) if structural disease is suspected. Treatment is based on etiology and may include allergen avoidance, pharmacotherapy (antihistamines, intranasal corticosteroids, anticholinergics), or surgery for structural causes.

Red flags: severe respiratory distress, swelling, or hypotension; unilateral or foul-smelling nasal discharge, persistent nasal congestion or facial pain, blood in nasal discharge, sudden loss of smell; headache or visual changes

Special populations: In children, foreign bodies, viral URIs, and allergic rhinitis are especially common. Consider adenoid hypertrophy or congenital anomalies. In older adults, senile rhinitis, medication-induced rhinitis, and neoplastic processes are more prevalent. In pregnant patients, note that hormonal rhinitis may result from mucosal edema. Immunocompromised patients have increased risk of unusual infections, fungal sinusitis, and neoplasms.

Further Reading

- Bernstein JA, Bernstein JS, Makol R, Ward S. Allergic Rhinitis: A Review. JAMA. 2024;331(10):866-877. doi:10.1001/jama.2024.0530
- Sur DKC, Plesa ML. Chronic Nonallergic Rhinitis. Am Fam Physician. 2018;98(3):171-176.
- Quillen DM, Feller DB. Diagnosing rhinitis: allergic vs. nonallergic. Am Fam Physician. 2006;73(9):1583-1590.
- Ellis AK, Corren J, Hussain Z, Feldweg AM. Allergic rhinitis: Clinical manifestations, epidemiology, and diagnosis. UpToDate. Updated June 16, 2024. Accessed July 26, 2025. [https://www.uptodate.com/contents/allergic-rhinitis-clinical-manifestations-epidemiology-and-diagnosis]
- Settipane RA, Kaliner MA. Chapter 14: Nonallergic rhinitis. Am J Rhinol Allergy. 2013;27 Suppl 1:S48-S51. doi:10.2500/ajra.2013.27.3927
- Dougherty JM, Alsayouri K, Sadowski A. Allergy. In: StatPearls. Treasure Island (FL): StatPearls Publishing; July 31, 2023.
- Wallace DV, Dykewicz MS, Bernstein DI, et al. The diagnosis and management of rhinitis: an updated practice parameter. J Allergy Clin Immunol. 2008;122(2 Suppl):S1-S84. doi:10.1016/j.jaci.2008.06.003

Seasonal Allergies

Introduction

Seasonal allergy, also known as hay fever or seasonal allergic rhinitis, is an IgE-mediated inflammatory response of the nasal mucosa to airborne allergens such as pollen from grasses, trees, and weeds, as well as outdoor molds. Typical symptoms include sneezing, nasal congestion, rhinorrhea, and itching of the nose, throat, and eyes. The timing and severity of symptoms often vary based on climate, geography, and specific allergen exposure. Understanding the differential diagnosis is crucial, as several other rhinitis disorders can present with similar symptoms but require different management approaches.

Checklist DDX

Serious/life-threatening: severe asthma exacerbation triggered by seasonal allergens, anaphylaxis (rare but possible with pollen-food allergy syndrome or severe atopy), angioedema

Common: seasonal allergic rhinitis (hay fever), perennial allergic rhinitis (triggered by year-round allergens such as dust mites, pet dander, and indoor molds), nonallergic rhinitis (including vasomotor, hormonal, drug-induced, and occupational subtypes), viral upper respiratory tract infection (common cold), bacterial sinusitis

Commonly misdiagnosed: nonallergic rhinitis (vasomotor, hormonal, drug-induced, occupational), local allergic rhinitis (LAR, with negative systemic allergy testing), structural causes (nasal septal deviation, polyps), mixed rhinitis (overlap of allergic and nonallergic forms), rhinitis medicamentosa (rebound from decongestant overuse), primary ciliary dyskinesia (in children), chronic sinusitis

Systematic DDX

- **Vascular**
  - Vasculitis involving the nasal mucosa (e.g., granulomatosis with polyangiitis)
- **Infectious/inflammatory**
  - **Viral:** upper respiratory tract infections (common cold, influenza, RSV, COVID-19)
  - **Bacterial:** acute or chronic sinusitis
  - **Allergic:** seasonal (pollen, outdoor mold), perennial (dust mite,

animal dander, indoor mold), local allergic rhinitis (LAR, with negative skin/serum IgE but positive nasal provocation), mixed rhinitis (both allergic and nonallergic mechanisms)
  - **Nonallergic rhinitis:** vasomotor (triggered by irritants, weather changes), hormonal (pregnancy, hypothyroidism), drug-induced (NSAIDs, beta-blockers, ACE inhibitors, oral contraceptives), rhinitis medicamentosa (overuse of topical decongestants), nonallergic rhinitis with eosinophilia syndrome (NARES), occupational rhinitis (latex, flour, chemicals), emotional rhinitis (stress, anxiety), exercise-induced rhinitis
- **Neoplastic**
  - Nasal tumors (benign or malignant, e.g., inverted papilloma, lymphoma, carcinoma) can present with nasal congestion, obstruction, or discharge
- **Dysfunction**
  - **Systemic disorders:** hypothyroidism (causing mucosal edema and congestion), primary ciliary dyskinesia (rare, especially in children), immunodeficiency (predisposing to chronic sinusitis)
- **Injury/trauma**
  - Nasal trauma or foreign body (especially in children) may cause persistent or unilateral nasal symptoms
- **Compression/obstruction**
  - Nasal polyps, septal deviation, adenoid hypertrophy (children), or other anatomical variants causing chronic symptoms
- **Anomalies of development/aging**
  - Congenital nasal anomalies, senile (age-related) rhinitis
- **Toxic-metabolic**
  - Medication-induced rhinitis (various drugs), environmental/occupational exposures (smoke, strong odors, air pollution, chemicals)
- **Everything else**
  - **Emotional/psychosocial:** anxiety, stress (emotional rhinitis)
  - **Food-related:** pollen-food allergy syndrome (oral allergy syndrome)
  - **Environmental:** high outdoor allergen exposure, poor indoor air quality

Notes

General considerations: A thorough history—including symptom timing, seasonality, triggers, associated allergic symptoms (ocular, throat, skin), response to therapy, and family history—guides diagnosis. Physical exam should assess for nasal mucosal edema, pallor, or polyps Differentiating between allergic and nonallergic rhinitis is crucial, as management strategies differ. Allergy testing (skin prick or serum-specific IgE) helps confirm diagnosis, but local allergic rhinitis may require nasal provocation testing. Avoidance of known allergens and environmental modifications are first-line, while pharmacologic therapy (intranasal corticosteroids, oral/nasal antihistamines, leukotriene receptor antagonists) is the mainstay for moderate-to-severe symptoms. Immunotherapy is considered for refractory or severe cases.

Red flags: unilateral symptoms (nasal obstruction, discharge), severe or persistent nasal obstruction with anosmia, recurrent epistaxis (nosebleeds), systemic symptoms (fever, weight loss, night sweats), poor response to standard therapy

Special populations: In children, adenoid hypertrophy, chronic sinusitis, foreign body, and primary ciliary dyskinesia are more common. Allergic rhinitis may be underdiagnosed in young children. In older adults, age-related (senile) rhinitis, polypharmacy (medication-induced rhinitis), and neoplastic causes are more common. In pregnant patients, hormonal rhinitis can be seen due to estrogen-mediated mucosal changes; medication use requires special consideration.

Further Reading

- Bernstein JA, Bernstein JS, Makol R, Ward S. Allergic Rhinitis: A Review. JAMA. 2024;331(10):866-877. doi:10.1001/jama.2024.0530
- Quillen DM, Feller DB. Diagnosing rhinitis: allergic vs. nonallergic. Am Fam Physician. 2006;73(9):1583-1590.
- Blanca-Lopez N, Campo P, Salas M, et al. Seasonal Local Allergic Rhinitis in Areas With High Concentrations of Grass Pollen. J Investig Allergol Clin Immunol. 2016;26(2):83-91. doi:10.18176/jiaci.0018
- Wallace DV, Dykewicz MS, Bernstein DI, et al. The diagnosis and management of rhinitis: an updated practice parameter. J Allergy Clin Immunol. 2008;122(2 Suppl):S1-S84. doi:10.1016/j.jaci.2008.06.003
- Ellis AK, Corren J, Hussain Z, Feldweg AM. Allergic rhinitis: Clinical manifestations, epidemiology, and diagnosis. UpToDate. Updated June 16, 2024. Accessed July 26, 2025. [https://www.uptodate.com/contents/allergic-rhinitis-clinical-manifestations-epidemiology-and-diagnosis]
- Greiwe JC, Bernstein JA. Allergic and Mixed Rhinitis: Diagnosis and Natural Evolution. J Clin Med. 2019;8(11):2019. Published 2019 Nov 19. doi:10.3390/jcm8112019
- Avdeeva KS, Fokkens WJ, Segboer CL, Reitsma S. The prevalence of non-allergic rhinitis phenotypes in the general population: A cross-

sectional study. Allergy. 2022;77(7):2163-2174. doi:10.1111/all.15223
- Leader P, Geiger Z. Vasomotor Rhinitis. In: StatPearls. Treasure Island (FL): StatPearls Publishing; July 10, 2023.
- Lund V. Allergic rhinitis--making the correct diagnosis. Clin Exp Allergy. 1998;28 Suppl 6:25-28. doi:10.1046/j.1365-2222.1998.0280s6025.x

Increased/Recurrent Infections

Introduction

Increased or recurrent infections refer to multiple, unusually frequent episodes of infections in an individual, exceeding the expected rate for age and environment. This pattern can reflect an underlying defect in immune function, anatomical abnormalities, chronic disease, or environmental exposures. Prompt recognition and systematic evaluation are critical – recurrent infections may signal serious or life-threatening conditions, cause significant morbidity, and impact quality of life. Understanding the differential diagnosis informs further work-up and management, ultimately improving patient outcomes.

Checklist DDX

Serious/life-threatening: severe sepsis, endocarditis, neutropenic sepsis, necrotizing fasciitis, occult/deep infections, HIV/AIDS, severe primary immunodeficiencies (e.g., severe combined immunodeficiency)

Common: recurrent viral upper respiratory tract infections, recurrent urinary tract infections (especially in women and children), chronic sinusitis, chronic obstructive pulmonary disease (COPD) exacerbations, atopic disorders (asthma, allergic rhinitis), diabetes mellitus

Commonly misdiagnosed: primary immunodeficiencies (selective IgA deficiency, common variable immunodeficiency), secondary immunodeficiency (e.g., from medications, malnutrition), anatomical abnormalities (e.g., vesicoureteral reflux, cystic fibrosis), autoimmune conditions (systemic lupus erythematosus), medication side effects (immunosuppressants), malignancies (leukemia, lymphoma)

Systematic DDX

- **Vascular**
  - Sickle cell disease (functional asplenia), vasculitis with immune suppression
- **Infectious/inflammatory**
  - **Chronic inflammatory diseases:** rheumatoid arthritis, systemic lupus erythematosus (SLE), other autoimmune diseases
  - **Deep/occult infections:** persistent viral infections, organ/muscle abscess, spinal infection, bone infections

- **Neoplastic**
    - **Hematologic malignancies:** leukemia, lymphoma, multiple myeloma
    - Solid tumors, especially if causing obstruction or immunosuppression (e.g., post-transplant, advanced cancer)
- **Dysfunction**
    - **Primary immunodeficiency:** severe combined immunodeficiency (SCID), common variable immunodeficiency (CVID), chronic granulomatous disease (CGD), selective IgA deficiency
    - **Secondary immunodeficiency:** HIV/AIDS, immunosuppression from medications (e.g., corticosteroids, chemotherapy), malnutrition, diabetes mellitus, chronic renal or liver disease
    - **Chronic pulmonary disease:** COPD, bronchiectasis
    - **Other organ dysfunction:** chronic kidney disease, chronic liver disease, poorly controlled diabetes mellitus
- **Injury/trauma**
    - **Iatrogenic:** central line infections, implanted/invasive devices, surgery
    - **Trauma:** disruption of skin or mucosal barriers
- **Compression/obstruction**
    - **Urinary tract obstruction:** kidney stones, benign prostatic hyperplasia, neurogenic bladder
    - **Airway obstruction:** anatomical anomalies, foreign body
- **Anomalies of development/aging**
    - **Genetic disorders:** cystic fibrosis, primary ciliary dyskinesia, tracheoesophageal fistula
    - **Congenital heart defects:** congenital heart disease predisposing to endocarditis (e.g., ventricular septal defect, tetralogy of Fallot, valvular heart disease)
    - **Gastrointestinal malformations:** Hirschsprung's disease
    - **Age-related:** immature immune system in children, immunosenescence in the elderly
- **Toxic-metabolic**
    - **Metabolic disorders:** diabetes mellitus, malnutrition
    - **Medication effects:** immunosuppressive drugs, chemotherapy
    - Chronic alcoholism
- **Everything else**
    - **Environmental exposures:** high-risk settings (crowded living, healthcare facilities), poor hygiene, exposure to tobacco smoke or air pollution

- **Lifestyle factors:** alcohol abuse, IV drug abuse, sexual activity (especially in women with recurrent UTIs), use of spermicides
  - **Psychosocial:** poor access to healthcare, homelessness

Notes

General considerations: A careful, structured history and physical examination are essential – focusing on the pattern, site, and severity of infections, previous diagnostic work-up, medication use, family history, and environmental exposures. Laboratory evaluation may include complete blood count, immunoglobulin levels, HIV testing, and targeted imaging or specialty referral as indicated. Early identification of underlying immune deficiency, anatomical abnormality, or chronic disease allows for tailored management and reduces complications.

Red flags: unresponsive to antibiotics, recurrent infections involving multiple organ systems (respiratory, urinary, gastrointestinal), failure to thrive or poor growth in children, unexplained weight loss, history of unusual or severe infections (e.g., sepsis, invasive fungal disease), family history of recurrent or severe infections

Special populations: Children may experience frequent infections due to immune immaturity, but severe, persistent, or unusual infections should prompt evaluation for primary immunodeficiency or anatomical defects. Older adults are at increased risk due to immunosenescence, comorbidities, and polypharmacy. Pregnant women with recurrent infections may have unique risks (e.g., urinary tract infections due to anatomical changes). Immunocompromised individuals (e.g., transplant recipients, those on biologic agents) require a lower threshold for evaluation. Social determinants (overcrowding, poor sanitation, substance abuse) may contribute in both children and adults.

Further Reading

- Justiz Vaillant AA, Qurie A. Immunodeficiency. In: StatPearls. Treasure Island (FL): StatPearls Publishing; June 26, 2023.
- Ballow M. Approach to the patient with recurrent infections. Clin Rev Allergy Immunol. 2008;34(2):129-140. doi:10.1007/s12016-007-8041-2
- Pasternack MS. Approach to the adult with recurrent infections. UpToDate. Waltham, MA: Wolters Kluwer; Updated October 18, 2022. Accessed July 26, 2025. [https://www.uptodate.com/contents/approach-to-the-adult-with-recurrent-infections]
- Butte MJ. Approach to the child with recurrent infections. UpToDate. Waltham, MA: Wolters Kluwer; Updated June 13, 2025. Accessed July 26, 2025. [https://www.uptodate.com/contents/approach-to-the-child-with-

recurrent-infections]
- Liyanarachi KV, Solligård E, Mohus RM, Åsvold BO, Rogne T, Damås JK. Incidence, recurring admissions and mortality of severe bacterial infections and sepsis over a 22-year period in the population-based HUNT study. PLoS One. 2022;17(7):e0271263. Published 2022 Jul 12. doi:10.1371/journal.pone.0271263
- Avery RK, Pasternack MS. Approach to adult patients with recurrent infections. Cleve Clin J Med. 1997;64(5):249-257. doi:10.3949/ccjm.64.5.249
- Aggarwal N, Leslie SW. Recurrent Urinary Tract Infections. In: StatPearls. Treasure Island (FL): StatPearls Publishing; January 20, 2025.
- Grant SS, Hung DT. Persistent bacterial infections, antibiotic tolerance, and the oxidative stress response. Virulence. 2013;4(4):273-283. doi:10.4161/viru.23987
- Ruffner, M. A., Sullivan, K. E., & Henrickson, S. E. (2017). Recurrent and Sustained Viral Infections in Primary Immunodeficiencies. Frontiers in Immunology, 8, 264423. https://doi.org/10.3389/fimmu.2017.00665

Concluding Remarks

Long H. Tu

Beyond this Text, Contact, and Feedback

This text has primarily focused on differential diagnoses for common presenting symptoms. Similar approaches could be adopted for less common presentations or exam findings not covered here. These concepts will also have parallels in subspecialty care as well as in the analysis of lab, imaging, and other testing results. In many ways, this book represents the sort of resource I wish I had at the end medical school and beginning of intern year. I hope it serves as a valuable tool in your journey to becoming a thorough and thoughtful clinician, especially when contributing to the diagnostic process.

This work is the result of collaborative efforts among more than two dozen co-authors. While every effort has been made to ensure correctness and concordance with the available literature, minor imperfections or omissions may be difficult to eliminate completely. For feedback or suggestions on improving future editions, please feel free to send me a message at long.tu@yale.edu. It would be great to hear from you!

www.ingramcontent.com/pod-product-compliance
Lightning Source LLC
Chambersburg PA
CBHW071236160426
43196CB00009B/1081